Preface

The provenance of this volume of essays is twofold. We editors, all at roughly the same stage in our careers, were contemplating our impending retirement. We wondered about writing a combined memoir that would address the highlights and frustrations of the more than four decades of clinical practice, teaching, and research. The prospect was exciting and intriguing, covering as it would scientific discoveries of all kinds, biological and psychological, advances of treatment, conceptual breakthroughs, and fiery intellectual debates on an inexhaustible range of topics. We also wanted to face up to psychiatry's negative side: perennial indecisiveness about the profession's boundaries—whether to promote an ambitious social vision or confine its activities strictly to the medical clinic; the limitations of a narrow approach to human suffering, dominated by arbitrary diagnosis; the retreat from the hope of a deinstitutionalized, community-based psychiatry; the divide between biological treatments and psychotherapy; the technical and ethical complexities of psychiatric research; and the low priority given to psychiatry, especially but far from exclusively in less developed countries. We would also have to deal with ethical challenges facing the profession, such as maintaining the basic human rights of severely disturbed patients while at the same time recognizing that many of them are unable to act independently without risk of harming themselves or others.

A second rationale for producing such a memoir was a shared perception of deficiencies in training experienced by our junior colleagues. Increasingly, they lack a developmental perspective for their patients and are taught to concentrate almost exclusively on the present and the immediate future with an emphasis on the questionable procedures of 'risk assessment'. In addition, as they embark on their odyssey they have—in our view—a relatively meagre knowledge of the contemporary history of psychiatry, especially at the level of oral and personal experiences.

We then posed the question: would it not be to the advantage of trainees to hear directly from the 'elders' of the profession—their observations, feelings, and fantasies about psychiatry from graduation as psychiatrists through to retirement? They could learn of our initial foray into the clinical setting, and the sense of excitement as we began to get to know our patients—their tantalizing life stories and inner mental lives—as well as our anxiety as to whether we were sufficiently equipped to help, let alone cure them.

The 1960s saw the end of the 350-year era of the asylum. However enlightened an innovation in mental health care this was in its inception as the Enlightenment took over from a religious context for conceptualizing mental illness, it had failed to rehabilitate most of its occupants. This was due to a lack of core scientific knowledge, inadequacy of rational treatments, and the degeneration of asylum conceived as caring and benevolent, to one of custodial regimentation. The early 1960s offered reason for cautious optimism, as stigma began to recede, more effective medicines were discovered, and psychosocial concepts and therapies devised. A collective memoir, we surmised, had the potential to provide a balanced picture of these changes, highlighting their benefits, as well as unanticipated and unwelcomed consequences.

Appealing as the memoir idea seemed, were we adequately equipped to write an authoritative and comprehensive narrative? Would our perspective on a half-century of developments and limitations be broad enough? Though we disliked the increasing fragmentation and subspecialization of medicine, from which psychiatry has not been immune, we had to acknowledge that there were many subjects where each of us had no direct experience or expertise. Then came the obvious solution: why not recruit renowned and respected colleagues who, like ourselves, were nearing the end of their active career? We would invite them to reflect on the area of psychiatry to which they had devoted their energies, culminating in much-lauded contributions. Our new aim was for a text comprising a set of *perspectives* written in essay form by an esteemed group of colleagues. That is what we now offer.

Having arrived at this overall objective, we settled on the following goals:

1 To promote the curiosity of mental health professionals about key developments in psychiatry over the past half-century and thus deepening their understanding of the historical context within which they work;

2 Within Santayana's rubric of 'Those that do not learn from the past are destined to repeat it', to sensitize the next generation of mental health professionals to the role they might play in advancing the state of knowledge about mental illness and its treatment during the course of their careers;

3 To offer an unparalleled collection of the perspectives of internationally recognized colleagues who have made notable contributions in specific domains;

4 To offer the interested laity an opportunity to gain a balanced account of psychiatry's evolution since the 1950s and its likely prospects in the 21st century; and, finally,

5 To serve as a valuable archival resource for scholars.

In the light of these goals, we identified two principal groups of readers. First, psychiatrists and allied mental health professionals, such as psychologists, psychiatric social workers, psychiatric nurses, and occupational therapists, both trained and in training. Secondly, the lay public who are commonly puzzled about what contemporary psychiatry has accomplished and what it may offer in the future. Many people harbour a prejudice towards, and fear of, the profession, derived from its commonly distorted portrayal in the media and possibly from personal experience of being a patient, or knowing a relative or friend who has received psychiatric care.

Having determined our purpose and identified our principal readership, we encountered the tricky issue of what topics to cover; the possible range was overwhelming. Readers will inevitably have misgivings about omissions but we feel confident they will not find fault with what we *have* included. Suffice to say that we resisted targeting individual diagnostic groupings—we believe that there are far too many of them and it would serve little purpose covering the evolution of each.

We are chary of drawing sweeping generalizations, programmes, or predictions from our colleagues' essays. They speak for themselves, and readers will draw what conclusions they may. Nevertheless a number of themes, for good or ill, stand out that any future mental health professional will want to take into account.

The first well-documented theme is the move in psychiatry since the mid-20th century from a broadly psychosocial approach to a narrower neuroscience-oriented perspective. The locus of interest and glamour has moved from societal ills and their impact on mental health to unravelling the intricacies of brain functioning. This new domain of neuroscience, vastly exciting as it is, risks focusing on the brain in isolation from other salient fields in psychiatry. We believe, and our view is supported by several of our contributors, that the opportunity now exists to see the brain-in-context, and explore how its genetic, biochemical, and structural features cannot be separated from lived experience, and the world of relating at the level both of the family and of the overall social environment.

A second, related theme lies in the burgeoning science of neurogenetics. Molecular biology was in its infancy when we started out, with genetics still confined within a largely Mendelian paradigm. The new field of epigenetics means that the search for, say 'the schizophrenia gene', is seen as illusory, and promises to unravel how nature and nurture are fascinatingly intertwined, aetiologically and clinically.

A third theme is the shifting power relations within psychiatry. Our generation was the first for whom the provenance of mental illness was not presided over by Asylum Superintendents, God-like figures (invariably men) who exercised near-feudal power over the inmates and staff of the mental hospital. The ethos of the psychiatric world in which we qualified was that of liberation from the atmosphere of institutional care that was at the same time nurturing and stifling. Psychiatrists attempted to cling to their hegemony, still claiming to be natural leaders of the mental health team, but that too has become a nostalgic vestige. Patients are no longer subjugated souls, but 'consumers' with the rights that attend a business-like relationship with their 'providers'. Psychiatrists compete on a levelled professional playing field with a range of mental health professionals and can no longer assume that they are *primus inter pares*; they must justify their status and salaries on merit.

Another striking change has been in the arena of therapeutics. In our psychiatric infancy treatments were broad-brush and non-specific: neuroleptics for psychosis; antidepressants for mood disorders; psychoanalysis for neuroses; and abstinence for addicts. Since then scientific advances and the influence of the multibillion-dollar pharmaceutical industry have contributed to a proliferation of diagnoses and attempts to find specific medications or psychotherapies to treat them. This trend leaves us wondering if something has been lost and in need of rediscovery. There is an urgent need for a whole-person medicine that engages patients not in terms of quasi-mechanistic dysfunction, but rather at the level of personal experiences, and agency.

With that *cri-de-coeur* we will desist. The future of our profession is uncertain. If a comparable text were to be compiled in the middle of the 21st century how would it look? Will psychiatry even exist as a medical speciality? Will it have merged with neurology? Will it confine itself to the minutiae of brain function leaving the world of emotions and relationships to psychology, nursing and social work? Or will psychiatry, we hopefully, but perhaps vainly suggest, finally have taken its place as the queen of the medical specialities, uniquely able to integrate the biological, psychological, social, and cultural, and to connect with the lived existence and meanings of its patients?

Only time will tell how the story of psychiatry will unfold. In the meanwhile, we hope that the perspectives provided by our contributors to this volume will assist younger colleagues in fulfilling their professional role as effectively as possible, and to keep in mind the essential lessons, both positive and negative, to be learned from the past.

We leave the last word, so apposite to our current purpose, to Thomas Hardy from his poem, 'An Ancient to Ancients':

> Much is there waits you we have missed;
> Much lore we leave you worth knowing,
> Much, much has lain outside our ken:
> Nay, rush not: time serves: we are going …

Sidney Bloch
Stephen A. Green
Jeremy Holmes

Acknowledgements

Psychiatry: Past, Present and Prospect has self evidently been a collaborative effort. By all accounts, our esteemed colleagues did not find the task entirely straightforward. What we did *not* want was a standard review of the scientific literature. Instead, what we hoped for, and believe has been achieved, was a confluence of personal and professional pathways, giving a unique perspective of the evolution of psychiatry in their area of expertise since the 1950s. The complexity and novelty of this writing assignment reflects in part the unprecedented nature of the volume and the objectives we set and which we have described in the preface. We are immensely grateful to our contributors for their deft efforts in helping to accomplish those goals.

We are also indebted to our colleagues at Oxford University Press: Martin Baum, Charlotte Green, Kathleen Lyle, Eloise Moir-Ford, Abigail Stanley, and Peter Stevenson. Not only was their enthusiasm for the project palpable from the outset, but they also carried out their editorial tasks effectively and efficiently. OUP's decision to seek the judgements of no less than five reviewers about our proposal provoked a degree of anxiety in us but turned out to be a bonus in that we benefited substantially from their suggestions. We thank them for their encouragement and diligence.

Contents

Contributors

Aaron T. Beck
Emeritus Professor of Psychiatry
and Director, AT Beck Psychopathology
Research Centre, University of
Pennsylvania, Philadelphia, USA;
Albert Lasker Award for Clinical
Medical Research, 2006

Anne E. Becker
Maude and Lillian Presley Professor of
Global Health and Social Medicine;
Vice Chair, Department of Global
Health and Social Medicine, Harvard
Medical School; Co-editor-in-chief,
Culture, Medicine and Psychiatry

German E. Berrios
Emeritus Chair of the Epistemology of
Psychiatry, University of Cambridge;
Formerly Consultant and Head of
Neuropsychiatry, Addenbrooke's
Hospital, Cambridge, UK;
Editor, *History of Psychiatry*

Vishal Bhavsar
Academic Clinical Fellow,
Department of Psychosis Studies,
Institute of Psychiatry,
King's College London, UK

Sidney Bloch
Emeritus Professor of Psychiatry,
University of Melbourne;
Honorary Psychiatrist,
St Vincent's Hospital, Melbourne;
Formerly Editor-in-Chief, *Australian
and New Zealand Journal of Psychiatry*

David J. A. Dozois
Professor of Psychology, Department
of Psychology and Department of

Psychiatry, University of Western
Ontario, London, Canada

Stephen A. Green
Clinical Professor of Psychiatry,
Georgetown University
School of Medicine,
Washington DC, USA

Max Fink
Emeritus Professor of Psychiatry
and Neurology
Stony Brook University School of
Medicine, SUNY, New York,
USA

Dusan Hadzi-Pavlovic
Senior Hospital Scientist,
Black Dog Institute,
Prince of Wales Hospital;
Conjoint Senior Lecturer,
School of Psychiatry,
University of New South Wales,
Sydney, Australia

Edwin Harari
Consultant Psychiatrist, St. Vincent's
Hospital, Melbourne; Clinical Associate
Professor of Psychiatry,
University of Melbourne, Australia

Jeremy Holmes
Visiting Professor of Psychological
Therapies, University of Exeter;
Formerly Consultant Psychiatrist
and Medical Psychotherapist, Devon
NHS Partnership, UK

Steven E. Hyman
Distinguished Service Professor
of Stem Cell and
Regenerative Biology,
Harvard University;

Director, Stanley Centre for Psychiatric Research, Broad Institute of MIT and Harvard; Formerly Director, U.S. National Institute of Mental Health, Washington DC; USA

Jerome H. Jaffe
Clinical Professor of Psychiatry, University of Maryland School of Medicine, Baltimore; Adjunct Professor, Johns Hopkins University Bloomberg School of Public Health, Baltimore; Formerly Director, Addiction Research Centre, National Institute of Drug Abuse, Washington DC; USA

Arthur Kleinman
Esther and Sidney Rabb Professor of Anthropology, Harvard University; Professor of Medical Anthropology and Professor of Psychiatry, Harvard Medical School; and Victor and William Fung Director, Harvard University Asia Centre, Boston, USA

Julian Leff
Emeritus Professor, University College and Kings College London; Formerly Director MRC Social and Community Psychiatry Unit, University of London, UK

Don R. Lipsitt
Clinical Professor of Psychiatry, Harvard Medical School; Emeritus Chair, Department of Psychiatry, Mount Auburn Hospital,Cambridge, USA; Founding Editor, *General Hospital Psychiatry*

Dana March
Assistant Professor, Department of Epidemiology, Joseph L. Mailman School of Public Health, Columbia University, New York, USA

Peter McGuffin
Emeritus Professor of Psychiatric Genetics; Formerly Director and Dean MRC Social, Genetic and Developmental Psychiatry Centre, Institute of Psychiatry, King's College London, UK

Philip B. Mitchell
Scientia Professor and Head, School of Psychiatry, University of New South Wales; Research Fellow, Black Dog Institute, Sydney, Australia

Paul E. Mullen
Emeritus Professor of Forensic Psychiatry, Monash University; and formerly Director, Victorian Institute of Forensic Mental Health, Melbourne, Australia

Robin M. Murray
Professor of Psychiatric Research, Institute of Psychiatry, King's College London; Honorary Consultant Psychiatrist, South London and Maudsley NHS Foundation Trust, London, UK

Catherine Oppenheimer
Formerly Consultant Psychiatrist, Oxfordshire and Buckinghamshire Partnership Mental Healthcare Trust, Oxford, UK

Michael Rutter
Professor of Developmental Psychopathology, MRC Social, Genetic and Developmental Centre, Institute of Psychiatry, King's College London, UK

Norman Sartorius
Formerly Director, Division of Mental Health, World Health Organization; Formerly President, World Psychiatric Association; President, Association for the Improvement of Mental Health Programmes, Geneva, Switzerland

Arieh Y. Shalev
Emeritus Professor of Psychiatry,
Hebrew University of Jerusalem, Israel;
Professor of Psychiatry, New York
University, New York, USA;
Founder-Editor, Israel Journal of
Psychotherapy

Danny H. Sullivan
Assistant Clinical Director, Victorian
Institute of Forensic Mental Health;
Adjunct Senior Lecturer, Monash
University; Melbourne, Australia

Ezra Susser
Professor of Epidemiology and
Psychiatry, Mailman School of Public
Health, Columbia University;
Formerly, Chair, Department of
Epidemiology, Mailman School
of Public Health,
Columbia University,
NY, USA

George Szmukler
Professor of Psychiatry and
Society, and formerly Dean,
Institute of Psychiatry,
King's College London, UK;
Honorary Consultant
Psychiatrist, South London
and Maudsley NHS
Foundation Trust

Psychiatry and neuroscience

Steven E. Hyman

Introduction

The human brain underlies cognition, emotion, and behavioural control. As such it is necessarily the substrate of all psychiatric disorders—except in the view of philosophical dualists, if any remain. Psychiatry has thus been a beneficiary of progress in neuroscience and other basic fields of inquiry ranging from genetics to psychology that elucidate brain function. Neuroscience, the interdisciplinary field that studies the brain (and nervous systems, more broadly), is enjoying a period of expansion in scope (1) and significant scientific success predicated on remarkable new tools, new discoveries, and new forms of organization that support large-scale collaborations and data sharing (2–4). Nonetheless, psychiatry has lagged behind many other medical fields in its ability to translate basic research findings into understanding disease mechanisms and generating new treatments. Moreover, it can justly be said that psychiatry has reached a scientific crossroads marked by the increasingly obvious limitations of its diagnostic classifications (5,6), and by a decades-long failure to improve upon the efficacy of existing treatments. This state of affairs is not simply an academic matter. Much of the pharmaceutical industry has de-emphasized or terminated work on psychiatric disorders based on longstanding failures to make significant advances (7,8). Treatment development based on devices such as deep brain stimulation (DBS) (9) and on applications of cognitive neuroscience to psychotherapy (10) has moved forwards, but, without understanding disease mechanisms, it is not clear how substantial progress can be accomplished. Clinicians, policy-makers, patients, and families are confronted by vast unmet clinical need for people with such maladies as autism, schizophrenia, bipolar disorder, depression, obsessive-compulsive disorder, and other forms of psychiatric disorder that, in aggregate, are leading contributors to global disease burden (11). The scientific question facing psychiatry is how to revitalize research that will lead to better diagnoses and treatments.

For the class of diseases that go by the inaccurate and anachronistic (because implicitly dualistic) term of mental disorders, there are significant obstacles to understanding pathogenesis or succeeding at mechanism-based treatment development. Most notably these include the remarkable complexity of the human brain, its relative uniqueness with respect to animals that could serve as disease models, its relative inaccessibility to direct investigation, and a lack of robust neuropathological or biochemical correlates of symptoms as occurs in neurodegenerative disorders, such as Alzheimer's disease (AD) and Parkinson's disease (PD). Even for AD and PD, which exhibit clear neuropathology and for which we know many mutations that produce rare Mendelian genetic forms, the development of treatments that alter disease progression has proven challenging.

The brain is arguably the most complex object of scientific inquiry (with all due respect to our colleagues in physics and astronomy). The brain expresses approximately 80% of our full complement of genes, a far higher proportion than any other organ or organ system. Most organs are constructed of a relatively limited number of types of cells. In contrast, the human brain contains thousands of distinct types of neurons, the principal cells involved in the processing of information and the generation of outputs such as thought and behaviour. Each cell type is distinguished by the complement of genes that it expresses, i.e. reads out from its DNA into ribonucleic acid (RNA), and by how it processes RNA and proteins (which are translated from a subset of RNA molecules) into diverse molecular species. Ultimately the precise patterns of gene expression that define each cell type are reflected in such recognizable characteristics as their different neurotransmitters, receptors, ion channels, and other signalling molecules. In aggregate the cells of the brain possess a staggeringly rich and complex molecular vocabulary within which each cell type has its own identity. In addition to their distinct molecular composition, each type of neuron has a characteristic morphology, location in the brain, and stereotypic connections to other neurons. They are distinguished from other cell types by their connectivity via synapses, specialized connections that permit precise chemical neurotransmission. Neurons in the brain make, on average, approximately 1000 synapses with other neurons, but the patterns are highly diverse. Each of the large Purkinje cells of the cerebellum may contain 200,000 synapses. The other major cell type in the nervous system, the glia, have more complex functions than merely supporting neurons. For example, astrocytes, one type of glial cell, may participate in synaptic communication.

Overall the human brain contains approximately 100 trillion synapses that form local and large-scale circuits. The synapses, and thus the circuits in which they participate, are not unchanging features of the neural landscape, but undergo frequent remodelling or 'plasticity' in response to developmental processes, external stimuli including lived experience, hormones, drugs, and disease. Plasticity in synapses and circuits is responsible for the encoding of memories and for behavioural adaptations to the environment. Abnormal or maladaptive plasticity also plays an important role in the pathogenesis of many psychiatric disorders, whether highly genetically influenced as in schizophrenia and autism (12) or more strongly influenced by experience as in depression that can follow upon adversity or in post-traumatic stress disorder (PTSD). Treatments for psychiatric disorders, whether psychotherapies, medications, or neuromodulatory interventions such as DBS, must ultimately influence synapses and circuits since activity in the circuits produces all experience, thought, emotion, motivation, and behavioural control. This might sound terribly reductive unless one contemplates the extraordinary complexity and exquisite connectivity of the human brain, indeed one of the most profound mysteries of science.

The maladies that come under the purview of psychiatry involve dysfunction of many basic brain functions that humans share with other animals, which can result, for example, in abnormal sleep and circadian rhythms, appetite, energy, and motivation. Psychiatric disorders are distinguished, however, by disturbances in brain functions that are either unique to humans or significantly expanded in evolution by comparison with our near primate relatives. Thus many psychiatric symptoms affect higher cognition, emotional regulation, decision-making, and executive function that are poorly modelled in animals (13). Our limited ability to model cardinal features of psychiatric illness in animals creates a particularly high scientific hurdle because, for ethical as well as pragmatic reasons, the living human brain is not readily accessible to direct study. Even if brain biopsies were somehow imaginable for psychiatric disorders, they might provide limited information since these are not 'cell autonomous' diseases but the result of abnormal patterns of neural activity across widely distributed circuits.

Notwithstanding the extraordinary scientific challenges that confront psychiatry, the question for people affected by mental illness is how to make significant progress in diagnosis and treatment. In this essay I shall present an admittedly selective perspective of the historical path by which psychiatry has arrived at its current scientific crossroads, and a guardedly optimistic view of how the field might move forwards. Progress will require fresh thinking about disease classification, which exerts strong influence over translational and clinical research, new strategies to understanding aetiology and pathogenesis, and novel approaches to treatment development. If my account is correct, then the answers must lie in science. Specifically, I would argue that psychiatry has focused too narrowly (although of course, not exclusively) on pharmacological and endocrinal models of disease, and would do well to embrace broader aspects of neuroscience and other fields of modern biology. It is also worth noting that the continued separation of psychiatry and neurology (a topic beyond the scope of this essay), by inhibiting the free flow of ideas about diseases of the nervous system, remains highly unfortunate for both scientific progress and clinical practice (14).

Neuroscience

Modern neuroscience began to coalesce as a recognizable field in the 1960s based initially on efforts to bring together scientists who had been studying the anatomy, physiology, and biochemistry of the nervous system within their own 'silos' (15). Soon thereafter psychologists with an interest in brain mechanisms and clinical scientists joined this increasingly interdisciplinary endeavour. As molecular biology, neurogenetics, computational biology, and bioengineering matured, more of their practitioners began to identify themselves as neuroscientists and to link up with departments and graduate programmes in neuroscience. Of course fundamental studies of the nervous system had been performed as early as the late 19th century by such pioneering scientists as Camillo Golgi and Santiago Ramón y Cajal. The latter was the main author of 'neuron theory', the foundational idea that communication within the nervous system occurs between distinct, morphologically polarized neurons, rather than across a continuous network of conjoined cells. During the early and mid-20th century basic findings included the ionic basis of the action potential (Hodgkin and Huxley), chemical neurotransmitters (Loewi and Dale), and the physiological basis of synaptic transmission (Fatt and Katz). However, these investigators lacked ready means of scientific interaction (15).

In 1962, the biologist Francis Schmitt created an interdisciplinary, cross-institutional Neuroscience Research Program based at the American Academy of Arts and Sciences that held symposia and published influential proceedings (16). In 1967, Stephen Kuffler at the Harvard Medical School founded the first neurobiology department. The Society for Neuroscience (SfN) was founded 2 years later. Fourteen hundred scientists attended its inaugural conference; since that time its membership has increased to over 40,000 (1). The SfN was founded as a North American society but its membership has always been international; neuroscience societies and organizations have proliferated globally as the field has expanded and matured.

In addition to its interdisciplinary character, several other factors are central to effective studies of the brain. Processes in the nervous system operate at multiple spatial and temporal scales, so understanding often demands the integration of information from diverse technologies and perspectives (17). Proceeding from 'micro' to 'macro' scales within the brain, an understanding of normal function and of disease must recognize the contributions of molecules, cells, synapses, and local and large-scale circuits. At the next level of organization, cognition, emotion, and behaviour can be viewed as complex emergent properties of activity in large-scale circuits. Finally, while the mechanisms by which our brains produce consciousness—our subjective mental lives—remain unknown, no serious thinker questions the brain's fundamental role in the underlying processes.

As in any biological system, causal influences that act upon the brain function from 'top down' and 'bottom up'. Acting bottom-up, sensory experiences are first captured by specific molecular detectors expressed by specialized sensory neurons. For example, opsin molecules on retinal neurons called rod and cone cells capture light. In the visual system, the brain analyses incoming information in complex circuits (entirely inaccessible to introspection) within the retina, thalamus, and cerebral cortex. This circuitry separately analyses the position of an object in space (the 'where' pathways) from its characteristics (the 'what' pathways). Within the latter, different circuits analyse the contours of an object, such as its colour, whether it is moving, and in what direction. All such information is synthesized by higher-level neural circuits that also integrate vision with information from other sensory modalities to produce the coherent picture of the world that we experience and that guides behaviour.

Bottom-up sensory processes are modulated from the top down. For example, some top-down control derives from circuits that have not only been shaped by evolution to recognize stimuli with survival relevance (e.g. danger and rewards), but also shaped by experience. All day humans are bombarded by an enormous amount of sensory information, but based on effective top-down influences, pay attention to only the small fraction that is 'relevant' or salient. Competing stimuli that would serve as distractions tend to be suppressed. In conditions such as attention deficit hyperactivity disorder (ADHD) such top-down processes work poorly and 'distracters' intrude upon important tasks. In depression and anxiety disorders, a different kind of pathological top-down process seems to be at work: stimuli with a negative valence tend to command attention at the expense of neutral or positive stimuli. Beyond paying attention, additional mechanisms determine what aspects of experience get encoded in memory, based on such factors as the salience of the experience and on prior experience. A top-down set of influences of interest to psychiatry is temperament influences not only the nature of responses to stimuli, but what pertains to a person to begin with.

Observing brain activity in humans

Non-invasive neuroimaging technologies have emerged as sets of tools permitting measurement of brain structures and providing surrogates of neural activity. These technologies have made it possible to observe the living, functioning human brain, even if indirectly. However, much of the psychiatric neuroimaging literature remains correlational. The demonstration of causal mechanisms often requires the kind of invasive perturbations that can only be performed in animals. Nonetheless, combined with other technologies, such as genetics, neuroimaging has begun to provide clues to disease phenotypes and may eventually contribute to diagnostic tests and biomarkers.

In animal models it is possible to measure the activity of synapses and circuits with electrophysiological recordings and newer technologies including advanced microscopy. In living human beings neural activity is mostly studied indirectly using older tools such as electroencephalography (EEG), and more recently with magnetoencephalography (MEG) and various forms of non-invasive neuroimaging. These technologies cannot observe neural activity directly, but rely on detectable outputs that correlate with activity such as electrical and magnetic fields for EEG and MEG respectively, or other proxies of neural firing such as changes in blood flow or metabolism for neuroimaging. Current non-invasive tools lack the fine spatial resolution of the recording electrodes that can be used in animals; EEG, MEG, and functional imaging modalities therefore reveal activity only in large ensembles of neurons.

The EEG detects endogenous electrical signals produced by the flow of ions across neural membranes when the brain is active. MEG detects the tiny magnetic fields produced by the flow of electrical current in neural processes. Each of these technologies has millisecond temporal resolution, the timescale of much neural activity. However, they have poor spatial resolution and are thus complemented by various forms of neuroimaging, which have better spatial resolution; on the other hand, their temporal resolution is of the order of a second—very slow compared to neural activity. Neuroimaging relevant to psychiatry includes structural magnetic resonance imaging (MRI), diffusion tensor imaging (DTI), functional magnetic resonance imaging (fMRI), and positron emission tomography (PET). The signal measured in all forms of MRI is energy released; radio waves are pulsed through the brain when it is placed in a strong magnetic field. Its resolution has progressively improved based on the ability to use stronger magnetic fields. MRI used to measure brain structure has also benefited from computer algorithms that can correct for different head shapes and sizes and reliably measure the contours and volumes of specific anatomical structures like cerebral cortical thickness or hippocampal volume. Using structural MRI with such computational tools has demonstrated that prefrontal and temporal cortical grey matter loss is characteristic of schizophrenia. Similarly, measurement of hippocampal volume is a useful biological marker even in the presymptomatic stage. DTI is an MRI-based technology that makes it possible to study the white matter tracts that connect different brain regions. It exploits the fact that water molecules do not move randomly in the brain but tend to be constrained by fibre tracts. DTI reveals, for example, white matter damage following traumatic brain injury (TBI) that may not be visible through other means.

Beyond observations of the structure of the brain, functional imaging permits the study of the living human brain at work. fMRI is the predominant current technology both because of its good spatial resolution and its apparent safety. In contrast, PET requires the administration of radioactivity, albeit at very low levels. The most common implementation of fMRI technology depends on blood oxygen level dependent (BOLD) contrast as the marker of neural activity. As neurons fire, they (and surrounding glial cells) require more blood flow in order to exchange carbon dioxide for oxygen and to obtain glucose. Oxygenated haemoglobin and deoxygenated haemoglobin behave differently in the magnetic fields employed by MRI technology. Although the cellular mechanisms that couple activity to the generation of the BOLD signal are not fully clear, there is evidence that it is a good proxy for neuronal firing.

Cognitive neuroscientists and clinical investigators have used fMRI to map the circuitry involved in diverse cognitive and emotional tasks in health and disease. One well-studied example is the neurobiology of fear learning and how it changes in anxiety disorders. The amygdala is a complex nucleus (grey matter structure) within the temporal lobes that plays a significant role in the processing of emotionally salient stimuli. Among its functions, the amygdala responds to threats and is necessary in encoding into memory information about fear-inducing stimuli, including their context. When healthy people participate in fear conditioning experiments in the laboratory (e.g. associating an aversive stimulus, such as a mild shock or a fear-inducing photograph, with a previously neutral stimulus) the amygdala is activated for a brief period. In concert with this activation, the medial prefrontal cortex, which suppresses aspects of amygdala function, shows a reciprocal decrement in activity. In patients with PTSD, the amygdala becomes active at a lower threshold and remains so for longer. Moreover, fMRI shows that the medial prefrontal cortex is less active than in healthy people. Fear conditioning is a basic survival process conserved in evolution. Thus, these human investigations were predicated on antecedent animal experimentation. However, fMRI has also been used to map aspects of higher cognition that cannot be readily studied in animals.

Confronting complexity

The diversity of spatial and temporal scales, the complexity of building blocks (and their interactions) at each scale, and the multiplicity of causal influences converging on all outputs of the nervous system, require thoughtful experimental design and model-building. Reductionist strategies (i.e. breaking problems down into tractable pieces or working in simple model systems) are often required if there is to be meaningful progress. Such reduction of complexity in the service of feasibility, for example, motivated the use of simple invertebrate systems (the sea slug *Aplysia californica*) by Eric Kandel in his Nobel prize-winning studies of the molecular and cellular bases of memory—even though his ultimate goal has been to understand human memory (18,19). Applying such strategies in the service of progress does not imply that reduction is an ultimate goal of neuroscience. Reducing certain aspects of behaviour to molecular biology and chemistry might provide investigational tools relevant to therapeutics. However, a rich explanation of behaviour demands the integration of multiple levels of analysis. If we ask questions about behaviour, answers at the molecular level will not be useful, even if certain molecules play important roles. Thus, the attribution of depressive disorders to low serotonin levels, as found in pharmaceutical marketing material, would be anathema to reputable neuroscientists despite the roles of this neurotransmitter (20,21).

We must also appreciate that theories, hypotheses, and textbook explanations of many aspects of brain function are based on radically incomplete knowledge. Indeed, scientific understanding of psychiatric disorders remain crude. Diagnostic systems are still phenomenological (5,6) and well-validated biological markers for purposes of diagnosis or to judge efficacy of treatments remain challenging goals of research. In unusual cases, significant insights into the biology of certain psychiatric maladies have been obtained through 'bottom-up' approaches, as when rare, highly penetrant genetic mutations that cause syndromes associated with autism have been used to generate transgenic mouse models (22). Insights have also been gleaned looking 'top down' with diverse modalities of neuroimaging, often in combination with cognitive neuroscience or pharmacology (23–25). For instance, the use of neuroimaging together with bio-chemical measures to generate biomarkers in AD is promising (26), as is its combination with cognitive neuroscience to produce treatment biomarkers for the cognitive symptoms of schizophrenia (27). Nonetheless, understandings of pathogenesis, which demand both molecular information and better disease definitions, have progressed slowly and fitfully for autism, schizophrenia, bipolar disorder, depressive disorders, obsessive-compulsive disorder, and other morbid states, and remain far from complete.

As alluded to, the challenges come in part from the inherent nature of psychiatric disorders. For example, while anatomical abnormalities have been identified in schizophrenia based on neuroimaging and post-mortem studies, the kind of robust biochemical pathology observed in AD and other neurodegenerative disorders is not evident. Some rare forms of autism are caused by mutations in single genes but the vast majority of cases (and essentially all cases of other psychiatric disorders) appear, at least hitherto, to be genetically complex, making it difficult to identify molecular clues to pathogenesis. This is true even for disorders in which genes, in aggregate, play a large role.

A dialectic of progress followed by intellectual retrenchment

In the mid-20th century, neuroanatomy, neurophysiology, and neuropathology yielded notable empirical discoveries and conceptual advances that shaped modern ideas of how emotion is processed in the brain (28,29). Despite the relevance of such findings to understanding the biology of psychiatric disorders, they did not explain specific symptoms and impairments. Historically, interest in brain anatomy and physiology within the psychiatric research community arrived later, with the emergence of non-invasive neuroimaging methods as described above. The discovery in schizophrenia of enlarged cerebral ventricles (30) and deficits in prefrontal cortical function (31) elicited great interest among both clinicians and researchers, not only because these represented replicable brain abnormalities associated with a psychiatric disorder, but also because they could be correlated with a particular subset of symptoms, namely cognitive impairment. However, it was an earlier and truly astonishing series of psychopharmacological discoveries that began to move psychiatry from a nearly exclusive focus on the psyche in the mid-20th century to a far greater focus on the brain (see Mitchell and Dusan Hadzi-Pavlovic, this volume, pp. 335–54).

Discoveries in psychopharmacology benefit patients and capture psychiatric thinking

Beginning with John Cade's investigations of lithium in the late 1940s (32), a rapid succession of therapeutic discoveries initiated revolutionary changes in psychiatric practice and ignited a growing interest in biology (reviewed in 33). Astute observation of unexpected actions of chemical compounds led to their use in treatment of several severe psychiatric disorders for which specific treatment had previously been lacking. The first antipsychotic drug, chlorpromazine, synthesized in 1950, was initially tested as a pre-anaesthetic for use in surgery. The first tricyclic antidepressant, imipramine, was synthesized as a potential antipsychotic drug (which it proved not to be) as a result of chemical modifications of the three-ring structure of chlorpromazine. The first monoamine oxidase inhibitor antidepressant (MAOI), iproniazid, was originally developed to treat tuberculosis, for which it had no benefit, but was observed to improve the mood of depressed sanatorium patients. By 1957 the antidepressant properties of imipramine and iproniazid had been investigated and demonstrated. While there have been controversies over the degree to which antidepressants are efficacious and under what circumstances (34,35), early trials and clinical experience focused on more severely depressed patients, and made a convincing case that mental illnesses could be treated with at least some specificity by drugs affecting the brain. Subsequent studies of the action of antipsychotic and antidepressant drugs helped lead to the identification of molecular components of synapses, including neurotransmitter receptors and reuptake transporters that functioned as the targets of the different drugs.

This revolutionary series of discoveries gave rise to speculation that the monoamine neurotransmitters (noradrenaline, dopamine, and serotonin) targeted by the new antidepressant and antipsychotic drugs might be involved in pathogenesis. The idea that treatments identify disease mechanisms is invariably tarred by the *post hoc ergo propter hoc* fallacy. In fairness, however, hypothesized noradrenaline or serotonin deficits or dopamine excess were often introduced with appropriate caveats, and many proponents recognized the need for evidence independent of treatment effects (36). The hypothesis that depression might be caused by low levels of noradrenaline, serotonin, or both arose not only from the therapeutic action of drugs (tricyclics and MAOIs) that increased synaptic levels of these monoamines, but from the observations concerning reserpine, a drug that had been used as an antihypertensive and antipsychotic drug that depleted neurons of all monoamine neurotransmitters (noradrenaline, dopamine, and serotonin). Reserpine was associated with sadness, sedation, and, in a minority of cases, the onset of depression, and for such reasons fell out of clinical use. In contrast, psychostimulant drugs such as amphetamine that elevated levels of monoamines in synapses produced, at least transiently, elevations in mood and energy. Despite these apparent pharmacological clues, numerous attempts over ensuing decades failed to find monoamine-related biochemical abnormalities in depressed patients, even while the mechanism of action of antidepressants was recognized as far more complex than could be simply attributed to monoamine neurotransmitter levels (37). In subsequent decades, pursuit of a version of the monoamine hypothesis focused on the genetics of serotonin systems, specifically a common variant in the gene encoding the serotonin reuptake transporter, but no convincing results have emerged and, indeed, depression is more influenced by development and environment than by genes. The maximum heritability for depression is estimated at 35%, but even within this aggregate figure, it appears that many genes contribute small increments of risk.

Since the 1960s, much evidence has suggested that stress or significantly adverse events trigger a proportion of episodes of major depression. In depressive episodes, neuroendocrine systems release stress hormones including cortisol (38). It has subsequently emerged that marked early life stress alters neuroendocrine functioning in the long term and increases the risk of depression (39). Although the syndrome of depression differs markedly from the stress response, there is significant overlap. For example, both stress and depression may affect sleep, appetite, and cognitive functions such as attention. Based on these similarities, many animal models of depression involve administering stress. This line of research has proven fruitful but the resulting animal models have neither elucidated a convincing mechanism for depression nor identified novel drug treatments that have made it into clinical practice. Overall, the pathogenesis of depression and the mechanism of action of antidepressants, beyond their initial effects on the nervous system, have not been solved.

In the case of schizophrenia a dopamine excess hypothesis was undergirded by the observation that amphetamine, which increases synaptic monoamines, including dopamine, can produce or exacerbate psychosis when used continuingly at a high dose. Moreover, drugs that block D2 dopamine receptors (all approved antipsychotics) ameliorate psychotic symptoms. Perhaps the most direct evidence for dopamine abnormality is the observation, first made using single photon emission tomography (SPECT) and confirmed with PET, that amphetamine causes greater dopamine release in people with schizophrenia than in control subjects (25). But these findings do not explicate the panoply of symptoms that characterize schizophrenia, which include not only the positive (psychotic) symptoms that respond to D2 dopamine receptor antagonist antipsychotics, but also negative (deficit) symptoms and cognitive impairments that do not.

The dopamine hypothesis has been supplemented by a hypothesis involving impaired glutamate neurotransmission, spurred by the finding that N-methyl-D-aspartate (NMDA) glutamate receptor channel blockers, such as phencyclidine (PCP) and ketamine, could induce psychotic-like symptoms in humans and, even at lower doses, impaired cognition. Interestingly, findings from large-scale genetic studies suggest that diverse components of excitatory synapses that utilize glutamate play roles in both autism and schizophrenia pathogenesis. However, neither the dopamine nor glutamate hypotheses in their current forms represent the complete story, given schizophrenia's likely developmental origins leading to pathology in multiple brain circuits. Thus, abnormal dopamine or glutamate neurotransmission, while possibly playing roles in the formation of symptoms, may occur downstream of initiating as yet unknown developmental events.

These neurotransmitter- and hormone-based hypotheses of depression and schizo-phrenia are plausible enough to have captured substantial research attention. Frustrat-ingly, however, despite decades of investigation, none of them has advanced sufficiently to explain the cause or the abnormalities of brain function.

The retreat of the pharmaceutical industry

As described above, despite large markets and the limited efficacy of existing treatments (40), the pharmaceutical industry has, since 2010, rapidly de-emphasized psychiatry or abandoned the field altogether. This may represent complex commercial decisions, but there is widespread doubt that adequate knowledg is available to develop better drugs that will gain regulatory approval. Specifically, no clear path exists to drugs with novel mechanisms of action that will provide subtantial benefit in terms of core features of autism or cognitive symptoms of schizophrenia, or that will prove more efficacious than drugs such as the antidepressants which action noradrenaline and serotonin neu-rotransmission (7,40). Given that no antidepressant is superior in effect to imipramine or the MAOIs, and no antipsychotics are better than clozapine (a drug first used in the 1960s), the dominant focus on monoamine systems has become sterile. Essentially all progress in antidepressants has come through the development of drugs, such as the selective serotonin reuptake inhibitors (SSRIs), that are safer and have fewer side ef-fects than their predecessors but are no more effective. In the case of antipsychotics, the second-generational group again has yielded no greater benefits and even a new set of side effects. Unfortunately, there is a dearth of validated molecular targets with which to replace the old monoamine warhorses. By validation I am referring to existence of a proven biological mechanism by which the molecular target of a candidate drug can influence disease mechanisms. Even if such targets were to be discovered, it will be dif-ficult to know whether the drug binds its intended target in the human brain. One labo-rious but convincing method of ensuring so-called target engagement is via PET. While it has been used in ways analogous to fMRI to study brain activity using markers of glucose utilization or of blood flow, PET is the tool of choice to label specific models in the brain. Doing so requires the synthesis of a drug known to bind a specific molecular target, such as a neurotransmitter receptor or enzyme, with the addition of a positron-emitting isotope. Ensuring that the chemistry of the added isotope does not impair the desired binding is a challenge. When this approach succeeds, the PET ligand, namely the molecule that binds a receptor, can be administered to a human subject and a range of doses tried. The goal is for the candidate to compete with, and displace, the PET ligand, thus causing a dose-dependent decrease in the radioactive signal detected in appropriate brain regions. This methodology has the added advantage of determining the required drug dosage.

The challenge of animal models for psychiatric disorders

The scarcity of validated targets is not the only problem that inhibits investment by the pharmaceutical industry in psychiatry. A serious hurdle is the limitations of ani-mal models for most psychiatric disorders. In all of medicine, animal disease models play crucial roles in studying pathogenesis and testing the toxicity and efficacy of drug candidates. The paramount criterion for the validity of a disease model is whether it is produced by the same mechanism as the relevant human condition and reproduces much, if not all, of its pathophysiology. For example, genetic animal models can be produced by replacing mouse genes with adequately penetrant human disease genes by infecting an animal with a relevant pathogen, or in the case of many cancers, by placing human cancer cells in an immunodeficient mouse. Lacking knowledge of aetiology or pathophysiology, validated animal models of depression, schizophrenia, bi polar disorder, and many other conditions are elusive. It is not clear that entirely useful animal models could be produced even with relevant information about pathogenesis given that psychiatric disorders involve, in part, brain structures and functions (e.g. the prefrontal cortex) uniquely advanced in humans. Of course animal research has been central for basic neurobiology and of relevance to psychiatry, yielding disease-relevant information concerning neural circuits conserved in evolution from rodents to humans. Such circuits underlie certain basic emotions such as reward and fear, and cognitive functions like memory (41). However, the utility of rodent models is limited in studying many of the circuits and functions of the prefrontal cortex, a critical region for psychiatry given its role in executive function. Many circuits in humans are rudimentary or absent in our ubiquitous rodent models; for instance, rodent cortices lack gyri and sulci that markedly expand the surface area of the human cerebral cortex. In addition, patterns of gene expression in the human prefrontal cortex differ substantially even from those in chimpanzees, our closest evolutionary relatives.

Many animal-based assays developed to identify possibly therapeutic drugs in psychiatry have become falsely conflated with disease models. Widely used assays in rodents, such as the forced swim (Porsolt test) and tail suspension test to detect antidepressants, or amphetamine administration to detect antipsychotic drugs, originated as empirical attempts to predict new drugs with actions that would mimic those of the prototypical drugs of the 1950s like imipramine or chlorpromazine. A widely recognized problem with deploying assays based on existing drugs is that they may fail to detect new mechanisms to treat disease. Unfortunately, this has proved to be the case in psychiatry. Indeed, the molecular targets of all commonly used psychiatric drugs are the same as those of their 1950s prototypes.

The challenge of defining indications for treatment and developing biomarkers

In addition to the problems related to target identification and animal models, another gap in knowledge inhibiting investment in treatment discovery and development is the phenomenological diagnostic system that characterizes psychiatry and the associated lack of biological markers for disease or treatment response. Although progress in neuroimaging, genetics, and other forms of investigation may ultimately provide objective markers, these have not yet been identified. Pharmaceutical companies are dissuaded from developing new drugs if they must rely on descriptive DSM diagnoses (as described later) that almost certainly identify heterogeneous syndromes as official indications for treatment development. Similarly, lacking objective markers to gauge treatment response, they have been forced to rely on subjective rating scales such as the

Hamilton Rating Scale used for depression, which makes clinical trials almost prohibitively difficult. Depression, like many other psychiatric conditions, is characterized by waxing and waning symptoms that can readily confound the results of treatment trials.

The history of psychiatric diagnosis is very much tied to history of treatment. In concert with the discovery of the effects of lithium, antidepressants, antipsychotics, and benzodiazepines, there was resurgent interest in diagnosis that produced concerted efforts in the 1960s and 1970s. The latter was motivated in no small part by the need to match patients with the most appropriate interventions, and also by a wish to define psychiatric disorders in ways that were thought to be compatible with biology. The Department of Psychiatry at Washington University, St. Louis separated itself from the psychoanalytic mainstream and returned to Emil Kraepelin's diagnostic concepts. He had asserted that, as in the rest of medicine, psychiatry could identify specific disorders, likely of biological origin, based on careful descriptions of symptoms and course. He illustrated this approach by carefully differentiating what he called dementia praecox (later renamed schizophrenia) from manic-depressive illness (later called bipolar disorder). In a seminal article that launched an era of research on psychiatric diagnosis in the 1970s, Robins and Guze (42) argued that it was possible to achieve reliable and valid diagnoses based on clinical description, laboratory study, exclusion of other disorders, follow-up observations, and family research. Given the lack of biological markers, their work, like that of Kraepelin, was based entirely on clinical description but had profound influences that brought psychiatry closer to both biology and other fields of of medicine.

The descriptive approach championed by the St Louis research group came to dominate psychiatric diagnosis because of its central role in the third edition of the widely influential *Diagnostic and Statistical Manual of Mental Disorders* (DSM) (43), published in 1980. In the service of reliability, the manual used operationalized criteria in a manner that had been pioneered by the St. Louis group in the early 1970s (44). With the sole exception of mental retardation (which was defined as a quantitative deviation from the normal based on IQ) all disorders in the DSM-III, DSM-IV (45), and DSM-V (the last published in May 2013) were defined as categories that could be distinguished from health and from one other. On the assumption that it was possible to identify homogeneous categories for the purposes of research and treatment, DSM-III created a fine-grained subdivision of psychopathology that resulted in a remarkably large number of specific diagnoses. DSM-III advanced psychiatry by providing a common diagnostic language but, paradoxically, its very success in this regard has led to questioning of its phenomenological and categorical approach to classification.

Through the identification of homogeneous patient groups, Robins and Guze (42) argued that their careful descriptive approach would lead not only to reliable diagnoses (i.e. the agreement of different raters), but also to valid entities (the identification of 'natural kinds'). In fact, descriptive psychiatry as represented in the last three editions of the DSM is a poor reflection of nature (5,6). Robins and Guze did not foresee the remarkable heterogeneity of psychopathology, which has been progressively elucidated applying new genetic technology (see McGuffin, this volume, pp. 22–44) (12). Nonetheless, with the benefit of hindsight, DSM-III applied descriptive psychiatry and set the stage for the emergence of major clinical and scientific problems. The abundance of diagnostic silos has led to a high degree of comorbidity that is, in the main, the result of inappropriate subdivision of pathological entities sharing risk factors or neural mechanisms. Similarly, the overly narrow silos have forced scrupulous clinicians to use the 'not otherwise specified' (NOS) subtype, which lacks informational content. Scientifically, the DSM categories have not mapped onto the results of family and genetic studies, and assert arbitrary diagnostic thresholds.

Pathological states based on quantitative deviations from health have long been well known in medicine; these include such conditions as hypertension and type 2 diabetes mellitus. By contrast, Kraepelin, the St. Louis school, and the DSM system all treated psychiatric disorders as discontinuous categories in a manner analogous to infectious disease, such as pneumococcal pneumonia or tuberculosis. The implicit idea (occasionally explicit) in the literature of descriptive psychiatry is that a valid disorder is a homogeneous category produced by one or, at most, a limited set of related aetiologies. In fact, psychiatric disorders—like most common, enduring medical conditions—are heterogeneous and genetically complex (12); that is, a disease phenotype can result from multiple genetic pathways interacting with many non-genetic factors, with no gene either necessary or sufficient for the disorder. Psychiatric disorders that have been studied in detail also appear to be polygenic, meaning that a large number of genes contribute to risk. With the exception of some rare forms of autism, genes that confer risk for psychiatric disorders act in a statistical rather than a deterministic fashion.

Well-studied conditions such as autism (46), schizophrenia (47,48), and bipolar disorder appear to be remarkably polygenic. Gottesman and Shields (49) presciently raised the possibility as early as 1967 that schizophrenia is polygenic, but unfortunately their work had little influence on model-building for many years. Empirically, the contribution to risk conferred by variation in DNA sequences (1) is both inherited and *de novo* (2,46); reflects both common and rare sequence variants (3); affects protein coding genes and regulatory sequences; and involves (4) single nucleotide variants (SNVs) and—at least for a proportion of cases of autism, schizophrenia, and other neurodevelopmental disorders—larger copy number variants (CNVs). There is far greater sharing of genetic risk factors across different diagnoses (50) than was expected, not dissimilar to what has emerged across various forms of inflammatory bowel disease and several autoimmune disorders.

In sum, the relationship between genetics and nosology remains opaque (51,52) but, as is the case of many polygenic diseases, psychiatric disorders are better captured as quantitative deviations from health on multiple dimensions than as discontinuous DSM-style categories. For example, symptoms and, in some cases, laboratory findings associated with autism (53), schizophrenia, and mood disorders are normally distributed in the population with no clear natural demarcations that would justify a categorical break. The implications for science, clinical practice, and treatment development are profound. For example, it is not sensible to try to develop biomarkers for current DSM categories that in retrospect should have been seen as transiently useful fictions. Prominent attempts to start *ab initio* include the Research Domain Criteria (RDoCs) initiative of the National Institutes of Health (NIMH) (54), which foresees diagnoses that are entirely dimensional. In its initial iteration this project attempts to start with brain circuits for which patterns of cognition, emotion, and motivation relevant to psychiatry are adequately known; for example, fear, reward, and prefrontal cortical circuitry, the last involved in executive function.

A diagnostic system must also have clinical utility; in that regard, rough and ready categories can be extremely useful (55). Fortunately, imposing such categories on an underlying structure of quantitative dimensions has been shown to work well in many areas of medicine. For example, 'bins' relevant to treatment are superimposed on multiple dimensions that define hypertension (these include systolic and diastolic blood pressure) and dyslipidaemias (these include measures of total cholesterol, LDL cholesterol, HDL cholesterol, and triglycerides). Psychiatry is hardly alone in having to rethink nosology for the purposes of improving treatment. There is a dawning recognition in oncology that patterns of the particular somatic mutations within a tumour (i.e. the acquired genetic lesions that drive oncogenesis), are likely to be more important in selecting drug treatments for a cancer than its tissue of origin. As such, lung or breast cancer is turning out to be not one disease, but many, and treatment selection is increasingly made on the basis of molecular mechanisms.

The age of 'omics'

Given the challenges we have described above, a critical question for psychiatry is how to develop new hypotheses that can inform neurobiological investigations relevant to disease mechanisms and treatment. How can psychiatry escape the tunnel vision created by its descriptive straitjacket and over-reliance on old pharmacological and endocrinal models of disease. Across all of biology, gaps in knowledge are being addressed through large-scale, unbiased (hypothesis neutral) modes of discovery that can complement and ultimately enrich hypothesis-driven science. As with reductionist strategies, the databases, 'parts lists', and tools produced by such approaches must ultimately be integrated into multi-level explanatory models. While not a panacea, large-scale unbiased approaches can, along with a deeper engagement with neuroscience, help renew psychiatric research.

Genomics, the systematic determination and analysis of the complete DNA sequence of an organism (i.e. its genome) was the first area of biology to coalesce around large-scale, systematic efforts to generate shared data. The Human Genome Project (HGP) provided organization and support to sequence entire genomes, including an initial reference sequence of the human genome. In addition to DNA sequence information *per se* a key result of the HGP and parallel efforts in industry was investment in technologies to increase the speed and accuracy of DNA sequencing and to decrease its cost (56). Indeed, the cost has declined a million-fold over a mere decade, making it possible to determine the DNA sequences of thousands of human genomes, as well as those of many animal species, and even to obtain nearly complete sequences from the remains of ancient humans such as Neanderthals (57). In parallel with sequencing technologies, increasingly fast and powerful computing and vast, inexpensive data storage capacities have made modern genomics possible.

Technologies and intellectual approaches developed for genomics have facilitated great strides in the ability of human genetics to analyse complex traits, including risk of genetically complex common diseases. At the population level, a trait such as disease risk may result from many different rare DNA variants acting in different individuals to produce a similar phenotype, from the interaction of many different common sequence variants each contributing a small effect, or a combination of the two. This means that to achieve the statistical power to discover variations in DNA sequences contributing to disease risk, we need to study large numbers of patients and control subjects in various research designs. New technologies have made this both feasible and affordable. Thus progress is accelerating in identifying the genetic architecture of heterogeneous and polygenic disorders like autism, schizophrenia, and bipolar disorder. Given our ignorance of the disease mechanisms in psychiatry, it is critical that genetic strategies remain agnostic concerning biological hypotheses. Research has revealed many previously unimagined genetic loci conferring risk of disorder (12,46), and far greater sharing of risk-conferring genes across diagnoses (58). Hitherto, systematic approaches (59) have also failed to confirm many reports from past small studies based on biological hypotheses. Although disappointing, the frailty of such hypotheses has reaffirmed the need for humility in confronting brain complexity, and underscored the central role of unbiased methodology.

By analogy with genomics, systematic attempts to describe and analyse all members of a class have received the fashionable suffix of 'omics'. Although they are on the increase, big, costly, technology-driven projects, beginning with the HGP, have often been controversial (60,61) because of the concern they will divert resources from smaller laboratories engaged in hypothesis-driven science. It is also the case that not all 'big science' projects supported by governments and foundations have proved cost-effective. Yet it is increasingly clear that if we are to understand such complex matters as the mechanisms underlying mental disorders, we will need both large-scale unbiased discovery projects and hypothesis-driven science. The large databases and reagent collections derived from 'omics' research should ultimately provide a rich source of new hypotheses to drive inquiries into psychiatric conditions.

With the exception of some rare forms of autism, DNA sequence is not destiny when it comes to psychiatric disorders. This can be illustrated by the observation that in schizophrenia, bipolar disorder, major depression, and other psychiatric disorders monozygotic twin pairs (derived from a single fertilized ovum and sharing 100% of their DNA sequences) do not exhibit 100% concordance for the disorder. Indeed, in schizophrenia, which is highly genetically influenced, given a monozygotic co-twin with the disorder, the other member of the pair has only a 50% risk of full-blown schizophrenia. (The co-twin might show a degree of cortical thinning and cognitive impairment but never psychotic symptoms.) Specific environmental factors or chance might convert genetic risk into psychiatric disease. These environmental and stochastic factors might act by influencing the rates at which specific genes are transcribed into RNA. Especially when such factors act during embryogenesis, and perhaps early postnatal life, they may persist into adulthood by creating long-lived patterns in the proteins that package DNA in the cell nucleus. These patterns, which determine whether a particular gene is available to be transcribed, are captured by the term 'epigenetics'. Historically the study of epigenetic mechanisms was limited to prenatal development. The last decade has seen the application of epigenetics to postnatal life. For example, influential models of stress due to early maternal separation in rat pups (e.g. 62) have influenced the study of human development by suggesting that early adversity might act via epigenetic mechanisms to alter responses to stress for many years. This historically recent extension of epigenetics to become a possible mechanism by which postnatal experience causes persistent changes in physiology and behaviour is still at a stage where the significance of the evidence is a matter of debate.

The global study of gene expression (the transcriptome) or of proteins (the proteome) in cells or organisms adds a new level of complexity to 'omics', as the production and modification of RNA and proteins are regulated processes that differ according to cell types and conditions. Thus, unlike genomics in which each individual organism has a single unique set of DNA sequences (with the caveat concerning somatic mutations), each cell type, and each of the many types of neurons and glial cells in the brain, has its own transcriptome and proteome, which change as these cells are subjected to diverse signals and stresses. Relevant research demands efficient high-throughput technologies such as gene arrays (or 'chips') to study patterns of global gene expression; and mass spectrometry in the case of proteomics. Alongside these approaches, enquiry into the biology of mental disorders will benefit from future studies of the epigenome (global studies of epigenetic modifications), the metabolome (the complete set of metabolic intermediates in a cell under particular conditions), and the connectome (systematic wiring diagrams of the nervous system or systematic maps of brain activity).

Reconnecting with neuroscience: reprogramming cells, engineering circuits in vitro, connectivity maps, and optogenetics

In many areas of medical research, such as cancer biology, diseased cells can be obtained after surgical biopsy or resection. These cells can then be examined directly, made into cell lines that will propagate indefinitely, or injected into immunologically compromised mice to study tumour formation. Here lies another hurdle for psychiatric research. Brain biopsies for psychiatric disorders—unlike those for cancer, including brain cancer—are ethically unimaginable. Moreover, a localized sample of brain tissue might not be informative about disease mechanisms since psychiatric disorders are the result of abnormal physiology affecting widely distributed circuits and are not 'cell autonomous'. Nonetheless, the study of living human neurons is critical if we are to study genes that confer disease risk successfully. Part of the uniqueness of the human brain appears to be its patterns of gene expression in multiple regions of the forebrain. Therefore, even as psychiatry wrestles with the utility of animal models, it will be necessary to devise models based on human neurons to interrogate gene function and other domains of disease-relevant biology.

Remarkably, it is becoming feasible to study molecular and cellular aspects of psychiatric disorders with human neurons *in vitro* using stem cell technologies. One such approach makes it possible to generate pluripotent cells (cells that can generate any tissue in the body) from skin fibroblasts. This technology, which resulted in the award of the 2012 Nobel Prize to Shinya Yamanaka, initially used engineered viruses to carry genes that encoded four transcription factors (proteins that control gene expression) into fibroblasts that had been placed in culture. The resulting induced pluripotent stem cells (iPSCs) can then be used to manufacture diverse other cell types including neurons. The technology is moving rapidly, so that specific types of neurons have been produced, such as motor neurons. It is a pivotal goal to identify the specific neuronal cell types involved in psychiatric disorders and to be able to engineer those cells.

One major advantage of iPSC technology is that skin fibroblasts can be taken both from control subjects and from patients, and the cells can be fully genotyped. It is now readily possible to engineer disease-risk-associated DNA sequence variations into the genomes of the 'control' cells and to 'rescue' patient cell phenotypes by replacing risk-conferring DNA sequences with non-risk variants. Initial experiments relevant to psychiatry have compared neurons engineered from skin biopsies of patients with schizophrenia and neurons derived from control subjects and have reported phenotypic differences (63). It is early days in the adaptation of this technology to psychiatric disorders, but if successful, this might partially obviate the need for animal models.

While molecular and cellular approaches are critical to the pursuit of new medications, neural circuit activity underlies psychiatric symptoms and is therefore relevant to improved diagnosis, possibly to treatment biomarkers, and new non-pharmacological treatments ranging from DBS (9) to cognitive therapies (10,27). For all of these reasons, a high-resolution connectivity map of the human brain is a critical platform for psychiatric research to the same degree as a complete catalogue of genetic and epigenetic contributors to risk. Given that the brain has 100 trillion synapses underlying its connections, even achieving a rough wiring diagram poses a challenge. As in the case of genomics, however, new technologies combined with greater computing power and data storage capacity have made it possible to envision a serious effort in 'connectomics'. The ultimate goal of such efforts is connectomes—high-resolution maps of all neurons and their synaptic connections for entire organisms, including humans. Much of the micro-scale mapping at the level of cells and synapses has perforce begun with model organisms. Much of the initial focus for the human connectome has been at the macro-scale and dependent on an array of neuroimaging technologies including methods for mapping grey matter, white matter tracts, and activity.

The ultimate utility of connectivity maps for psychiatry requires functional maps superimposed on structural ones that, to date, in humans, have largely relied on PET and fMRI. As described earlier, however, functional imaging in humans is largely correlational. New technologies, most notably optogenetics, implemented in animals, have now made it possible to stimulate or suppress activity in particular neural cells and circuits and thus to test hypotheses about their functions. Engineered viruses carrying specific genes are injected into the brain, or genes are inserted by recombination into the germ line of animals. The genes carried into the brain are designed to be turned on only within specific neural cell types where they express light-activated ion channels. The pioneering work used a gene from algae that encoded a light-activated ion channel, rhodopsin, but other light-regulated channels have since been used that can produce neuronal firing or inhibition in response to specific wavelengths of light. The desired wavelength, introduced into the animal brain through fibre optic instruments, permits the activation or inhibition of specific cells and, thus specific circuits, on a millisecond timescale (2,64). The specificity of optogenetics is not only temporal but also spatial compared to previous stimulation methods, generally involving electrodes, which involved neighbouring axons in addition to those targeted intentionally. Optogenetics has already yielded salient new insights into the control of fear, reward, aggression, and many other functions relevant to psychopathology and, in many cases, can be extrapolated to humans.

Conclusion

Psychiatry has reached a crossroads; the understanding of disease processes has progressed very slowly, resulting in the suspension of the development of significant novel medications. The exit of the pharmaceutical industry from the psychiatric arena is a symptom of this stasis and, at the same time, an impediment to progress in treating psychiatric patients. The half-century stasis in therapeutics reflects, above all, the exceeding difficulty of studying heterogeneous, polygenic disorders. At the same time, seemingly unnecessary obstacles have also limited advances. These encompass the continuing acceptance of a diagnostic system that has palpably limited translational and clinical science, and a set of research paradigms rooted in the pharmacological discoveries of the 1950s that have resulted in many funding grants and publications but no deep understanding of disease mechanisms (7). Despite the challenges, this is not a time for pessimism. New technologies including large-scale unbiased genetic studies, the early development of stem cell technologies with all their implications for the study of disease, and advances in understanding neural circuits can, if effectively deployed, move psychiatry past the current crossroads.

References

1 http://www.sfn.org/index.aspx?pagename=about_SfN#timeline [Referenced 24 August 2012].

2 Fenno, L., Yizhar, O., and Deisseroth, K. (2011). The development and application of optogenetics. *Annual Review of Neuroscience* **34**, 389–412.

3 Fox, M. D., Synder, A. Z., Vincent, J. L., Van Essen, D. C., and Raichle, M. E. (2005). The human brain is intrinsically organized into dynamic, anticorrelated functional networks. *Proceedings of the National Academy of Sciences of the U S A* **102**, 9673–8.

4 http://www.alleninstitute.org [Referenced 16 August 2012].

5 Hyman, S. E. (2007). Can neuroscience be integrated into the DSM-V? *Nature Reviews Neuroscience* **8**, 725–32.

6 Hyman, S. E. (2010). The diagnosis of mental disorders: the problem of reification. *Annual Review of Clinical Psychology* **6**, 155–79.

7 Hyman, S. E. (2012). Revolution stalled. *Science Translational Medicine* **4**, 155cm11.

8 Insel, T. R. (2012). Next-generation treatments of mental disorders. *Science Translational Medicine* **4**, 155ps19.

9 Holtzheimer, P. E. and Mayberg, H. S. (2011). Deep brain stimulation for psychiatric disorders. *Annual Review of Neuroscience* **34**, 289–307.

10 Minzenberg, M. J., and Carter, C. S. (2012). Developing treatments for impaired cognition in schizophrenia. *Trends in Cognitive Science* **16**, 35–42.

11 World Health Organization (2008). *The global burden of disease*, 2004 update. Geneva: World Health Organization.

12 Sullivan, P. F., Daly, M. J., and O'Donovan, M. (2012). Genetic architecture of psychiatric disorders: the emerging picture and its implications. *Nature Reviews Genetics* **13**, 537–51.

13 Nestler, E. J., and Hyman, S. E. (2010). Animal models of neuropsychiatric disorders. *Nature Neuroscience* **13**,1161–9.

14 Martin, J. B. (2002). The integration of neurology, psychiatry, and neuroscience in the 21st century. *American Journal of Psychiatry* **159**, 695–704.

15 Cowan, W. M., Harter, D. H., and Kandel, E. R. (2000). The emergence of modern neuroscience: some implications for neurology and psychiatry. *Annual Review of Neuroscience* **23**, 343–91.

16 Schmitt, F. O., Melnechuk, T., Adelman, G., and Worden, F. (1966) *Neurosciences research symposium summaries, Vol 1*. Cambridge, MA: MIT Press.

17 Kopnisky, K. L., Cowan, W. M., and Hyman, S. E. (2002) Levels of analysis in psychiatric research. *Developmental Psychopathology* **14**, 437–61.

18 http://www.nobelprize.org/nobel_prizes/medicine/laureates/2000/kandel-lecture.pdf [Referenced 25 August 2012].

19 Pittinger, C. and Kandel, E. R. (2003). In search of general mechanisms for long-lasting plasticity: aplysia and the hippocampus. *Philosophical Transactions of the Royal Society London B Biological Sciences* **358**, 757–63.

20 Dayan, P. and Huys, Q. J. (2008). Serotonin, inhibition, and negative mood. *Public Library of Science Computational Biology* **4**(2), e4.

21 Dayan, P. and Huys, Q. J. (2009). Serotonin in affective control. *Annual Review of Neuroscience* **32**, 95–126.

22 Peça, J., Feliciano, C.,Ting, J. T. et al. (2011). Shank3 mutant mice display autistic-like behaviours and striatal dysfunction. *Nature* **472**, 437–42.

23 Thompson PM, Vidal C, Giedd JN et al. (2001). Mapping adolescent brain change reveals dynamic wave of accelerated gray matter loss in very early-onset schizophrenia. *Proceedings of the National Academy of Sciences of the U S A* **98**, 11650–5.

24 Barch, D. M., Carter, C. S., Braver, T. S. et al. (2001). Selective deficits in prefrontal cortex function in medication-naive patients with schizophrenia. *Archives of General Psychiatry* **58**, 280–8.

25 Laruelle, M., Abi-Dargham, A., van Dyck, C. H. et al. (1996). Single photon emission computerized tomography imaging of amphetamine-induced dopamine release in drug-free schizophrenic subjects. *Proceedings of the National Academy of Sciences of the U S A* **93**, 9235–40.

26 Westman, E.Muehlboeck, J. S., and Simmons A (2012). Combining MRI and CSF measures for classification of Alzheimer's disease and prediction of mild cognitive impairment conversion. *Neuroimage* **62**, 229–38.

27 Carter, C. S.,Barch, D. M.; CNTRICS Executive Committee (2012). Imaging biomarkers for treatment development for impaired cognition: report of the sixth CNTRICS meeting: Biomarkers recommended for further development. *Schizophrenia Bulletin* **38**, 26–33.

28 Nauta, W. J. (1946). Hypothalamic regulation of sleep in rats: an experimental study. *Journal of Neurophysiology* **9**, 285–316.

29 MacLean, P (1990). *The triune brain in evolution: role in paleocerebral functions*. New York: Plenum Press.

30 Johnstone, E. C., Crow, T. J., Frith, C. D., Husband, J., and Kreel, L (1976). Cerebral ventricular size and cognitive impairment in chronic schizophrenia. *Lancet* **2**, 924–6.

31 Berman, K. F. (1987). Cortical 'stress tests' in schizophrenia: regional cerebral blood flow studies. *Biological Psychiatry* **22**, 1304–26.

32 Cade, J. F.J (1949). Lithium salts in the treatment of psychotic excitement. *Medical Journal of Australia* 2: 349–52.

33 Mitchell, P. B. and Hadzi-Pavlovic, D (this volume).

34 Kirsch, I., Deacon, B. J., Huedo-Medina, T. B., Scoboria, A. Moore, T. J., and Johnson, B. T. (2008). Initial severity and antidepressant benefits: a meta-analysis of data submitted to the Food and Drug Administration. *Public Library of Science Medicine* 5(2), e45.

35 Horder, J., Matthews, P., and Waldmann, R (2011). Placebo, Prozac and PLoS: significant lessons for psychopharmacology. *Journal of Psychopharmacology* 25, 1277–88.

36 Schildkraut, J. J. and Kety, S. S. (1967). Biogenic amines and emotion. *Science* 156, 21–37.

37 Hyman, S. E. and Nestler, E. J. (1996). Initiation and adaptation: a paradigm for understanding psychotropic drug action. *American Journal of Psychiatry* 153, 151–62.

38 Sachar, E. J. (1967). Corticosteroids in depressive illness: I. A reevaluation of control issues and literature. *Archives of Geneneral Psychiatry* 17, 544–53.

39 Heim C, Newport D. J., Heit, S. et al. (2000). Pituitary-adrenal and autonomic responses to stress in women after sexual and physical abuse in childhood. *JAMA* 284, 592–7.

40 Khin, N. A., Chen, Y-F., Yang, Y., Yang, P, and Laughren, T. P. (2011). Exploratory analyses of efficacy date from major depressive disorder trails submitted to the US Food and Drug Administration in support of new drug applications *Journal of Clinical Psychiatry* 72, 464–72.

41 Fernando, A. B. P. and Robbins T. W. (2011). Animal models of neuropsychiatric disorders. *Annual Review of Clinical Psychology* 7, 39–61.

42 Robins, E. and Guze, S. B. (1970). Establishment of diagnostic validity in psychiatric illness: Its application to schizophrenia. *American Journal of Psychiatry* 126, 983–7.

43 American Psychiatric Association (1980). *Diagnostic and statistical manual of mental disorders (3rd edn)*. Washington, DC: American Psychiatric Association.

44 Feighner, J. P., Robins, E., Guze, S. B., Woodruff, R. A. Jr, and Munoz, R. (1972). Diagnostic criteria for use in psychiatric research. *Archives of General Psychiatry* 26, 57–63.

45 American Psychiatric Association (1994). *Diagnostic and statistical manual of mental disorders (4th edn)*. Washington, DC: American Psychiatric Association.

46 Neale B. M., Kou Y., Liu L., Ma'ayan A. et al (2012). Patterns and rates of exonic *de novo* mutations in autism spectrum disorders. *Nature* 485, 242–5.

47 Lee, S. H., DeCandia, T. R., Ripke, S. et al (2012). Estimating the proportion of variation in susceptibility to schizophrenia captured by common SNPs. *Nature Genetics* 44, 247–50.

48 Gejman, P. V., Sanders, A. R., and Kendler, K. S. (2011). Genetics of schizophrenia: New findings and challenges. *Annual Review of Genomics and Human Genetics* 12, 121–44.

49 Gottesman, I. I. and Shields, J. (1967). A polygenic theory of schizophrenia. *Proceedings of the National Academy of Sciences of the U S A* 58, 199–205.

50 Lichtenstein, P., Carlstrom, E., Rastam, M., Gillberg, C., and Anckarsater, J. (2010). The genetics of autism spectrum disorders and related neuropsychiatric disorders in childhood. *American Journal of Psychiatry* 167, 1357–63.

51 Kendler, K. S. (2006). Reflections on the relationship between psychiatric genetics and psychiatric nosology. *American Journal of Psychiatry* 163, 1138–46.

52 Craddock, N., O'Donovan, M. C., and Owen, M. J. (2006). Genes for schizophrenia and bipolar disorder? Implications for psychiatric nosology. *Schizophrenia Bulletin* 32, 9–16.

53 Di Martino, A., Shehzad, Z., Kelley, C. et al. (2009). Relationship between cingulo-insular functional connectivity and autistic trats in neurotypical adults. *American Journal of Psychiatry* 166, 891–9.

54 http://www.nimh.nih.gov/research-funding/rdoc/index.shtml [Referenced 24 August 2012].

55 Kendell, R. and Jablensky, A. (2003). Distinguishing between validity and utility of psychiatric diagnoses. *American Journal of Psychiatry* **160**, 4–12.

56 Shendure, J. and Ji, H. (2008). Next-generation DNA sequencing. *Nature Biotechnology* **26**, 1135–45.

57 Green, R. E., Krause, J., Briggs, A. W. et al. (2010) A draft sequence of the neandertal genome. *Science* **328**, 710–22.

58 Talkowski, M. E., Rosenfeld, J. A., Blumenthal, I. et al. (2012). Sequencing chromosomal abnormalities reveals neurodevelopmental loci that confer risk across diagnostic boundaries. *Cell* **149**, 525–37.

59 Major Depressive Disorder Working Group of the Psychiatric GWAS Consortium (2013). A mega-analysis of genome-wide association studies for major depressive disorder. *Molecular Psychiatry* **18**, 497–511.

60 Collins, F. S., Morgan, M., and Patrinos A. (2003). The Human Genome Project: lessons from large-scale biology. *Science* **300**, 286–90.

61 Lichtman, J. W. and Sanes J. R. (2008). Ome sweet ome: What can the genome tell us about the connectome? *Current Opinions in Neurobiology* **18**, 346–53.

62 Meaney, M. J. and Szyf, M. (2005). Maternal care as a model for experience-dependent chromatin plasticity. *Trends in Neuroscience* **28**, 456–65.

63 Brennand, K. J., Simone, A., Jou, J. et al. (2011). Modelling schizophrenia using human induced pluripotent stem cells. *Nature* **473**, 221–5.

64 Deisseroth, K. (2012). Optogenetics and psychiatry: Applications, challenges, and opportunities. *Biological Psychiatry* **71**, 1030–2.

Essay 2

The past, present, and future of psychiatric genetics

Peter McGuffin

Introduction: prelude and fugue

The retrospective timescale of half a century, taken throughout this book, is a particularly apt one for psychiatric genetics. In 1959 a landmark event occurred in the United Kingdom that had wider implications for the subject's development internationally. The Medical Research Council (MRC) Psychiatric Genetics Unit at the Institute of Psychiatry in the University of London was founded under the directorship of Dr Eliot Slater. It was housed on the campus of the Institute of Psychiatry/Maudsley Hospital in a building that became known as the 'Genetics Hut'. Austere and modest in its scale, it nevertheless became internationally famous, at least among the tiny band of researchers on psychiatric genetics that then existed around the world.

Although it was the first university-embedded unit of its type in the United Kingdom, the Hut's intellectual roots traced back to Germany where, in 1917, the German Research Institute for Psychiatry (Deutsche Forschungsanstalt für Psychiatrie) in Munich was founded and directed by Emil Kraepelin. He established a genealogical and demographic department in his institute and appointed as the head a pioneer of psychiatric genetics, Ernst Rudin. His department contained a number of talented researchers working on family and twin studies, including Bruno Schulz, Hans Luxenburger, and Franz Kallmann, who shared with Rudin an enthusiasm for the science but not his politics. Rudin was an enthusiastic supporter of the National Socialist (Nazi) party and an influential adviser concerning its policies in eugenics and 'racial hygiene', whereas Luxenburger was at one point banned from teaching at the university because of his open criticism of Nazi ideologies. Eliot Slater, who began a fellowship with Rudin in 1934, became outraged by his political views. While in Munich he fraternized with Jewish intellectuals and married one of them, the poet Lydia Pasternak, sister of Boris the celebrated writer. (Their daughter, Catherine Oppenheimer, is a contributor to this volume.) Slater returned to London in 1936 and began the task of founding psychiatric genetics as a new discipline in the United Kingdom. In the same year Kallmann, who was half Jewish, fled to the United States where he was offered a position as the first head of a new medical genetics department at the New York State Psychiatric Institute, essentially founding psychiatric genetics in the United States. Other visitors to the Munich department in the mid-1930s included a young Dane, Erik Strömgren, who went on to become the pre-eminent Scandinavian psychiatric researcher of his generation.

In the wake of World War II, the discrediting of Nazi eugenics policy also tainted psychiatric genetics, which died out in Germany. Thus the Munich genealogy department provided both the prelude to psychiatric genetics in Europe and North America and a flight from the subject in Germany that was to last for over 30 years.

The era of twin and adoption studies

The idea that mental illness has a tendency to run in families is almost certainly an ancient one. There are patient case records dating back to the early 19th century in the museum of the hospital where I do my clinical work, London's Bethlem Royal Hospital, showing that doctors then were already attempting to record systematically whether their patients' disorders were hereditary. Of course diseases can run in families because of a shared environment that might include anything from exposure to toxins or infectious agents to shared upbringing and lifestyle. Normal traits, behaviours and characteristics run in families too. For example, a study that I carried out 20 years ago in Cardiff with my then registrar (1) showed that the 'risk' of attending medical school among the first-degree relatives of Cardiff medical students was 80 times that of the general population. We further showed that the pattern of inheritance was compatible with a Mendelian recessive gene. We published our results not to convince colleagues that there was a gene to clone, but rather to point out that it is dangerous to make simple genetic assumptions about a complicated trait.

Fortunately there are two types of 'natural experiment' that can come to our rescue in teasing out the effects of genes, 'nature' and within-family 'nurture'. These are twin studies and adoption studies. The English polymath Sir Francis Galton first suggested studying twins 'as a criterion of the relative powers of nature and nurture' in 1876 (2), but this was before much was known about the biology of twinning. It was Wilhelm Weinberg, a German obstetrician and pioneer of statistical genetics, who, at the beginning of the 20th century, made the first inference that there are two main types of twin: monozygotic (MZ) or identical twins who result from the splitting of a single egg and who have 100% of their genes in common, and dizygotic (DZ) or fraternal twins who result from the simultaneous fertilization of two eggs and have the same proportion of genes in common as siblings, i.e. 50%. In the 1920s twin studies began first by Siemens, a dermatologist (and again a German) investigating the inheritance of skin moles. This was followed by Luxenburger's study of schizophrenia, the first of its kind.

The basic idea of the classic twin method is that greater resemblance for a trait or disorder in MZ than DZ pairs reflects the influence of genes. However, this depends on an additional assumption about twins, that MZ and DZ pairs share the environment to roughly the same extent. This 'equal environments assumption' is open to criticism, particularly because half of DZ pairs are of opposite sex. For this reason many early twin studies were restricted to same-sex pairs; however, even in same-sex pairs MZ twins might be treated more alike by parents and be dressed alike, placed in the same class at school, have more friends in common than DZ pairs. As it turns out, studies have found that these sorts of environmental sharing do not much bias the results. Indeed, a repeated surprise finding emerging from twin studies of common traits is that the role of shared environment is often small.

A different potential source of bias in twin studies depends on how twins are selected for inclusion in the research. Very early twin studies of schizophrenia tended to focus on twins where at least one of the pair had been chronically hospitalized. They also often relied on the subjects being referred to the twin researcher by the doctor in charge of their case. Together these factors meant that early twin studies tended to include the most severe cases and the most conspicuous or memorable ones, and it is likely that this led to a bias in favour of concordant pairs (i.e. pairs where both had the disorder) and identical pairs, tending to inflate MZ–DZ differences and giving a 'more genetic' appearance. To overcome this problem Slater, in 1948, established a systematic way of ascertaining twins from the hospital-based register at the Maudsley and Bethlem Royal Hospital where every inpatient and outpatient, at their point of registration, was asked the question, 'Are you a twin?' Elsewhere, (e.g. the Scandinavian countries) it was possible to ascertain twins systematically via national registers and match these data with hospital case registers.

The 1960s saw the first flourishing systematic twin studies being carried out on a variety of disorders, but there was a particular focus of attention on schizophrenia which, at the time, was one of psychiatry's ideological battlegrounds. Earlier twin studies created suspicion in the minds of some that their authors had a hereditarian bias. There was even the idea advanced by Jackson (3), a psychoanalyst, that twins, particularly identical twins, may suffer from 'ego identity' problems more than singletons and would thus be particularly prone to psychotic disorder. In the later 1960s, a disparate group of critics often referred to collectively as 'anti-psychiatrists', such as the followers of R.D. Laing on the existentialist left and of Thomas Szasz on the radical right, questioned the very existence of schizophrenia as a 'real' disorder. Like other mental illness schizophrenia, according to Szasz, was just a myth.

In the United Kingdom social psychiatry had a powerful influence in the 1960s and 1970s and many viewed genetics as dismally deterministic. Indeed, Slater had the experience of a social psychiatrist colleague bursting into his office and 'whooping for joy' following the publication of a paper by the Finnish psychiatrist Pekka Tienari which purported to find zero concordance for schizophrenia in identical twins. However, Tienari's findings were in contrast to those of Slater's unit. A postdoctoral psychologist from the United States, Irving Gottesman, worked with Slater's long-time assistant, James Shields, to study schizophrenia using the Maudsley twin register. Their research (4) was notable for its careful methodology, including rating of twin data 'blindfolded' to the identity or zygosity of the subject by multiple diagnostic experts. They found over 50% concordance in monozygotic twins compared with just over 10% concordance in dizygotic twins. These figures were much in line with several other studies published at around the same time, including a follow-up study from Tienari who found that several co-twins from his earlier negative study had become ill, making the total pattern of results wholly consistent with a genetic effect in schizophrenia.

For those who remained unconvinced clinching evidence came from adoption studies. The first of these was by Leonard Heston (5) who was still a trainee psychiatrist in the United States when he obtained blindfolded diagnoses on two groups of adults who had been fostered or adopted away from their natural mothers in infancy. The first group consisted of 47 offspring of mothers with a diagnosis of schizophrenia who had given birth when they were inpatients in Oregon state mental hospitals at a time when state law dictated that such offspring be separated from their mothers within 72 hours. The second group of adoptees consisted of 50 age- and sex-matched controls whose mothers were free from psychiatric illness. The results were quite striking in that five of the offspring of schizophrenic mothers became schizophrenic whereas none of those with healthy biological mothers were so affected.

Soon after, a series of publications began appearing as a result of a collaboration between American and Danish psychiatrists, led by Seymour Kety, using Danish adoption and psychiatric registers. These were larger in scale and had the advantage of allowing a variety of study designs. The first was, like Heston's, an adoptees study looking at the biological offspring of schizophrenics compared with control adoptees, but this time a substantial number of the schizophrenic parents, about one third, were fathers. This meant that criticisms of Heston's study concerning the possible role of prenatal or perinatal maternal influences could be addressed. The second design was called an adoptee's family study; the starting point was adoptees who had become schizophrenic and whose biological and adoptive relatives were compared. The finding of a small sample of adoptees with biological parents but who had been raised by adopting parents one of whom became schizophrenic, permitted the third type of study design, the cross fostering study; these adoptees were compared with those in the schizophrenic biological parent group who were raised by normal parents. All three types of study pointed clearly in the same direction: What mattered in creating an increased risk of schizophrenia was sharing genes rather than sharing environment. This led Kety to remark, 'If schizophrenia is a myth, it is a myth with a strong genetic basis'.

Adoption and, even more importantly, twin studies continue to play a role in psychiatric genetics up to the present time, and have recently provided more sophisticated insights using modern statistical modelling techniques that capitalize on the availability of high-speed computers. However, in the 1960s and 1970s they were not able to show which genes were involved, or where they lay on the genome, the 23 pairs of chromosomes that carry our genetic material. Therefore, for many, studies that actually visualized chromosomes were a more exciting route to follow.

Cytogenetics and the joy of seeing chromosomes

The existence of chromosomes had been known since the mid-19th century. However, an understanding of their roles only began in the 1950s, as technology for visualizing them became developed. Most of the time chromosomes are extremely elongated structures contained in the cell nucleus invisible under a light microscope. However, when cells divide the chromosomes become shorter and more compact, aligning themselves in pairs. If cells are stimulated to divide, the cell division then chemically arrested and the cell broken down, it is possible to stain the chromosomes with a dye and visualize them under a microscope. Early cytogenetics depended on taking a photograph of stained chromosomes, cutting out the images of individual chromosomes with scissors, arranging the 22 pairs of ordinary chromosomes (or autosomes) in order of size by hand, picking out the sex chromosomes (X and Y) and re-photographing them to give a final image of the 23 pairs—a so-called karyotype.

This incredibly crude-sounding approach actually yielded astonishing break-throughs, the first of which was the discovery by Lejeune, in 1957, that Down's syndrome is caused by an abnormal karyotype most commonly involving an extra chromosome 21 (6). Discoveries of other so-called trisomies followed, including Klinefelter's syndrome (men with an extra X chromosome, hence XXY rather than the normal male XY), as well as discovery of deletion syndromes where a chromosome or part of a chromosome goes missing. A good example is Turner's syndrome where the appearance is female though there is only one X chromosome (X0) rather than the normal two (XX).

Both Klinefelter's syndrome and Turner's syndrome are of psychiatric interest. Men with Klinefelter's usually have lower IQ and, by some reports, an increased rate of schizophrenia. Women with Turner's syndrome have normal intelligence but tend to test poorly measuring performance rather than verbal reasoning. More recently they have been reported to have increased rates of autistic features, particularly when their single X chromosome is inherited from their mother (7). The cytogenetic discovery of greatest interest in the early years of cytogenetics concerned men with an extra Y chromosome (XYY). Jacobs reported finding that 3% of men in Carstairs, a Scottish secure psychiatric hospital for offenders, had XYY karyotypes (8). They were also unusually tall and had below average intelligence. But was the XYY syndrome, as it came to be called, really a newly discovered genetic cause of antisocial behaviour? A key question was how common was the XYY karyotype in the general population. Further research revealed its presence was somewhere between 1/1000 and 1/2000, which meant at least 1000 adult XYY men in Scotland (the total population at that time being about 5 million) were not in Carstairs Hospital. A subsequent study (9) remarkably screened nearly all non-institutionalized men in Denmark who were over 1.84 m in height, approximately 4000. Twelve had XYY karyotypes, five of whom (42%) had criminal records compared with 9% of non-XYY men. However, the records of the XYY men involved mainly minor offences, effectively refuting the idea the syndrome predisposes to violent criminality.

Cytogenetics continues to be refined in its methodologies and is now a vital branch of laboratory diagnostics in learning disability and medical genetics; however, the karyotypes that one can see using a light microscope proved to be less informative in psychiatic genetics than many had hoped for. Interestingly, there has been a resurgence of interest in cytogenetics as methods have been developed to detect much smaller, subtler, submicroscopic changes in chromosomes.

Statistical models and muddles

While early cytogenetics did not offer much explanatory power for the bulk of psychiatric disorder, a different set of technologies were beginning to be employed. Disorders such as schizophrenia and bipolar disorder were clearly not Mendelian, where genes are either dominant (when a single copy is sufficient to cause the disorder) or recessive (when two copies, one from each parent, are required). Family studies did not show clear-cut patterns of transmission as predicted by Mendel's first law, the law of segregation, where half the offspring of an affected parent show the disease in the case of dominant genes, and a quarter of the offspring of unaffected 'carrier' parents show

the disease due to recessive inheritance. Twin studies revealed incomplete concordance in identical twins, indicating that the non-genetic factors played a role. Therefore
the only way that such disorders could result from the effect of single genes would be
through incomplete penetrance, when an individual carries a disease genotype without
manifesting the disorder. Slater (10) was the first to put forward a plausible single-gene
model of schizophrenia by invoking this notion. He showed that, assuming the disorder is a lifetime risk in approximately 1% of the general population, a dominant gene
with a specified incomplete penetrance and a specified frequency and population could
explain the risks in various categories of relatives of individuals with schizophrenia. He
studied the hypothesis empirically, using a graphical method to solve the parameters
of his model.

In contrast, Gottesman and Shields (11), working in Slater's unit, put forward a more
radical 'polygenic' model based on the work of Falconer (12), a statistical geneticist.
He postulated that what is inherited in common disorders is a liability contributed by
multiple genes, each of small effect, so that in the general population the liability tends
to have a bell-shaped (or normal) distribution and only those individuals who live beyond the threshold at the upper tail of the curve actually become affected. Relatives of
affected individuals have an augmented liability so that more of them lie beyond the
threshold then do members of the general population. This model allows calculation
of a measure called 'correlation in liability' for various categories of relatives which, in
turn, can be used to estimate the heritability, the proportion of variation in liability to
the disorder that can be attributed to genes. There subsequently ensued a debate that
lasted for almost three decades as to whether the single-gene or polygenic model of
schizophrenia was correct. (Similar debates existed about other disorders, but again it
was schizophrenia that was the most hotly contested battleground.)

One of the problems about differentiating between single-gene and polygenic models
is that both are comparatively 'elastic' and therefore difficult to refute. More sophisticated types of modelling were developed in the 1980s as high-speed computers became
widely available. In the meantime an influential piece of evidence that argued against
the single-gene model was another graphical method demonstrating that many of the
available data points from family and twin studies of schizophrenia plotted outside
the envelope compatible with the biologically plausible range of single-gene parameters (13). The same result was later found for bipolar disorder (14). When speaking
to clinical audiences on the topic, I have often been asked about my confidence in
dismissing single-gene models when Slater's solution seemed so plausible. This led me
to re-examine Slater's original work. Interestingly, he never actually formally tested
whether his schizophrenia single-gene model was a satisfactory statistical explanation
of the data, and if one applies a simple chi-squared goodness-of-fit test the model can
be unequivocally rejected (1,15).

Biometrics and behaviour genetics

The debate over whether schizophrenia could be best explained by a single or polygenic
inheritance model provides a specific example of a type of controversy present since
the beginnings of genetics as a new branch of biology in the early 20th century—the

so-called 'Galton versus Mendel' controversy. Francis Galton was an English polymath born in 1822, the same year as Gregor Mendel, and far more celebrated than Mendel during his lifetime. Galton was the first to suggest the study of twins as a means of assessing the relative contributions of nature and nurture and in one of his most famous works, *Hereditary Genius*, he laid the foundation of behavioural genetics. Galton was interested in the resemblance between relatives for continuous traits, which he saw as being predominantly normally distributed (i.e. following a bell-shaped curve). He was the first to describe the phenomenon of 'regression to the mean' whereby parents with extreme characteristics (e.g. great height or mental ability) tend to have offspring who are closer to the average. Here he provided the beginning of a fundamental method in statistics, regression analysis, subsequently developed by his disciple Karl Pearson, who first devised the correlation coefficient as a measure of similarity between pairs of observations (e.g. continuous traits in pairs of relatives).

In contrast to the influential writings of Galton and his followers, Mendel's laws, originally published in 1866, remained almost completely ignored for the next 35 years. When 'rediscovered' they had a revolutionary effect, explaining transmission of present/absent characteristics, but were seen by Galton's followers, the biometric school, as largely irrelevant to the majority of human characteristics that are continuous. It was not until 1918 when Ronald Fisher showed that many genes of small effect, behaving in Mendelian fashion, could add up to produce a continuous trait that has a normal distribution (16). Fisher's rapprochement between Mendelian and Galtonian ideas, however, was contained within a mathematically dense and difficult piece of work that only really impressed the statistical *cognoscenti* who were rare among biologists. Subsequently Mendelian and biometric genetics progressed in parallel, often in a non-overlapping fashion, through much of the 20th century.

The mainstream of behavioural genetics was definitely in the biometric camp and, with regard to human behaviours, heavily influenced by interpretation of twin studies. The subject matter included both continuous traits, such as personality and cognitive ability as reflected in IQ tests, and present/absent traits, such as psychiatric disorder which could be considered as having an underlying continuous liability as in the Falconer-type model. As examples, Figure 2.1 shows concordances for a number of traits of psychiatric relevance. These data provide two important messages. The first is that all of the disorders shown have greater similarity in MZ than DZ twins, indicating genetic effects. The second is that no disorder shows complete concordance in MZ twins even though these are genetically identical, indicating that all the disorders have an environmental component. The environment can be conceptualized as having two main components: shared environment, that causes family members to resemble each other, and non-shared environment, that operates at the individual level and therefore contributes to differences between members of the same family. Thus it becomes possible with twin data to estimate the size of the contribution to the variation within a trait according to the additive genetic component, the heritability, and the variation attributable to shared and non-shared environment.

Such concepts about a partitioning variance had been around for several decades and were imported into human genetics originally from agricultural genetics, where knowing the heritability of milk yield in cattle or the size of tomato fruits has practical implications for selective breeding. A graphical method called path analysis, put forward by

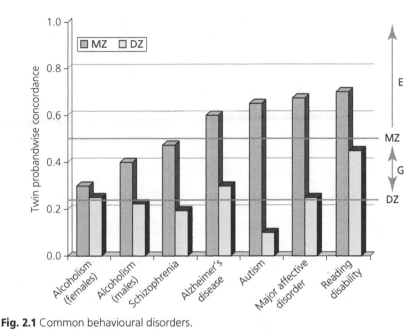

Fig. 2.1 Common behavioural disorders.

From R. Plomin, M. J. Owen, P. McGuffin, The genetic basis of complex human behaviors, in *Science*. 17 June 1994: Vol. 264 no. 5166 pp. 1733–1739. Reprinted with permission from AAAS.

the American geneticist Sewall Wright in the 1920s, lent itself perfectly to deriving the necessary equations to estimate the variance components. However, the technical advance that eventually allowed statistical model fitting based on twins to advance rapidly was the advent and widespread availability of high-speed computers in the 1980s. Some results using this approach, which is now known as structural equation modelling, are illustrated in Figure 2.2.

All of the traits and disorders shown here are heritable, that is they show significant additive genetic effects. 'Significance' is formally tested in structural equation modelling by eliminating, in turn, components from the model and seeing whether any make a difference that is significantly different from chance. By contrast, for most of the traits it is possible to drop the shared environmental component without worsening the fit, the exceptions being reading disability and IQ in childhood. It is surprising that the environment shared within families contributes little or nothing to family resemblance, but it is a finding that is completely consistent across the behavioural genetics literature, largely supported by studies of MZ twins reared apart. Twins separated soon after birth are rare, and the studies of them inevitably rely on unsystematic recruitment methods, including advertisements in the media, that could result in sampling biases. Nevertheless they tend to show that for measures such as personality tests twins reared apart are no less similar than twins reared together. Indeed, one early study actually found that twins reared apart had slightly more similar personalities than twins reared together (17). Various explanations of this phenomenon have been put forward, including the idea that twins in particular, but perhaps siblings in general, tend to

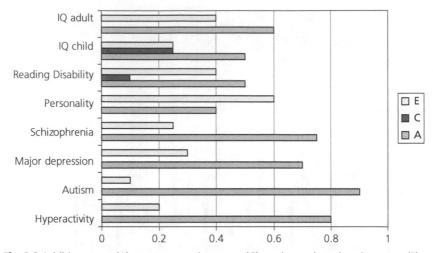

Fig. 2.2 Additive genes (A), common environment (C), and non-shared environment (E).

Data from P. McGuffin, B. Riley, and R. Plomin. (2001). Genomics and behavior. Toward behavioral genomics. *Science* 291(5507), 1232–1233.

consciously or unconsciously differentiate themselves from each other in their behaviours. Similarly it may be that parents' treatment of offspring, however hard they try to deal with them equally, inevitably includes different approaches to different members of a sibship, what behaviour geneticists have sometimes called contrast effects. It is also sometimes suggested that peers outside the family actually have greater effect on the behavioural development of children than their brothers or sisters. These hypotheses are all difficult to test, but what is clear is that, for characteristics such as IQ, the effects of shared environment are substantial in childhood (and cannot be dropped from the explanatory models), but diminish in adulthood and are overwhelmed by additive genetic effects in later life (18).

In addition to examining the genetic architecture of single traits, structural equation modelling provides ways of exploring the overlap between traits and the extent to which they share genetic or environmental underpinnings. This is of particular interest in psychiatry where there is frequently an admixture of symptoms from two or more disorders that, at least according to conventional classification schemes, are considered to be more or less distinct entities. A good example is depressive disorder and generalized anxiety. Here analysis of twin data from a population-based study in the United States showed that the genes contributing to anxiety and depression overlap entirely, and that phenotypic differences are contributed by environmental effects (19). Subsequent analyses (20) largely confirmed this finding, although suggested the existence of additional genetic effects specific to depression. A study that was more controversial when it was first published a decade ago took a similar approach to analysing twin data based on the Maudsley Hospital register (21). The authors addressed the issue of whether schizophrenia and bipolar disorder show overlapping causes. The results pointed to separate specific, as well as overlapping, genetic effects contributing to both disorders. These findings have been borne out by molecular genetic studies and a genetic overlap between schizophrenia and major affective disorders is now the accepted orthodoxy even though such proposition was almost heretical a decade ago.

Locating and identifying genes

Our ability to map genes depends upon the phenomenon called genetic linkage, whereby genes close together on the same chromosome disobey Mendel's second law, the so-called law of independent assortment. In his experiments on pea plants Mendel observed that pairs of characteristics are inherited independently of each other. He of course had no knowledge of chromosomes or of the physical basis of inheritance. A few years after Mendel's laws were rediscovered, the English biologists Reginald Punnett and William Bateson observed that there were sometimes departures from Mendel's independent assortment, and coined the term 'linkage' to describe them. Subsequently Thomas Hunt Morgan, an American who worked largely on the genetics of fruit flies, proposed that genes are carried on chromosomes. He further proposed that genes that are close together on the same chromosome tend not to be separated during meiosis, the type of cell division that results in the formation of sperms and eggs.

Meiosis is a rather complicated process during which pairs of chromosomes, one set derived from the paternal line and the other from the maternal line, come to lie alongside each other and exchange parts of their material. This process, called 'crossing over' or recombination, is essentially like shuffling the genetic deck of cards. It thus ensures that sexual reproduction optimizes genetic diversity with attendant evolutionary advantages. Morgan correctly inferred that recombination between pairs of genes will occur 50% of the time if they are carried on different chromosomes or are widely separated on the same chromosome. For genes closely aligned on the same chromosome, recombination rates of less than 50%, that is linkage, may be observed, with the rate of recombination approximately proportional to the distance between pairs of genes. Today we still measure genetic distance in gene mapping studies using units named after Morgan; the human genome is approximately 35 morgans (M) or 3,500 centimorgans (cM) in length. (Strictly this is the 'sex averaged' length of the genome since there is more crossing over in female meiosis than in male meiosis.)

Organisms that have a very short life cycle and where mating patterns can be manipulated by researchers (e.g. fruit flies) are ideal for studying linkage between pairs of genetically determined characteristics. Human beings, who have long life cycles and a preference for selecting their own patterns of mating, are much less suitable. Special statistical methods are required to help assess whether the rate of crossing over, or recombination, is significantly less than the expected rate of 50% that occurs in independent assortment. One of the first tests of linkage in humans was devised by Lionel Penrose, a psychiatrist and pioneer statistical geneticist (22). It was based on the rate of sharing of alternative forms ('alleles') of genes in pairs of siblings. Around this time geneticists were beginning to explore the relationship between diseases and genetic markers, that is Mendelian characteristics that are reliably measured, such as blood groups. The most useful genetic markers are 'polymorphic', with two or more alleles that are common in the population.

Tests such as the one devised by Penrose were useful for detecting the presence of linkage but not for estimating how much recombination is present; that latter provides a means of estimating the distance between the two points on a chromosome ('loci') where the two genes are located. Modern methods for estimating recombination, and hence genetic distance, are essentially derived from an approach put forward by Newton Morton in 1955 called the LOD (log of odds) score method. This is based upon plotting out a series of odds ratios (odds on linkage versus no linkage) between two characteristics over a range of possible recombination rates from zero (complete linkage) to 0.5 (independent assortment). The method uses the common log of the odds which gives LOD scores the useful property of simply being summed (rather than multiplied) over a collection of families to give a combined score, where the LOD score peaks provide the best estimate of recombination. Hence if one trait is a genetic marker of known location on a chromosome and the other is a disease it is possible to infer that the gene conferring susceptibility to the disease maps close to the marker.

The main problem about applying this approach to identify the genes involved in any disease, even ones that show simple Mendelian inheritance within families, is that until the mid-1980s the genetic markers that were available to researchers were few in number. They included ABO and various other blood groups, some enzymes that could be measured in red cells, various polymorphic plasma proteins and polymorphisms within the HLA system, the components of the major histocompatibility complex (MHC) that determines the success or rejection of tissue transplants. Despite this, optimistic researchers began collecting families multiply affected by disorders such as schizophrenia and bipolar disorder, with a view to employing these pre-DNA 'classical' markers to carry out linkage studies.

In my own study commencing in 1979 I was fortunate to obtain guidance and collaboration from world-class London-based laboratories directed by Peter Cook and Ruth Sanger at University College London and by Hilliard Festenstein at the Royal London Hospital. Nevertheless I was only able to explore about 30 different marker systems in 12 families. The study proved to be almost entirely negative but, with certain optimistic assumptions, I concluded that I had at least managed to exclude a major schizophrenia susceptibility locus from about 6% of the genome (23).

The advent of the 'new genetics'

The development that opened up the prospect of mapping disease genes was the discovery of a brand-new type of DNA-based genetic marker. Restriction fragment length polymorphisms (RFLPs) would allow the creation of a set of 'tags' to search the entire genome and track down all major genes leading to disease susceptibility. Briefly, RFLPs are detected by cutting up DNA with bacterial enzymes that recognize specific 'restriction sites', stretches of DNA that are recognized by specific enzymes and show variability in the population. If a restriction site is present at a particular point the DNA is cleaved. If the site is altered or absent, DNA is not cleaved. This leads to fragments of different sizes that can then be separated by placing them on a gel and passing an electric current through it, causing movement of fragments according to their length. The gel is then blotted onto paper and the DNA fragments identified with specific probes which, in the beginning, were radioactively labelled. The process is called Southern blotting, named after the Edinburgh scientist, Ed Southern, who first described it. This technology was so revolutionary that the editor of the *American Journal of Human Genetics* coined the term 'new genetics' to describe it (24). Researchers conducting linkage studies now had several hundred markers to work with; by the end of the 1980s detailed linkage maps of evenly spaced markers throughout the 23 pairs of chromosomes were available.

Not surprisingly, the first major successes involved less common diseases with simple Mendelian modes of inheritance; the prime psychiatric example was Huntington's disease, where the gene was located on chromosome 4 (25). Soon researchers were using RFLPs in attempts to track down genes contributing a major role in the risk of schizophrenia and bipolar disorder. Two high-profile studies were published in the journal *Nature*, each based on rather unusual populations, attractive for gene mappers. The first looked at a large extended family with many members affected by bipolar disorder or depression from a rural Old Order Amish community in Pennsylvania (26). There appeared to be strong evidence of linkage between affective disorder and markers on chromosome 11.

The following year a short report suggested involvement of chromosome 5 with schizophrenia in a family containing a maternal uncle and nephew pair both affected by the condition and showing an abnormality called translocation, where a piece of chromosome is broken off and attached to another. The nephew's mother was unaffected, but was a 'carrier' of the translocation (27). Subsequently Sherrington et al. (28) explored the chromosome 5 region with DNA markers in Icelandic families (like the Amish, from a partial genetic isolate), as well as some British families multiply affected by schizophrenia. They found significant evidence of chromosome 5 markers assorting with the disorder. Others were unable to replicate a schizophrenia finding, but this still left the possibility of heterogeneity of schizophrenia at the molecular level such that some forms were linked and others unlinked to the markers on the chromosome 5 region (15). Consequently enthusiasm for linkage studies in psychiatry persists, and interest in the new genetics of mental disorders continues.

Evidence of increasing interest, even before the publication of the two *Nature* papers, was reflected in the establishment of the first World Congress of Psychiatric Genetics in 1988. It was organized by a committee under the chairmanship of Tim Crow, arguably the most prominent biological psychiatrist in the United Kingdom at that time and a recent convert to the idea that schizophrenia was largely a genetic disorder. I was pessimistic that the conference would attract more than a handful of delegates, given the scepticism and hostility to genetics I experienced during my years as a trainee psychiatrist. My doubts were dispelled when more than 300 researchers attended with well over 100 offers of presentations.

Around the same time another agreeable surprise, funding of a network to explore the molecular neurobiology of mental illness (MNMI) by the European Science Foundation (ESF), occurred. This arose from a proposal by Roger Marchbanks, a biochemist in the United Kingdom, and myself. Psychiatric departments and genetics laboratories across Europe joined forces to collect data and analyse the DNA from large numbers of multiply affected families with schizophrenia and bipolar disorder. Previously, linkage studies in psychiatry were too small to detect anything other than fully penetrant

Mendelian genes. As previously mentioned, such genes were probably rare. The MNMI network was coordinated by a steering committee chaired by a leading French neurobiologist, Jacques Mallet, and included several rising figures in human genetics such as Leena Peltonen from Finland, Francois Clerget-Darpoux from France, and Kay Davies from the United Kingdom. Launched with a workshop that subsequently became an annual event, it can be viewed as a kick-start for molecular psychiatric genetics across Europe.

Soon after, the National Institute of Mental health (NIMH) funded a similar network in the United States. The ESF and NIMH began a collaboration, reaching agreement on basic issues such as a common diagnostic approach and an attempt to establish US–European diagnostic reliability (29).

Many linkage studies progressed in North America, Europe, Asia, and Australasia, made more feasible by a shift from RFLPs to a newer generation of DNA markers called microsatellites. They result from variation in the number of repeats of DNA bases (e.g. dinucleotides, or repeated runs of two bases) that occur throughout the genome. They are generally more polymorphic (or variable) than RFLPs and therefore provide more useful tags by which to track down genes within families. The discovery of microsatellites and methods of genotyping resulted in more useful, finer-grained linkage maps with which to search the genome.

The promise of 'positional cloning'

The justification for all the effort that was being put into linkage studies, not just in psychiatry but across the whole of medicine, was that 'positional cloning' provided a method of discovering the aetiology of disorders where knowledge of the underlying pathogenesis was scant or absent. The broad principle is that linkage allows a method of pinpointing the genes involved in disorders to specific chromosomal locations. It is then possible to move from location to identifying the gene itself, studying the sequence and structure and eventually looking at the variation in the protein that the gene encodes to discover how a miscoding contributes to the disease. With much of the 'new genetics' positional cloning was often trickier than the optimists had anticipated, even with single-gene disorders, but it eventually worked. In 1993, 10 years after the first report of linkage on chromosome 4, a paper announcing the cloning of the Huntington's disease gene was published (30). It immediately provided new insights into the biology of the disorder and a new mechanism of mutation that turned out to be particularly relevant for neuropsychiatric and neurological disorders. The Huntington's gene contained a repeated sequence of three DNA bases, an unstable trinucleotide repeat. Once expanded beyond a critical length of 40 repeats it becomes pathogenic and causes the protein that the gene encodes to have an abnormal structure.

The other advances of psychiatric relevance were in studies of families containing multiple early-onset cases of Alzheimer's disease (AD) where the disorder appeared to follow a Mendelian dominant pattern of inheritance. Three genes were identified, the amyloid precursor protein gene on chromosome 21 and two others that had similar structures to one another. They were presenilin 1 and presenilin 2. Carrying the relevant mutations in any one of these three genes was demonstrated to be enough to carry a virtual certainty of developing presenile dementia (31). However, early-onset forms of AD are very rare, whereas late-onset forms, particularly beyond the age of about 80 years, are extremely common. What then might be the relevance of genetics of the early rare forms to later common forms? The answer is probably very little (32). However, the discovery of another linkage signal on chromosome 19 (33) eventually led to discovery of an association between the apolipoprotein E gene (*ApoE*) and AD that proved to be an important risk factor for the common type of the disorder. Association is a related phenomenon to linkage but it is is observed in populations rather than in families. This occurs either because a marker itself has a direct effect on the risk of disease or because the marker is so extremely close to a disease susceptibility gene that the relationship between the marker and the gene remains undisturbed over many generations of recombination. In the case of *ApoE* the association with AD turned out to be with the alternative form of the gene, or allele, called *E4*.

Although it took much longer, the same general approach of searching for associations with genes within regions of the genome where there appeared to be a linkage signal resulted in the discovery of several novel genes associated with schizophrenia. Interestingly, all of them, which included neuregulin, dysbindin, and D amino acid oxygenase activator (DAOA), encoded proteins that are involved in the type of signalling in the brain that occurs via the chemical messenger glutamine (34).

Another gene involved in the liability to schizophrenia was discovered in a slightly different way. A large Scottish family with many members affected by schizophrenia, as well as other severe disorders, was discovered. Mental illness appeared to coincide with carrying a chromosome abnormality called a translocation in which there were breakages resulting in most of a chromosome 1 having a chromosome 11 fragment attached (35). The Edinburgh group studying this family went on to clone the breakpoint on chromosome 1 and identified a gene which they named 'disrupted in schizophrenia-1' (*DISC1*). At first many thought that this was a one-off family and that *DISC1* was unlikely to be generally relevant to schizophrenia. However, it turned out that when association studies were carried out comparing schizophrenic patients with healthy controls, the former group more often had a particular set of variants within the gene. It was subsequently shown that *DISC1* is not just relevant to schizophrenia but, as in the original Scottish family, variants in the gene are also associated with depression and bipolar disorder. Indeed, when researchers began to explore the new 'schizophrenia genes' in other conditions, associations with bipolar disorder again emerged, in line with the findings discussed earlier from the Maudsley twin study (21) that suggested a genetic overlap between the two conditions.

Gene–environment interplay and the nature of nurture

Until about a decade ago molecular genetic studies in psychiatry paid comparatively little heed to the environment. This was surprising, given earlier evidence from twin studies suggesting a sizeable environmental component in all common psychiatric disorders. On the other hand, the twin analyses make an assumption, likely an oversimplification, concerning gene–environment interplay; namely, that genes and environment simply add up to produce a clinical picture, the phenotype. However, behavioural genetic studies on animals have demonstrated that genes and their environment can interact in a multiplicative way, as genes may have an effect on sensitivity to the environment. A further complication is that genetic and environmental effects may be correlated. For example, parents usually provide their offspring with the environment in which they are reared as well as their genes, so that alcoholic parents may provide their offspring with early exposure to alcohol as well as a genetic predisposition to heavy drinking. Alternatively, some types of behaviour that have some genetic basis may influence the type of environment an individual selects. For example, a genetic predisposition to antisocial behaviour may elicit a response in others that encourages aggression or predisposes an individual to consort with peers who indulge in antisocial behaviours. Thus, once we take into account gene–environment interaction and covariation, aptly termed by my colleague Robert Plomin, 'the nature of nurture', 'pure' genetic or environmental effects are more difficult to distinguish than has traditionally been acknowledged.

Among the examples of studies using purely statistical 'premolecular' methods are those looking at adversity and depression in families and twins. A study during the 1980s revealed that not only did depression cluster in families, but so did adverse life events. Measuring life events in a relatively objective way, using a semi-structured interview, demonstrated that familial clustering was due to the same events affecting multiple members of a family. However, twin studies have shown that less objectively measured life events, collected by self-report questionnaires, are moderately heritable. Furthermore, the tendency to report life events and to report depressive symptoms appear to have overlapping genetic effects. In sum, the data, at least for subjective reports of adversity, suggest that the relationship with depression involves both gene–environment interactions and gene–environment correlations.

The first successful attempt to take this further by looking at a specific gene was published in 2003 in a landmark paper by Caspi et al. (36). They studied a cohort of nearly 1,000 individuals who had been followed from birth in Dunedin, New Zealand. When Caspi and colleagues looked at depressive symptoms in relation to objectively measured life events there was the expected clear relationship between the two. The novel aspect of the study was that the subjects were also genotyped for a common variation in the gene that encodes a protein called the serotonin transporter. This particular molecule is of great interest in neurobiology and neuropharmacology because it is the site of action of the most widely used type of antidepressants, the selective serotonin reuptake inhibitors (SSRIs). The variant that Caspi and colleagues studied was in a region, the promoter, that controls how active the gene is. The variant exists in two forms—a long (L) and a short (S) form—the L form resulting in higher gene activity than the S form. Subjects who had inherited the short form from both parents (SS) were significantly more reactive to life events than subjects who had inherited two copies of the long form (LL), while the so-called heterozygous individuals (LS) were intermediate in their response to life events.

One reason this paper is so often cited is because some researchers have been sceptical of the findings or failed to replicate them. However, if one reviews all the available data, the negative studies are entirely based on subjective self-report measures of life events which, as mentioned, are almost certainly 'contaminated' by genetic factors that overlap with those predisposing subjects to report depressive symptoms. There are also several lines of biological data suggesting that this serotonin transporter promoter variant has an effect on environmental reactivity (37). These include studies on rhesus macaque monkeys which have a similar variant and show a similar gene–environment interaction when exposed to the stress of separation from their mothers. In summary, we should not conclude that the serotonin transporter gene is 'the gene for' depression, but rather that it is one of many genes that contribute to the disorder. And, more specifically, the promoter variant is an example of a gene variant affecting sensitivity to the environment.

From candidate genes to genome-wide association

Studies of the serotonin transporter, and other genes in the same chemical pathway, are examples of candidate gene studies. Candidate genes are so called because they encode a substance thought to have relevance to a disease, for example, based on knowledge about the mode of action of the drug used to treat the disease. In candidate gene association studies researchers simply compare the frequency of variants in that gene in affected individuals versus a control group. Countless such studies were performed in depression, bipolar disorder, and schizophrenia during the 1990s, as RFLPs, microsatellites, and variants based upon a single base change (single nucleotide polymorphisms or SNPs) were discovered in potential candidate genes or their regulatory regions. Sadly, no consistent pattern emerged in any of these disorders until researchers honed in on 'positional candidates', such as neuregulin or dysbindin mentioned earlier, within regions identified by linkage studies of schizophrenia. Studies of gene–environment interactions also provided some consistency. However, what many genetic researchers really yearn to do is a genome–wide association study (GWAS) searching the entire genome of cases and comparing them with unaffected controls.

It has long been recognized that association studies have greater power than linkage to track down genes of small effect. They are therefore potentially ideal in complicated polygenic disorders. The downside of association studies is that in order for a genetic marker to tag a disease susceptibility gene it has to be within the gene itself or extremely close to it. Linkage can be used to track genes in families over distances as great as 10–15 cM and hence, if we remember that the genome is about 3500 cM long, only a few hundred markers are needed to span the genome. By contrast, association can only be detected over a distance of a small fraction of a centimorgan, so that hundreds of thousands of roughly evenly spaced markers are needed for a GWAS. The first big milestone on the path to being able to perform a GWAS was the completion of the sequencing of the human genome.

The nearly complete annotated human genome sequence was announced in 2000, with most of the gaps being filled in over the next 3 years. This was the culmination of the Human Genome Project, an international governmental project charitably complemented by the parallel project of a commercial enterprise called Celera that sought to patent the genome. In Janary 2001 *Science* and *Nature* devoted whole issues to the descriptions of the new and revolutionary findings, with accompanying articles discussing the likely uses and consequences. One of the uses was the subsequent delivery of a

SNP map and the demonstration that SNPs are plentiful enough to conduct a GWAS. A subsequent milestone was a major project called HAPMAP which explored the way in which pairs of SNPs are inherited together on the same chromosomes in differing human populations. The final milestone was the development of a technology enabling many SNPs to be typed in a single experiment. This involves SNP micro-arrays ('SNP chips') on which thousands of probes that detect SNPs within DNA are placed on either a glass slide or an array of tiny beads. The first micro-arrays produced contained around 10,000 SNP probes and current commercially available versions are able to detect over 1 million SNPs.

There was an early win with the GWAS approach. A important new gene was discovered by comparing individuals with macular degeneration, a common eye disease, to healthy controls. The first full-scale GWAS was the Wellcome Trust Case Control Consortium (WTCCC) study published in *Nature* in 2007. Groups of 2,000 cases each of seven diseases, one of which was bipolar disorder, were compared to 3,000 controls. The large samples were needed for two reasons. First, the disorders were common complex ones likely to involve many genes of small effect. Secondly, the micro-arrays used in the study detected half a million SNPs, leading to a huge multiple testing problem. The multiple testing problem is as follows. Typically in a case-control comparison a 'significant' result is one observed by chance one time in 20 or less, a 0.05 or less probability of a false positive. A researcher conducting half a million simultaneous experiments would therefore find 25,000 appearing to be significant using the 0.05 criterion, even if no difference between cases and controls exists. Hence, a highly stringent criterion of significance is required in GWAS which conventionally is taken as a probability of 5×10^{-8} or less.

The WTCCC study was a methodological landmark and produced important new findings in some diseases, including Crohn's disease and type I and type II diabetes. A parallel GWAS had been performed in the United States on bipolar disorder, and data were also emerging from studies in the United Kingdom and Ireland. One of the hazards of any association study is that different ethnic groups have different frequencies of genetic marker alleles and may have different frequencies of diseases. Therefore mixing together different populations can yield spurious results. Mindful of this problem, the American, British, and Irish studies focused only on white subjects of European origin. Nick Craddock from Cardiff University and Pamela Sklar from Harvard formed a consortium that combined the data on nearly 5,000 cases of bipolar disorder and an even larger set of controls (38). This study, stupendous in scale compared with almost anything in psychiatry preceding it, resulted in the discovery of two completely novel genes that had never previously been implicated in the aetiology of bipolar disorder, *ANK3* and *CACNA1C*. Each is an important ion channel gene, associated with the structures that sit on the surface of nerve cells and are involved in rapid transmission of messages involving passage of ions (e.g. sodium or calcium) across the cell membrane. This was a particularly compelling finding in bipolar disorder given that many of the mood stabilizer medications used in long-term treatment were originally developed as antiepileptic drugs and have the common property of stabilizing nerve cell membranes.

CACNA1C has subsequently been implicated in schizophrenia and unipolar depression and GWASs involving many thousands of subjects have identified new genes conferring susceptibility to schizophrenia, autism, AD, and bipolar disorder. Regrettably, although the sample sizes amassed for unipolar depression are even bigger than for other psychiatric diseases, no consistent 'hits' have emerged that can be replicated across different datasets. This perhaps suggests that depression, the commonest of the major psychiatric disorders, is actually more heterogenous than the rest, and collaborative efforts involving huge samples collected across the United States and Europe are currently taking place to attempt to discover more homogenous subgroups that might give more consistent signals. Meanwhile a recent positive and tantalizing finding emerging in unipolar depression is a possibility that a larger number of tiny pieces of genome go missing in people who developed depression than in those not depressed.

Copy number variants

Earlier on I described the excitement that occurred in the 1950s and 1960s when geneticists discovered that psychiatric syndromes were sometimes associated with having extra chromosomes, parts of chromosomes, or missing chromosomes that could be seen with the light microscope. Later, using more sophisticated techniques such as fluorescent *in situ* hybridization (FISH), smaller bits of missing chromosome could be detected. Half a century later much excitement has arisen with the discovery, largely as a by-product of GWAS technology, that much smaller submicroscopic stretches of DNA are detected as missing (deleted) or having more than one copy (duplicated). This type of copy number variation (CNV) is responsible for a large amount of the differences between individuals' genomes. Large CNVs, consisting of tens of thousands or even a few million DNA bases, are individually rare with frequencies in the general population of less than 100. However, many of them are dotted across the genome, so that the probability of anyone carrying at least one large CNV is high. A study in our laboratory estimated that about one in three healthy controls has at least one large deletion CNV, suggesting that the majority of large, rare CNVs are 'silent'. However, it does appear that the CNV 'burden', defined as the number of large CNVs or the number of CNVs that disrupt genes, is increased in a variety of psychiatric disorders, particularly schizophrenia and autism. Indeed, some rare CNVs have repeatedly been found in both disorders and confer a much higher risk (although never a certainty) of the disorder than the SNP variants in genes that have been uncovered by association studies. Thus it appears that the early advocates of major gene theories of schizophrenia were not entirely wrong and it is likely that the both schizophrenia and autism are contributed to both by common genetic variants of small effect and rarer variants of large effect, and that there is some genetic overlap between the two conditions.

The story is just beginning to unfold with depression. In a sample of around 3,000 cases of mainly recurrent and severe depression, our research suggests an excess of CNVs consisting almost entirely of deletions that disrupt coding regions of genes (exons). Interestingly, we see the largest difference between cases and controls who have been screened for never having had any psychiatric disturbance in their lifetime. Unscreened controls (who are ostensibly well but may have had psychiatric symptoms in the past) also have significantly fewer large CNVs than cases, but more than the 'super healthy' screened controls. This might suggest that having a lower CNV burden has something to do with a genetic basis for well-being or resilience.

Pharmacogenetics and pharmacogenomics: personalized pharmacotherapy?

One hope of the GWAS approach was that it would lead to the discovery of genes useful in predicting response to treatment and development of side effects. The general idea is a much older one and goes back more than half a century, before genome-wide studies were possible. Speculations began in the 1950s that rare and idiosyncratic adverse reactions to certain drugs had a genetic basis. The first discovery relevant to psychiatric patients was that one in 3,000 individuals receiving electroconvulsive therapy (ECT) were 'slow acetylaters'. They were slow to metabolize drugs like the muscle relaxant suxamethonium, and hence had a prolonged, potentially hazardous recovery from general anaesthesia. The medical geneticist Arno Motulsky subsequently suggested that a new branch of genetics dealing with drug response should have a bright future and coined the term pharmacogenetics. Since then many genetic variants involved in the breakdown of medications have been discovered, the biggest family involving the cytochrome P450 enzyme system in the liver. These show a large degree of variation, the extent varying between ethnic groups, which is thought to have evolved because of advantages possibly conferred by resistance to naturally occurring toxins. Many of the drugs used in psychiatry are broken down via cytochrome P-450 enzymes, such as the one encoded by a gene called *CYP2D6*, that shows a high degree of variation. Slow CYP2D6 metabolizers are much commoner that slow acetylaters, which may have relevance for the occurrence of side effects in people taking certain antidepressants.

Pharmacokinetics refers to the rate at which drugs are metabolized. Another source of potential genetic variability has to do with pharmacodynamics. This involves genes that produce variation in the site at which drugs act, such as the promoter variation in the serotonin transporter gene in relation to stress response. A number of studies show that patients who carried the double dose of the less active SS form responded less well to selective serotonin reuptake inhibitor antidepressants than patients who had at least one (more active) L form of this genetic variant.

Several other tantalizing findings have emerged from taking a candidate gene approach to pharmacodynamics; for example, some genetic variants seem to predict emergence or worsening of suicidal ideation during antidepressant treatment. Such findings require replication and more research before conclusions about clinical benefit can be drawn. Potentially more readily translatable results from elsewhere involve rare, more idiosyncratic types of effects. For example, carbamazepine—a drug used to treat epilepsy and sometimes as a mood stabilizer in bipolar disorder—causes a rash, joint pains, fever, and possibly death in a small proportion of patients. This reaction, the Stevens–Johnson syndrome, is associated in East Asians with a variant in the HLA genetic complex. The genetic finding is currently being explored as a possible basis of routine clinical genetic testing.

There have now been three genome-wide studies looking at response to antidepressants. Each produced a positive finding, but unfortunately no agreement exists across studies. This suggests that, contrary to expectations, no genes on their own will provide a clinically useful test. However, calculations based on genome-wide data allow an estimate of the heritability of antidepressant response, probably in the region of 30–40%, suggesting that a combination of genes might provide the basis of clinically useful tests. In summary, many areas in psychiatric genetics are turning out to be more complex than originally hoped or foreseen and, consequently, it is still too early to know whether personalized pharmacotherapy informed by genetic tests will become a reality.

The future and postgenomic psychiatry

The history of genetics over the past 50 years has been full of surprises accompanying the discoveries about the molecular basis of inheritance and the structure of the genome. Therefore I should be circumspect and conservative in rounding off of this essay by sticking to predictions concerning current research.

Beginning with pharmacogenetics and genomics, analysis that has occurred thus far has been fairly straightforward (e.g. looking across the genome for signals that predict therapeutic response or common side effects). In the near future I foresee researchers turning to integrative analysis that takes into account the complexity of what goes on when a disorder, such as depression, is treated. This would involve monitoring the blood level of drugs, as well as looking at what other markers reveal. This concerns not only whether certain gene variants are present or absent, but also the level of activity of genes. Such studies comprise transcriptomics (studies of the level of messages contained in RNA which convey information from the nucleus to the cell) and proteomics (studies of the levels of all proteins that can be detected in the blood). They would also consider the role of epigenetic mechanisms.

Epigenetics is likely to prove the next 'big thing' in pharmacogenetics, as well as across psychiatric genetics generally. An explanation of epigenetics is complicated, although the concept is relatively straightforward. My colleague Jonathan Mill has produced an excellent metaphor. When we go to hear an orchestra we see the conductor reading from a score, but more often than not the conductor's working score will not only contain what was written by the composer, but also marks the conductor has made to remind him of how he thinks the music should be interpreted. What we hear corresponds to the phenotype, and what the composer has written is the genotype—the conductor's marks correspond to the epigenotype. Epigenetics, then, is concerned with the marks, some of them reversible, that are placed on the genome by events that can include where a gene comes from (father or mother), exposure to early adversity, or exposure to a certain diet or drug. Broadly speaking, the marks involve the chemical processes of methylation and acetylation, and modification of histones, structures within chromosomes that enable DNA to be tightly coiled and packed into the nucleus of the cell. Methylation has the effect of switching off the message from a gene, as does tight coiling of DNA around histones. Removing methylation or uncoiling histones has switching-on effects.

To date, the study of epigenetics in psychiatry has just begun, but already there are strong hints that it reveal much—for example, why genetically identical, monozygotic twins differ in many respects such as being discordant for illnesses like schizophrenia or depression. And this is another area where technology is moving rapidly. For example, an ingenious adaptation of the bead array technology mentioned earlier in connection with GWAS now enables the methylome (i.e. methylation patterns across the entire genome) to be scanned in a single experiment, so we can expect results soon to come thick and fast.

Another set of methods that will soon advance our knowledge is referred to as next-generation sequencing. This enables very rapid reads of the genome sequence at comparatively small cost. Whereas the original sequencing of the complete human genome took more than a decade and cost billions of dollars, it is now possible to sequence anyone's genome for a few thousand dollars in about 3 weeks. It is already feasible to sequence all the coding regions within the genome that are expressed as proteins (the exome), and soon results of a study of 10,000 exomes, comparing cases and controls that include 3,000 patients with either schizophrenia or autism, will be available.

Perhaps large-scale sequencing studies should provide answers to several conundrums that are relevant to human genetics generally, not just to psychiatric disorders. For example, the exome is only a small fraction of the genome, carrying codes for proteins. This discovery that the coding region of the genome was so small, together with the finding of the Human Genome Project that there are only about 25,000 human genes, surprised many. It led to questions as to whether most of the genome was 'junk', and if so why? It soon became clear that the junk or non-coding DNA within genes in the so-called introns, does have a function in determining how different variants of the same proteins are made up in different tissues (called splice variants), and affecting stretches of DNA that are important in controlling levels of gene expression. In between genes there are elements of DNA that have been conserved through evolution, regions likely to have some function that may affect expression of genes at a distance. One particular type of non-protein-coding DNA is now known to code for short forms of RNA responsible for a phenomenon called RNA interference, a mechanism by which the signals sent by genes can be controlled.

In conclusion, many mysteries concerning the human genome remain, as do many clues concerning the role of non-coding DNA in controlling those parts of the genome that code for proteins. Such clues will need to be pursued, as will the part played by epigenetic phenomena in psychiatric disorder. Progress up to and since the sequencing of the human genome has generated huge amounts of data and information so that computational biology and the whole new science of bioinformatics is assuming an ever-increasing importance. Meanwhile, one of the earliest technological innovations of human genetics, the twin study, will continue to have a key place in psychiatric genetics. This will include continuing refinement of disease boundaries and overlaps, as well as use of concordant and discordant twins to explore new territories such as epigenetics.

References

1 McGuffin, P. and Huckle, P. (1990). Simulation of Mendelism revisited: the recessive gene for attending medical school. *American Journal of Human Genetics* **46**, 994–9.

2 Galton, F. (1876). The history of twins, as a criterion of the relative powers of nature and nurture. *Journal of the Anthropological Institute* 5, 391–406.

3 Jackson, D. (1960). *The etiology of schizophrenia*. New York: Basic Books.

4 Gottesman, I. and Shields, J. (1972). *Schizophrenia and genetics: a twin study vantage point*. New York: Academic Press.

5 Heston, L. (1966). Psychiatric disorders in foster home reared children of schizophrenic mothers. *British Journal of Psychiatry* **112**, 819–25.

6 Lejeune, J., Gautier, M., and Turpin, R. (1959). Etude des chromosomes somatiques de neuf enfants mongoliens. *Comptes Rendus Hebdomadaires des Séances de l'Académie des Sciences* **248**, 1721–2.

7 Skuse, D. H., James, R. S., Bishop, D. V. et al. (1997). Evidence from Turner's syndrome of an imprinted X-linked locus affecting cognitive function. *Nature* **387**, 705–8.

8 Jacobs, P. A., Brunton, M., Melville, M. M., Brittain, R. P., and McClemont, W. F. (1965). Aggressive behavior, mental sub-normality and the XYY male. *Nature* **208**, 1351–2.

9 Witkin, H. A., Mednick, S. A., Schulsinger, F. et al. (1976). Criminality in XYY and XXY men. *Science* **193**, 547–55.

10 Slater, E. (1958). The monogenic theory of schizophrenia. *Acta Genetica et Statistica Medica* **8**, 50–6.

11 Gottesman, I. and Shields, J. (1967). A polygenic theory of schizophrenia. *Proceedings of the National Academy of Sciences of the U S A* **58**, 199–205.

12 Falconer, D. (1965). The inheritance of liability to certain diseases, estimated from the incidence among relatives. *Annals of Human Genetics* **29**, 51–76.

13 O'Rourke, D. H., Gottesman, II, Suarez, B. K., Rice, J., and Reich, T. (1982). Refutation of the general single-locus model for the etiology of schizophrenia. *American Journal of Human Genetics* **34**, 630–49.

14 Craddock, N. (1995). Genetic linkage and association studies of bipolar disorder. PhD thesis, University of Wales College of Medicine, Cardiff.

15 McGuffin, P. (1991). Models of heritability and genetic transmission, in: Häfner, H. and Gattaz, W. (eds.) *Search for the causes of schizophrenia*, pp. 111–25. Berlin: Springer-Verlag.

16 Fisher, R. (1918). The correlation between relatives on the supposition of mendelian inheritance. *Philosophical Transactions of the Royal Society of Edinburgh* **52**, 399–433.

17 Shields, J. (1962). *Monozygotic twins, brought up apart and brought up together*. London: Oxford University Press.

18 McClearn, G. E., Johansson, B., Berg, S. et al. (1997). Substantial genetic influence on cognitive abilities in twins 80 or more years old. *Science* **276**, 1560–3.

19 Kendler, K. S., Neale, M. C., Kessler, R. C., Heath, A. C., and Eaves, L. J. (1992). Major depression and generalized anxiety disorder. Same genes, (partly) different environments? *Archives of General Psychiatry* **49**, 716–22.

20 Thapar, A. and McGuffin, P. (1997). Anxiety and depressive symptoms in childhood— a genetic study of comorbidity. *Journal of Child Psychology and Psychiatry* **38**, 651–6.

21 Cardno, A. G., Rijsdijk, F. V., Sham, P. C., Murray, R. M., and McGuffin, P. (2002). A twin study of genetic relationships between psychotic symptoms. *American Journal of Psychiatry* **159**, 539–45.

22 Penrose, L. (1952). The general purpose sib-pair linkage test. *Annals of Human Genetics* **17**, 120–4.

23 McGuffin, P., Festenstein, H., and Murray, R. (1983). A family study of HLA antigens and other genetic markers in schizophrenia. *Psychological Medicine* **13**, 31–43.

24 Comings, D. E. (1980). Prenatal diagnosis and the 'new genetics'. *American Journal of Human Genetics* **32**, 453–4.

25 Gusella, J. F., Wexler, N. S., Conneally, P. M. et al. (1983). A polymorphic DNA marker genetically linked to Huntington's disease. *Nature* **306**, 234–8.

26 Egeland, J. A., Gerhard, D. S., Pauls, D. L. et al. (1987). Bipolar affective disorders linked to DNA markers on chromosome 11. *Nature* **325**, 783–7.

27 Bassett, A. S., McGillivray, B. C., Jones, B. D., and Pantzar, J. T. (1988). Partial trisomy chromosome 5 cosegregating with schizophrenia. *Lancet* **1**, 799–801.

28 Sherrington, R., Brynjolfsson, J., Petursson, H. et al. (1988). Localization of a susceptibility locus for schizophrenia on chromosome 5. *Nature* **336**, 164–7.

29 Williams, J., Farmer, A. E., Ackenheil, M., Kaufmann, C. A., and McGuffin, P. (1996). A multicentre inter-rater reliability study using the OPCRIT computerized diagnostic system. *Psychological Medicine* **26**, 775–83.

30 The Huntington's Disease Collaborative Research Group (1993). A novel gene containing a trinucleotide repeat that is expanded and unstable on Huntington's disease chromosomes. *Cell* **72**, 971–83.

31 Liddell, M. B., Lovestone, S., and Owen, M. J. (2001). Genetic risk of Alzheimer's disease: advising relatives. *British Journal of Psychiatry* **178**, 7–11.

32 Gerrish, A., Russo, G., Richards, A. et al. (2011). The role of variation at AbetaPP, PSEN1, PSEN2, and MAPT in late onset Alzheimer's disease. *Journal of Alzheimers Disease* **28**, 377–87.

33 Pericak-Vance, M. A., Bebout, J. L., Gaskell, P. C., Jr et al. (1991). Linkage studies in familial Alzheimer disease: evidence for chromosome 19 linkage. *American Journal of Human Genetics* **48**, 1034–50.

34 Harrison, P. J. and Owen, M. J. (2003). Genes for schizophrenia? Recent findings and their pathophysiological implications. *Lancet* **361**, 417–19.

35 St Clair, D., Blackwood, D., Muir, W. et al. (1990). Association within a family of a balanced autosomal translocation with major mental illness. *Lancet* **336**, 13–16.

36 Caspi, A., Sugden, K., Moffitt, T. et al. (2003). Influence of life stress on depression: moderation by a polymorphism in the 5-HTT gene. *Science* **301**, 386–9.

37 McGuffin, P., Alsabban, S., and Uher, R. (2011). The truth about genetic variation in the serotonin transporter gene and response to stress and medication. *British Journal of Psychiatry* **198**, 424–7.

38 Ferreira, M. A., O'Donovan, M. C., Meng, Y. A. et al. (2008). Collaborative genome-wide association analysis supports a role for ANK3 and CACNA1C in bipolar disorder. *Nature Genetics* **40**, 1056–8.

Essay 3

Fifty years of applied clinical research: schizophrenia as an example

Vishal Bhavsar and Robin M. Murray

Introduction

Researching the causes and treatment of a clinical condition involves the use of many conceptual and methodological approaches to obtain valid knowledge; these include nosology, neurobiology, psychology, epidemiology. This is evident in the study of schizophrenia which was one of the first mental illnesses to be conceptualized as a medical disorder. We will therefore use schizophrenia as an example of how progress has been made

Schizophrenia is one of the major contributors to psychiatric morbidity across the world. We do not know the 'cause' of schizophrenia, but since the 1980s we have understood the illness as emerging partly as a result of disordered brain development in early life, under the influence of an array of interacting genetic and environmental influences. Individuals who suffer the illness experience distressing symptoms that affect a number of aspects of brain function, including thinking, perception, and mood. It can confer considerable disability, and managing the illness involves a range of approaches, including medication as well as psychological and occupational therapies.

In this essay, we discuss the history of research into schizophrenia since the 1960s. There were many challenges to overcome. Firstly, the lack of a clear organic basis at the beginning of our period created the context for a huge turnover of ideas about what constituted the condition and where the pathology was located. Secondly, the tremendous social impact of the illness and the ethical difficulties involved in detaining patients against their will led to criticism from both within and outside psychiatry. Thirdly, given the detrimental impact on physical, psychological, social, and occupational functioning, schizophrenia attracted interest from a wide range of disciplines, ranging from neuroscientists interested in neuronal circuitry to anthropologists examining the person's social world.

Schizophrenia research has been driven by two contrasting approaches. On the one hand, the acquisition of new data concerning the causes has been derived from comparing schizophrenia populations with normal populations or by studying cohorts of patients prospectively. On the other hand, research has been pervaded by a seemingly unquenchable need to question the definition and scope of the diagnosis itself. While initially characterized as a single psychiatric disease, schizophrenia is now seen as a syndrome comprising three main symptom 'dimensions' (delusions, hallucinations, and disorganized speech and behaviour) that may be measured separately. Increasing interest in the dimensional nature of psychosis and its likely biological basis has helped to create more of a consensus among researchers in the 21st century. As we shall see, however, the shape of research at the beginning of our study period presented a far more disparate picture.

The middle of the 20th century

By the 1950s, views on schizophrenia had become markedly divergent on the two sides of the Atlantic. European psychiatry had in general stayed true to the medical concept of schizophrenia outlined by Emil Kraepelin and Eugen Bleuler, as illustrated by the most influential textbook of the period (1). This model treated schizophrenia as an illness like any other in general medicine, with a pattern of characteristic symptoms that resulted from a single cause or aetiology. By contrast, American psychiatrists tended to align with psychoanalysis, informed by sociological and environmental explanations, as an 'organizing model' (2); this was driven by the ideas of Adolf Meyer who was responsible for accommodating Kraepelinian diagnostic categories into the context of psychogenic 'reactions'. Meyer held deep doubts about schizophrenia as a medical condition, arguing instead that the diagnosis was often assigned to cases where the psychological dynamics of the reaction were not sufficiently understood. The influence of psychoanalysis was widespread in the United States, with the vast majority of senior academics aligning themselves with this school (3). Consonant with this, the early editions of the *Diagnostic and Statistical Manual* published by the American Psychiatric Association, DSM-I (4) and DSM II (5), reflected a dynamically rooted understanding of mental illness, with assessment and treatment based on the interpretation of symptoms in the context of the patient's experience.

Psychiatry under attack in the 1960s

The 1950s saw a great change in the treatment of schizophrenia. The effectiveness of chlorpromazine was serendipitously discovered in 1952, and it was soon introduced to regular practice. By the end of the decade, a range of antipsychotics had become available across the developed world. Their use began to facilitate the move from custodial care in asylums towards treatment in the community.

A more difficult decade then ensued. Key publications in the early 1960s placed at their centre not the causes of mental disorder but the status of psychiatrists themselves. The most widely read books attacked psychiatrists, psychiatry, and the places in which they worked, the mental hospitals. R.D. Laing's *The Divided Self* (6) was pre-eminent. Apart from its analysis of schizophrenia as a disorder of ontological (in)security, Laing denied that schizophrenia was 'non-understandable', and positioned the family at the heart of the cause. Moreover, he concluded that psychiatry was guilty of promulgating a medical model which was poorly defined and nothing more than a covert form of social control. The psychiatric response to Laing's attack was largely antagonistic, revealing a fragmented, theoretically diverse community of practitioners often at odds with each other. Laing's critique of a central disease construct came at a bad time for the discipline.

There was indeed a crisis of legitimacy for psychiatry in the 1960s, brought about by populist criticism of practice not only from Laing but also from Thomas Szasz and Michel Foucault, all of whom attracted a wide lay readership. Although labelled as 'anti-psychiatrists', Laing and Szasz continued to practice clinically. Two powerful challenges faced conventional psychiatry. First, there was the explicit denial of schizophrenia as an entity accessible to scientific analysis. To this end, the anti-psychiatry group approached the condition using methods drawn from philosophy, sociology, and anthropology, with each discipline defining schizophrenia in its own way, if at all. Secondly, the criticism of psychiatry took place in the context of vigorous attacks on other structures—such as the military–industrial complex, conventional sexual mores, and organized religion—that were all regarded as instruments of social control.

Standardizing diagnosis

A major problem undermining the response of orthodox psychiatry to its critics was existence of several competing concepts of schizophrenia. As a result, a patient might be diagnosed as schizophrenic by one psychiatrist but as having affective psychosis by another. Diagnostic practice varied considerably across countries. The traditionally narrow concept of European psychiatry continued much as before, whereas the analytically based view in the United States had become much broader. This disparity became only too obvious with the findings of the US–UK Study in which trained psychiatrists in the two countries viewed videotapes of clinical interviews (7). A much larger proportion of patients were diagnosed as schizophrenic by American than by British psychiatrists. Subsequently, an international study was carried out by the World Health Organization which showed, ironically, that the only countries with a diffuse concept were the United States and its cold-war enemy, the USSR.

These examples of diagnostic inconsistency were a gift to psychiatry's critics, such as Rosenhan who persuaded mentally healthy volunteers to present to psychiatric units in the United States simulating psychotic symptoms and then when they were admitted to hospital, to act normally—some of these 'pseudopatients' remaining inpatients for months. It seemed much easier to get into psychiatric units than out of them (8)! Rosenhan's publication in the prestigious journal *Science* attracted a somewhat frenzied response from the psychiatric community; Robert Spitzer labelled his work 'pseudoscience', and even felt it left a 'bad aftertaste'! Nevertheless, academic psychiatrists redoubled their efforts to standardize methods of interviewing and diagnosing patients, aimed at differentiating between different disorders. This had begun with the introduction of Schneider's 'first rank symptoms', a list of phenomena thought to be characteristic of schizophrenia, into British psychiatry in the 1960s and their subsequent integration into a standardized interview developed by John Wing and his colleagues in the United Kingdom (9). First rank symptoms included particular types of auditory hallucinations and experiences of thoughts being inserted or removed from the mind. Robins and Guze, from the European-influenced bastion in Washington University,

St. Louis, adopted a parallel approach by devising the so-called Research Diagnostic Criteria. These developments ushered in what was later termed the neo-Kraepelinian phase of schizophrenia research; this model, of a single clinical syndrome with phenomenologically distinct subcategories, appealed to researchers keen on a reproducible construct of schizophrenia that would be viable for empirical enquiry.

The notion that the third edition of the *Diagnostic and Statistical Manual* (DSM-III) transformed American psychiatry is well known, but explanations of the process involved are more diverse. Its publication in 1980 was variously described as 'a victory for science' and a triumph of 'facts over ideology' (10,11). DSM-III amounted to the 'medicalization' of psychiatry, as manifest in an explosion of the number of diagnoses. Increasing criticism of analytically based psychiatric practice by health insurance companies, which were not keen to fund long-term psychotherapies, was another factor that drove the reorientation of psychiatry in the United States. Finally, and often overlooked, is the fact that standardized criteria were being adopted throughout medicine, albeit with less ensuing ruction. Under the influence of Robert Spitzer, its coordinator, the DSM-III manual presented a reinvigorated version of Kraepelinian theories of classification on the basis of patterns of symptoms, course, and outcome. Importantly, criteria for schizophrenia were more focused on delusions and hallucinations, and less on difficulties that were also part of other disorders, like depression and anxiety (12).

In summary, the fragmentation of thinking about schizophrenia in the 1960s was an obstacle to the development of scientific knowledge. Subsequent progress has depended to a considerable extent on standardized definitions initiated from the late 1960s onwards. Gradually, the many models of schizophrenia were replaced by a more standardized conception. However, there was a major snag in that although reliability was established, the lack of an objective test has impeded the aim of determining whether the diagnosis is valid, that is, represents a genuine disease.

Neuropharmacological advances

Abnormal perception, classically in the form of auditory hallucination of hearing voices, has been recognized as a hallmark of schizophrenia since the first descriptions of the disorder. After the Swiss pharmacologist Albert Hoffman discovered the hallucinogenic properties of lysergic acid diethylamide (LSD) in 1943, drug-induced psychoses were proposed as a model for schizophrenia. Considerable research was undertaken into hallucinogens, the most surprising concerning an elephant which was injected with LSD; sadly, Tusko trumpeted a few times, collapsed, and died an hour later. The pervasive interest in hallucinogens, both within the research community and in society at large, extended the attractive possibility that patients with schizophrenia might be 'walking hallucinogenic factories'. Friedhoff and Van Winkle defined the presence of a 'pink spot' in the urinary chromatography of schizophrenia patients in an acute psychiatric ward in 1962, to the great excitement of researchers hoping to find a neurochemical basis for the illness. A 1967 editorial in the *BMJ* was equivocal over the significance of the 'pink spot' data but, perhaps in a nod to American psychodynamic models, advocated 'stop[ping] investigating schizophrenics *en masse* and concentrat[ing] on individuals'. One of the most studied hallucinogens was dimethyltryptamine (DMT) which had been isolated from substances used by Amazonian Indians in their religious ceremonies. Although DMT was reported to be more frequently present in the urine of schizophrenic patients than controls (13), interest in endogenous hallucinogens gradually waned, mainly because the psychosis they produced was more visual in character than in schizophrenia which is characterized by voices rather than visions.

However, an important outcome of the expansion of neuropharmacology was the development of the dopamine hypothesis of psychosis which rested on two strands of evidence. Firstly, Connell (14) and others demonstrated that the abuse of amphetamines, drugs which were known to increase the availability of dopamine at the synapse, could induce psychosis. The second strand derived from neurochemical studies of the actions of antipsychotic drugs. Carlssen and Lindquist (15) analysed the plasma levels of monoamine metabolites and found that chlorpromazine enhanced the turnover of monoamines, while Van Rossum (16) suggested that dopamine receptor blockade was linked to antipsychotic effects. Creese and Snyder (17) demonstrated that the effectiveness of antipsychotics correlated with their strength of binding at the dopamine-2 (D2) receptor. Crow and Johnstone (18) reported that of the two chemical forms of the antipsychotic flupenthixol, only the form that was active at the D2 receptor had a beneficial effect on psychosis. Thus, by the end of the 1970s, the dopamine hypothesis was established as the leading pathogenic theory of schizophrenia.

Traditional genetics

The possibility of a heritable component in the causation of schizophrenia has had a long history. In 1932, Bruno Schulz, working in Kraepelin's department, found that 8% of more than 200 brothers and sisters of patients diagnosed with schizophrenia also suffered from the condition. However, the involvement of German psychiatrists, such as Ernst Rudin, in drawing up guidelines for the euthanasia program of the mentally ill in Nazi Germany, discredited this area of enquiry for many years. Indeed, in the United States in the postwar period, the familiality of schizophrenia was attributed variously to intrafamilial communication style, marital relationship structure, or particular social circumstances. Genetics was strictly off limits! A few researchers continued the genetic line of research, notably Erik Stromgren in Denmark, and Eliot Slater in the United Kingdom. Both had trained in Germany in the early 1930s but subsequently distanced themselves from their former colleagues who collaborated with the Nazis. By the 1960s, Slater had established a vigorous research unit at the Maudsley Hospital in London, and, as psychiatric genetics hardly existed in the United States, a trail of American researchers came to study with him.

One of the first, Irving Gottesman, examined schizophrenic twins attending the Maudsley and showed that the greater genetic similarity of monozygotic over dizygotic twins resulted in much higher concordance rates (i.e. both twins ill) in the former than the latter (19). Subsequently, Gottesman and Shields (20) pooled data on all available twin studies and generated overall concordance rates of 46% for monozygotic twins and 14% for dizygotic pairs. Increased rates were also found in a small sample of monozygotic twins who were reared apart. Leonard Heston, another American researcher who studied with Slater, carried out the first adoption study and demonstrated that the children of schizophrenic mothers who were adopted retained an increased risk of developing the disorder. Meanwhile, back in the United States, Seymour Kety, a neuroscientist, established a highly productive collaboration with Fini Schulsinger in Copenhagen and produced a series of articles on Danish-American adoption studies which put the role of a genetic contribution beyond doubt; they found higher prevalence of schizophrenia in the biological, but not adoptive, relatives of schizophrenia patients. The Dorado Beach conference in 1967 brought together many of the twin and adoption researchers and put genetic research back on the map.

The Finnish adoptive family study, carried out by Pekka Tienari, was the first to systematically investigate the impact of family rearing on schizophrenia, and showed an interaction between genetic predisposition and family rearing environment in influencing risk for the disorder. Since that time, large epidemiological studies have identified a number of risk factors for schizophrenia that act in early life, including child abuse, and experience of trauma, all of which appear to interact with genetic risk.

As in other areas of schizophrenia research, genetic researchers began to diagnose schizophrenia using operational definitions of schizophrenia. Thus, Kendler and Diehl (21) divided family studies into those carried out before and after 1980 and found that the later research still found evidence for a genetic basis to the disorder. Similarly, Anne Farmer (22) applied operational criteria to Gottesman and Shields's aforementioned twin study. The family, twin, and adoptive evidence pointing to high heritability held up even with these more stringent criteria. It was nevertheless clear that schizophrenia had a complex inheritance pattern not explainable in mendelian terms and the aetiology was more complex (23). Gottesman and Shields were the first to postulate a 'multifactorial' model of inheritance, involving multiple genes and environmental effects.

Schizophrenia as a brain disease

If there was one overarching 'paradigm shift' in schizophrenia research, it was from a psychodynamic understanding based on patterns of reaction, to regarding the condition as a brain disease. Intrinsic to the shift was the search for organic pathology. Early studies of brain structure such as those of Alzheimer (24) and Haug (25) had been disappointing. However, the study that sounded the death knell for analytical views was the 1976 study of Johnstone and her colleagues (26). This first CT imaging, case-control study demonstrated ventricular enlargement of the lateral ventricles in people with schizophrenia compared to normal control subjects. Initial responses ranged from the view that the patients could not have had schizophrenia since it was known to be a functional psychosis (i.e. one that by definition has no structural basis), to the view that the changes were secondary to antipsychotic treatment itself, with the neurologist David Marsden commenting in a letter to *The Lancet* that 'long-term neuroleptic therapy could explain some of the cerebral atrophy and related cognitive impairment . . .'. However, the findings were replicated by Reveley and her colleagues (27) who found larger ventricles in twins with schizophrenia than in their non-schizophrenic co-twins, indicating that this aspect of brain structure in schizophrenia was not under genetic control.

By the mid-1980s most psychiatrists were convinced that schizophrenia was a brain disease under a high degree of genetic control. It could be diagnosed reliably by using operational criteria, among which the DSM-III gained ascendance, due not to any intrinsic superiority over the International Classification of Diseases (its World Health Organization counterpart) but rather to the power and influence of the American Psychiatric Association. However, this reductionist view did not prove popular among other mental health professionals or patients' groups. There was a recrudescence of anti-psychiatry attacks, particularly by British psychologists; one of them, Mary Boyle wrote a widely read book entitled *Schizophrenia: a Scientific Delusion?*. Other critics like Steven Rose (28), an influential biologist able also to take a sociological quasi-Marxist perspective, protested that the genetic evidence was less than convincing.

The rise and rise of the neurodevelopmental model

The idea that psychosis may have a developmental origin is not new. The Scottish psychiatrist Thomas Clouston coined the term 'developmental psychosis' in 1873 when he pointed to the frequency of a family history and minor physical abnormalities (MPAs) in a group of insane patients. To his dismay, his work was overshadowed by that of Kraepelin who also had noted MPAs in schizophrenic patients but termed this 'degeneracy', and fitted the observation to his view that the illness was a form of dementia. The latter view held sway across Europe, with schizophrenia regarded as an adult-onset degenerative disease marked by a progressive decline in brain functioning from the very point of its onset. As we have noted earlier, this view was reinvigorated by the neo-Kraepelinian movement in the United States and by the work of Crow and Johnstone in the United Kingdom.

However, the 1980s saw a renewed interest in two old observations—that obstetric complications were common in schizophrenic patients (29), and that they were more likely to be born in the late winter and spring. These points could not readily be accommodated within the prevailing Kraepelinian degenerative model, and drove increased interest in the role of antenatal development which crystallized around the neurodevelopmental model of schizophrenia in the mid-1980s.

The neurodevelopmental hypothesis was proposed in 1987 by Weinberger (30) in the United States and Murray and Lewis (31) in the United Kingdom. Evidence originated from a variety of threads of research. Reports accumulated that rates of obstetric difficulties were higher in individuals who went on to develop schizophrenia, with important systematic reviews published in the mid-1990s. Neuropathological reports of abnormalities in the hippocampus in schizophrenic brain, that were attributed to disrupted neuronal migration, lent substantial support to the developmental model; sadly, these were not replicated. There was also much interest in the idea that prenatal exposure to influenza might increase risk of schizophrenia. Ecological relationships were found between timing of epidemics and births of individuals who developed the illness, but it was difficult to prove a causal link in individual patients, and as time progressed negative findings accumulated.

In spite of these setbacks, the neurodevelopmental hypothesis marched on, fuelled by cohort studies which showed subtle developmental delays, solitariness, and intellectual deficits in preschizophrenic children. Part of the success of the neurodevelopmental hypothesis can be attributed to its elasticity. For example, it exists in several forms: some investigators point to the effect of pre-and perinatal hazards on early brain development; others to deviations of brain maturation in adolescence (32). Taken as a whole, there is a wide range of possible points within development when causative 'lesions' might arise. Another factor was, of course, the failure of the main alternative idea that schizophrenia was a degenerative illness. Neurodegenerative disorders are classically marked by gliosis, a proliferation of glial cells, in affected areas of the brain. Repeated investigations of the brains of patients with schizophrenia failed to find such changes. Initially, there was also a failure to find progressive brain changes in patients using CT and early MRI studies but, as we will see later, this view has been revisited.

Two aspects concerning the rise of the neurodevelopmental model are of more general relevance to understanding how research has progressed. First, technological advances have often held the key—for example, the discovery of deviations in ventricular size and brain volumes was dependent on the use of more reliable and sensitive methods of brain imaging. Secondly, the more precise delineation of normal patterns of child development was necessary for the elaboration of subtle differences between normal individuals and those with schizophrenia.

The neurodevelopmental view has grown somewhat more sophisticated; hypotheses involving a single static perinatal brain lesion have been left behind, and models which allow for disruptions to neural development throughout childhood and adolescence have gained acceptance. The logical conclusion has been the increased interest in factors which contribute to the onset of psychosis (33).

Most contemporary scientific debate now occurs between different versions of the model (early versus late developmental lesions), rather than whether the model itself is valid or not. The model is thought to fit much of the accumulated experimental data, and has also proved to be a rich source of experimental ideas. Indeed, so central has the model become that proposals have even been made to reconfigure diagnostic categories of schizophrenia along neurodevelopmental lines.

New ways of imaging the brain

The arrival of structural MRI studies enabled the confirmation of earlier CT findings, demonstrating reduced volumes of the whole brain and of grey matter in schizophrenia, but also pointing to abnormalities in particular areas, especially the frontal and temporal lobes. Studies in the 1990s identified reductions in volume in the dorsolateral prefrontal cortex and in temporal lobe structures such as the hippocampus, amygdala, and superior temporal gyrus. Voxel-based morphometry, a more precise imaging method that accounts for the differences in brain anatomy between normal individuals, helped to increase the resolution of brain structural imaging even further.

Functional MRI imaging (fMRI), which allows visualization of differences in brain physiology between patients and normal controls, presented further opportunities. fMRI identified differences in frontal lobe activity between conditions of rest and carrying out specific tasks; this led initially to the idea that schizophrenic patients showed 'hypofrontality' or reduced activity in the frontal lobe, compared to control subjects.

Researchers then examined the physiological correlates of psychotic symptoms. For example, Shergill and colleagues found that when patients hear voices they activate Broca's area in the same way that normal individuals do when speaking aloud or when saying words to themselves (i.e. internal speech). When normal people are saying words to themselves (e.g. reciting a poem silently), signals appear to be transmitted from Broca's area to areas in the temporal lobes concerned with interpreting external speech (the auditory cortex), telling it to ignore the internal words. However, in the case of those suffering auditory hallucinations, the auditory cortex and associated subcortical areas remain active and process the words as if they are coming from an external source. Thus, one could say the brain is 'fooled' into thinking that the words are external.

fMRI studies have provoked a move away from focusing on purely regional abnormalities towards an approach based on disordered connectivity between parts of the brain (34). The idea that 'dysconnectivity' could result in psychotic symptoms dates from experimental observations first made in the mid-1990s, when Friston and Frith (35) conceptualized their findings as suggesting that psychotic symptoms could be related to problems in the connections between frontal and temporal brain regions. The new method of diffusion tensor imaging, which allows the quantification of the integrity of white matter tracts connecting the different brain areas, added support to the dysconnectivity hypothesis by proposing an anatomical basis to this.

With the turn of the century came renewed interest in the question of whether there might be a neurodegenerative component to schizophrenia, and that there was a spectrum of changes in schizophrenia, ranging from neurodevelopmental to neurodegenerative. Pantelis's MRI study in 2003 was among the first to find changes in the brains during the onset period of the first episode. Subsequently, it was established that grey matter volume was lost faster in people with schizophrenia than could be accounted for by normal ageing. Some investigators have suggested that this is part of a neurodegenerative process, others that it is not intrinsic to schizophrenia but secondary to such factors as stress and elevated cortisol levels, and continuing cannabis abuse. More alarmingly, recent studies suggest that prolonged high-dose antipsychotic medication may also contribute.

Epidemiology, not just head counting

A key benefit of the development of both standardized interview methods and diagnostic criteria was the ability to explore epidemiological risk factors systematically across populations for the first time. As part of a 10-year study, the World Health Organization (WHO) applied the same diagnostic procedure to patients in research sites in seven countries. The incidence ranged between 16 and 40 cases per 100,000 per year but notably, the range diminished to between 7 and 14 cases per 100,000 per year, when more stringent diagnostic criteria were used. The findings marked the beginning of a debate that was to have important implications for later research. At its heart was the question how to interpret the variation in incidence in different parts of the world. The WHO investigators themselves suggested that the figures indicated a rough uniformity, and some biologically oriented researchers emphasized what they saw as lack of variation and therefore evidence of a primarily genetic cause. Other commentators thought the variations were more significant and later research found clearly differing rates in various populations such as males and females, migrants, and between those living in cities and the country (higher in the urban group). These variations supported the role of environmental factors in the development of schizophrenia. A meta-analysis by McGrath and his colleagues convinced most researchers that considerable variation existed.

Irving Gottesman's 1991 volume, *Schizophrenia Genesis*, addresses noteworthy aspects of the research landscape of the time. He discusses the relative merits of European and American epidemiological findings, and regards the former as more meaningful because of their more conservative diagnostic practices and comprehensive national registers. Indeed, European countries in general, and Scandinavian countries in particular, have contributed more than their fair share of advances in the epidemiology of psychosis.

That geographical location could be relevant to variations in the incidence of schizophrenia had been first posited in 1936 by sociologists Robert Faris and Warren Dunham, who found a correlation between the social structure of Chicago and the rate of serious mental illness. After a gap of 60 years, prospective cohort studies in Sweden, Denmark, and Holland reported that urban birth, and indeed city-dwelling, was associated with later development of schizophrenia. Of course urban living must be a proxy for other variables—social adversity, social fragmentation, and isolation have all been proposed—but the answer remains elusive.

Odegaard's 1932 finding of increased rates of schizophrenia among migrants was reexamined in different populations. Increased incidence among African-Caribbeans in the United Kingdom was a firm finding by the late 1980s, although the first large-scale study was not carried out until two decades later (36). A meta-analysis showed that incidence was increased in most migrant groups, but especially in black people from developing countries who had migrated into predominantly white European countries.

Interest in social factors was furthered by longitudinal population studies. Thus, Danish investigators showed that the number of years children spent in a city, and the number of changes in residence made in adolescence, increased the risk. Adversity in childhood such as maltreatment and physical or sexual abuse also appeared to increase risk, as do adverse life events, especially of a victimization type.

Since the early 2000s, considerable attention has been paid to the role that 'drugs of abuse' play in contributing to schizophrenia. It has long been known that abuse of amphetamine, methamphetamine, and cocaine, which increase synaptic dopamine, can precipitate a clinical picture similar to that of paranoid schizophrenia. For a while, controversy raged over whether abuse of the seemingly safer cannabis could do the same. However, a consensus has emerged that its heavy use does have a consistent, though modest, effect in elevating the risk of both isolated psychotic symptoms and schizophrenia-like psychoses.

Evidence that factors such as urbanicity and cannabis have effects on promoting the risk of minor psychotic symptoms as well as of schizophrenia fed the idea of a continuum of subclinical psychotic symptoms extending into the general population (37). Studies in many countries have shown that minor features exist on a continuum of severity in the general population, and that transient psychotic experiences are not uncommon. Liability to psychosis came to be viewed in Europe in the same way as liability to hypertension or obesity, i.e. essentially a normal distribution with a threshold imposed at the point at which it seemed useful to intervene (38); however, some American psychiatrists continued to adhere to a model of schizophrenia as a discrete disease.

The new genetics

Advances in genetics in the 1980s provoked much hope for clarifying the nature of the genetic component in schizophrenia; researchers spoke with optimism of how molecular genetics held many of the answers they were looking for. The new methods offered the prospect of identifying genetic abnormalities in affected pedigrees, sequencing relevant genes, locating genetic sequences associated with illness, and developing targeted interventions. The reality of the 'genetics revolution' has been somewhat different. While reports of the discovery of genes for schizophrenia were plentiful, few of these findings were replicated. Indeed, in the 1990s it was said that the only field of human endeavour to produce as many false positives as schizophrenia genetics was the search for alien spacecraft!

Causal genes for schizophrenia proved elusive perhaps by virtue of small sample sizes, inconsistent research methodology, and uncertainty about the biological basis of the clinical phenotype. The 1990s saw a steady stream of positive findings which other centres failed to replicate. Hopes of identifying major genes faded and geneticists became more modest in their ambitions. However, cytogenetics implicated several chromosomal loci. For example, an Edinburgh group identified a balanced translocation between chromosomes 1 and 11 which was associated with schizophrenia and other mental illnesses in a single large family. Mutations identified in *DISC1* were also shown to associate with electrophysiological, cognitive and other deficits that overlap with the schizophrenia phenotype. The gene product of *DISC1* was identified, and localized to various regions of the brain. The *DISC1* story is an object lesson in how the molecular genetic approach can proceed systematically. Unfortunately, it appears to pertain to only a very small number of cases.

Much effort has been devoted to the study of biological markers for schizophrenia—for example patterns of brain electrophysiology, fMRI, or cognitive performance. In particular, interest has grown in identifying 'endophenotypes', or measurable parameters that are associated with and inherited alongside the illness. These are sometimes termed intermediate phenotypes because they are thought to be on the pathway between genes and the clinical phenotype. The study of intermediate phenotypes continues to hold promise but has not yet delivered much.

Whole-genome scanning, the increasing ease of carrying out candidate gene studies, and the arrival of the genome-wide association study (GWAS) which examines all genes in an individual, have given genetic researchers fresh heart. GWAS compare the complete genetic profile of a group of people with the illness with the genetic profile of normal controls in order to identify areas of the genome associated with illness. Such advances and larger sample sizes eventually led to the identification of eight replicable susceptibility genes. It appears now that schizophrenia is polygenic, with at least 100 susceptibility genes, each of tiny effect.

New antipsychotics and renewed interest in dopamine

Modern psychiatrists regard schizophrenia as a treatable illness with recovery of function and freedom from symptoms observed in up to 50% of cases. We have the antipsychotics, for the most part, to thank for this. The treatment of patients at the beginning of the 1960s centred on the use of the 'typical' antipsychotics such as chlorpromazine and haloperidol. These agents made possible the first historical reduction in numbers of inpatient psychiatric beds across the Western institutional system, and were influential in the growing popularity of the biological over the psychoanalytic model of schizophrenia.

The number of antipsychotic medications multiplied in the 1960s and 1970s but these were all dopamine blockers and many were derived from those previously identified. In an attempt to overcome lack of patient compliance, injectible long-acting antipsychotics whose administration could be supervised were introduced, but these benefited only a subgroup of patients. Little new happened until the reintroduction of clozapine in the late 1980s. This medication had been synthesized in Switzerland in 1958 and had the advantage of not giving rise to the distressing movement disorders such as tardive dyskinesia found in those treated with the first-generation group of antipsychotics. Unfortunately, it had been withdrawn in a number of European countries in 1974, when a group of Finnish patients died of agranulocytosis, a hitherto unrecognized adverse reaction to the drug. It was reintroduced in the United States in 1990, following a rigorous re-evaluation, with careful rules on regular blood monitoring for patients on the drug. It had been shown to bring benefit to about 40% of those hitherto regarded as unresponsive to treatment.

Clozapine has an effect on many types of brain receptors, and this broad receptor-binding profile gave rise to the concept of 'atypical antipsychotics', whose action was thought to extend beyond dopamine receptor blockade. The first new 'atypical' agent, risperidone, was soon followed by olanzapine and other atypical drugs throughout the 1990s, tailing off into the first decade of the 21st century. These new agents were initially marketed as superior to their predecessors for positive symptoms (hallucinations and delusions), but less so for for negative symptoms (e.g. lack of motivation and self-neglect) and least effective for cognitive impairment. None of these claims proved to be true, but they did have improved tolerability. Early overoptimism has given way to a more balanced view. A contemporary consensus, largely derived from two large independently funded controlled trials, CATIE and CUTLASS, holds that 'typical' and 'atypical' agents are equally effective but differ in their side effects: atypical agents are less likely to cause tremors and other movement problems but are more likely to induce obesity and diabetes. These differences in side-effect profile have important implications for what kinds of patient should be prescribed which drug—patients with heart disease or diabetes may be more likely to benefit from a typical agent.

As we have already noted, the knowledge that typical antipsychotics block the D2 dopamine receptor gave rise to the dopamine hypothesis of schizophrenia. However, information about the part played by dopamine was constrained by the available scientific methods in the early years, and it took three decades before direct evidence supporting this was found. Laruelle's 1996 study brought neurochemical imaging into the limelight as a valuable technique for elucidating mechanisms. This form of imaging showed that during an acute episode excess release of dopamine occurred in the striatal part of the brain. A key theoretical leap has been the assertion that this release of dopamine in the striatium is responsible for giving emotional resonance, or 'salience', to aspects of the external and internal world. Thus, increased dopamine transmission could lead to inappropriate salience being attached to objects or events in the environment, ultimately leading to the development of unusual beliefs and perceptions, and psychosis.

Other developments in treatment

Deinstitutionalization

The life of many people with severe schizophrenia at the beginning of the 1960s was manifest in institutional containment and the (il)liberal prescribing of antipsychotic medications. The asylums had begun to shrink in the 1950s and this trend accelerated from the 1960s under the joint influence of antipsychotics and a drive towards community care. The 1961 publication of Ervin Goffman's book *Asylums* gave a further impetus to this process. Goffman, a sociologist, analysed the experiences of patients admitted to psychiatric institutions, building on fieldwork in the huge St Elizabeth's Hospital in Washington DC. He explored their world in an attempt to better understand the process of 'institutionalization', forming the view that mental institutions rendered their inmates 'dull and inconspicuous' and caused them to lose their sense of identity and social role along with any hope of regaining social skills. For Goffman, asylums were marked by their rigid social structures and hierarchies, designed to keep problematic behaviours at bay.

Many mental health professionals agreed with Goffman that asylums provided poor care and had adverse consequences. Over the next three decades, a large-scale reduction in the number of psychiatric beds took place in most Western countries. Although patients generally preferred to live in the community rather than in a mental hospital, little research was done into the actual process of deinstitutionalization. However, Julian Leff's 1997 study, 'Care in the community: illusion or reality' in the United Kingdom demonstrated that restructuring of inpatient services and provision of psychiatric care in the community could be safe and cost-effective (see Leff, this volume, pp. 96–116)

There were, however, adverse effects of the shift. First, it became clear that many in the community did not approve of the process of deinstitutionalization and of the mentally ill residing in their neighbourhood; indeed, the tabloid press was often frankly antagonistic and demonized the sufferers. Secondly, deinstitutionalization resulted in some of those previously admitted to asylums simply being transferred to smaller homes or to prisons, a process termed 'transinstitutionalization' in the United States. Thirdly, in some countries (e.g. the United Kingdom) it became difficult to obtain a hospital bed even for the most severely psychotic patients. Fourthly, the remaining inpatient units concentrated very disturbed people so that the atmosphere could become non-therapeutic. Female patients sometimes felt frightened and those in an early stage of psychosis were distressed by being put in wards alongside chronic relapsing patients.

Service changes

Concerns for the well-being of female patients in mixed wards eventually led to the reintroduction of single-sex wards in the United Kingdom at the turn of the century, thus reversing what had been thought to be the innovation of mixed wards 30 years earlier. Interest in prevention led to the creation of specialist services dedicated to the early treatment of individuals with psychosis, with research into their efficacy. These developments have been driven by three factors. First, the developmental understanding led to increased interest in illness onset. Secondly, clinicians recognized that early intervention could reduce distress and disability, in line with primary and secondary preventive approaches applied in other areas of medicine. Thirdly, a view that prompt treatment of psychotic symptoms could lessen the chance of disability in the long term; this view has been cogent in convincing politicians to fund early intervention services although definitive evidence is yet to be found.

At-risk services seek to prevent the development of psychosis rather than simply treat the psychosis once it has emerged. In many ways this initiative has been a logical extension of early intervention programs. From the research perspective, 'at risk' services have allowed clearer elucidation of the process underlying the transition to psychosis. However, debate has arisen over the ethics of offering antipsychotic medication to people with mental states who are deemed '"at risk" for psychosis but without established psychotic features'. 'At risk' services have therefore tended to offer social, occupational, and psychological treatments rather than antipsychotic medication.

Social and psychological treatments

Early forays into social treatment centred on the role of high expressed emotion (EE) in the families of individuals with psychosis. It was a concept that originated in the work of George Brown and others in the 1960s, and attempts to capture the quality of the relationship that a given carer has with the patient, through an interview between the researcher and the main carer (see Leff, this volume, pp. 96–116). Elevated EE scores were found to predict poor outcome, whereas reduction in EE led to improvement. Relapse rates have also been found to be higher in individuals in high EE environments. However, in spite of numerous positive trials, this approach has not been frequently used in regular practice, perhaps because many patients do not have families available and willing to participate.

Fortunately, a new and enthusiastic workforce began to appear on the scene. Psychologists had not contributed much towards the care of schizophrenic patients other than to criticize the concept and the supposed barbarity of drug treatment. However, from the 1990s, cognitive therapy began to be applied to address not only the anxiety and depression that many patients with schizophrenia suffer but also the psychotic symptoms themselves. A series of studies by mainly British psychologists showed overall benefits, though modest ones. Trials of cognitive remediation, which aims to improve aspects of cognitive functioning such as attention, memory, and planning, have also followed, with early reports of some success.

Definitions, diagnoses, and dimensions

It is clear that research into schizophrenia has made major strides since the 1960s. By adopting diagnostic criteria free of theoretical assumptions in the 1970s, our understanding of schizophrenia has been able to accommodate a spectrum of findings concerning risk factors from the genetic to the social, and allowed a greater consensus than was the case in the preceding ideologically driven decade. However, one limitation to progress in ascertaining the causes has been the changing conceptualization of the illness itself. Questions about what schizophrenia 'is', have influenced aetiological research. For example, the marked narrowing of DSM criteria in the United States fed into an almost exclusively biological view, whereas a greater interest in social factors in Europe may have been related to the broader concept used in the WHO classification. Furthermore, not long after standardization of diagnosis with most clinicians and researchers using either the DSM or the WHO classification, criticism began to emerge. For example, Berrios (39) noted that definitional changes had not improved the validity of schizophrenia as a category, but simply reflected the changing consensus. Interestingly, there has been a retreat from the idea that schizophrenia is a single disease since the mid-1990s. Although many American psychiatrists still tend to regard it as a single illness with biological causes, their European counterparts have increasingly considered it merely as a syndrome, a group of symptoms occurring together. Indeed, a clamour for a more dimensionally driven understanding of psychosis in general has broken out, partly in response to criticisms of a categorically based definition. For example, Ian Brockington, one of Britain's foremost nosologists, cried, almost in despair:

> It is important to loosen the grip which the concept of 'schizophrenia' has on the minds of psychiatrists. Schizophrenia is an idea whose very essence is equivocal, a nosological category without natural boundaries, a barren hypothesis. Such a blurred concept is 'not a valid object of scientific enquiry' (40).

Perhaps it was frustration with the inconsistencies and changeability of schizophrenia diagnoses that led researchers to the idea that, instead of a single illness, schizophrenia was a constellation of different symptoms occurring to differing degrees in different people. These questions were approached statistically, using factor analysis to determine whether psychotic symptoms can be reduced to five or six dimensions (e.g. distortion of reality, negative symptoms, disorganization, mania, and depression). In itself, this has changed the way in which the concept of schizophrenia has been seen by clinicians and studied by researchers. Clinicians have increasingly prescribed medication for individual dimensions according to their impact on functioning, for example prescribing mood stabilizers for the mood dimension, and antipsychotics for delusions and hallucinations. Researchers have broadened their vistas to recruit people including non-schizophrenia patients with individual psychotic symptoms, and minor psychotic symptoms, in the general population. How best to integrate such views in research and clinical work is hotly debated—one proposal is that major psychotic diagnostic categories should be retained, but complemented by ratings on dimensions such as positive and negative symptoms and disorganization.

Conclusions

As historical reviewers, it is difficult to shake off the perspective of the contemporary psychiatric clinician, familiar with operational criteria in both clinical and research settings. Undoubtedly, research into schizophrenia has expanded from a small, circumscribed but highly contentious arena in the 1960s, and also become more coherent. While the development of contemporary diagnostic criteria may not represent a true paradigm shift in the Kuhnian sense, it has been clearly the most significant milestone in the last half-century. Across all types of studies from genetics to social research, basic epidemiological principles of comparing operationally diagnosed cases with matched controls have been applied.

The pioneering phenomenologically driven psychiatrists, such as Bleuler and Schneider, developed the nosological entities that were to be operationalized in the DSM and International Classification of Diseases (ICD) systems as the two major mental illnesses, schizophrenia and bipolar affective disorder. However, Kraepelin did not envisage diagnostic criteria based on clinical interview as the outcome of his endeavours, and instead believed that the physical basis of psychosis would eventually be identified. Instead, his early medical formulations of dementia praecox were based on course, outcome, and a group of co-occurring, non-specific symptoms. The commitment in DSM-III to the neo-Kraepelinian understanding of schizophrenia re-committed psychiatry to this view, and for 25 years, researchers laboured with this perspective.

Thus, for the last quarter of the 20th century, explanations of schizophrenia based solely on brain disorder and genetics held centre stage. However, the turn of the century has shown a renewed interest in psychosocial factors. There have, of course, been seismic shifts in social models of causation over the last five decades, from those focusing on family and communication dynamics, via a more biologically sensitive social adversity model, towards an integrated understanding of schizophrenia as a complex phenotype involving both biological and social determinants. A key aspect of the shift has been the thinking about social adversity as a causal factor rather than a mere epiphenomenon (41).

In general, these approaches have demonstrated that the importance of particular causal factors varies from individual to individual. While it is clear that that much research progress has been made, the extent to which it has impacted on the clinic remains more limited. We have seen how the development of new insights concerning pathogenetic mechanisms has depended on advances in technology such as structural, functional, and neurochemical imaging. However, none of the biological markers identified by imaging or electrophysiology has been able to detect, or rule out, the presence of schizophrenia with sufficient reliability to be useful diagnostically. Advances in treatment have been modest and sometimes driven by serendipity rather than expansion of basic knowledge.

There remain many critics of the concept of schizophrenia and indeed there is much to criticize. In considering these, it is important to consider that Emil Kraepelin would probably have been surprised that what he latterly considered a provisional diagnostic category has endured for so many years. Most investigators continue to consider it as just that, and the term is likely to endure only until we have a fuller understanding of the aetiology of the different types of psychosis.

As we conclude this essay, the story of schizophrenia research over the last half-century is one of advancing understanding of aetiology and pathogenic mechanisms, theoretical consolidation, and yet recently increased awareness of the limitations of conventional medical approaches. The biomedical approach continues to have an important role to play in identifying genetic and neurodevelopmental influences on the disorder, but its limitations have given rise to exciting efforts to conceptualize aspects of social life that were previously outside the purview of medicine, and integrate them into how we think about the causes of this damaging illness. It is notable that far fewer resources have been spent on the investigation of environmental risk factors than on genetics and biological approaches. Researchers have come to realize that gene–environment interactions are bound to be central to causality. Thus future research which sets out to systematically test environmental risk factors and their interaction with genetic variations should bring important insights, and allow us to think in new ways about treatment.

References

1 Mayer-Gross, W., Slater, E., and Roth, M. (1955). *Clinical psychiatry*. London: Cassell.

2 Hayes, R. and Horwitz, A. V. (2005). DSM-III and the revolution in the classification of mental illness. *Journal of the History of the Behavioral Sciences* 41(3), 249–67.

3 Murray, R. M., Oon, M. C., Rodnight, R, Birley, J. L., and Smith, A. (1979). Increased excretion of dimethyltryptamine and certain features of psychosis: a possible association. *Archives of General Psychiatry* 36(6):644–9.

4 American Psychiatric Association (1952). *Diagnostic and statistical manual*. Washington, DC: American Psychiatric Association.

5 American Psychiatric Association (1968). *Diagnostic and statistical manual* (2nd edition). Washington, DC: American Psychiatric Association.

6 Laing, R. D. (1969). *The divided self*. London: Tavistock.

7 Cooper, J. E. (1972). *Psychiatric diagnosis in New York and London: a comparative study of mental hospital admission*. Oxford: Oxford University Press.

8 Clare, A. (1976). *Psychiatry in dissent*. London: Tavistock.

9 Wing J. K., Birley J. L. T, and Cooper J. E. (1967). Reliability of a procedure for measuring and classifying 'Present Psychiatric State.' *British Journal of Psychiatry* 113, 499–515.

10 Klerman, G., Vaillant, G., Spitzer, R., and Michels, R. (1984). A debate on DSM-III: The advantages of DSM-III. *American Journal of Psychiatry* 141, 539–53.

11 Sabshin, M. (1990). Turning points in twentieth-century American psychiatry. *American Journal of Psychiatry* 147, 1267–74.

12 Kendell, R. E. (1975). *The role of diagnosis in psychiatry*. Oxford: Blackwell Scientific Publications.

13 Murray R. M., Oon M. C., Rodnight R, Birley J. L., and Smith A. (1979). Increased excretion of dimethyltryptamine and certain features of psychosis: a possible association. *Archives of General Psychiatry* 36(6), 644–9.

14 Connell P. H. (1958). *Amphetamine psychosis*.London: Oxford University Press.

15 Carlsson, A.and Lindqvist, M. (1963). Effect of chlorpromazine or haloperidol on formation of 3-methoxytyramine and normetanephrine in mouse brain. *Acta Pharmacologica et Toxicologica* 20, 140–4.

16 Van Rossum, J. (1967). The significance of dopamine-receptor blockade for the action of neuroleptic drugs. In Brill, H., Cole, J., Deniker, P., Hippius, H., Bradley, P. B. (eds) *Neuropsychopharmacology, Proceedings of the 5th collegium internationale neuropsychopharmacologicum*. Amsterdam: Excerpta Medica, pp. 321–9.

17 Creese, I, Burt, D. R., and Snyder, S. H. (1976). Dopamine receptor binding predicts clinical and pharmacological potencies of antischizophrenic drugs. *Science* 192(4238), 481–3.

18 Johnstone, E. C., Crow, T. J., Frith, C. D., Carney, M. W., and Price, J. S. (1978). Mechanism of the antipsychotic effect in the treatment of acute schizophrenia. *Lancet* 1(8069), 848–51.

19 Shields, J. and Gottesman, I. I. (1972). Cross-national diagnosis of schizophrenia in twins. The heritability and specificity of schizophrenia. *Archives of General Psychiatry* 27(6), 725–30.

20 Gottesman, I. I. and Shields, J. (1982). *Schizophrenia. The epigenetic puzzle*. Cambridge: Cambridge University Press.

21 Kendler, K. S. and Diehl, S. R. (1993). The genetics of schizophrenia: a current, genetic-epidemiologic perspective. *Schizophrenia Bulletin* 19, 261–85.

22 Farmer, A. E., McGuffin, P., and Gottesman, I. I. (1987). Twin concordance for DSM-III schizophrenia. Scrutinizing the validity of the definition. *Archives of General Psychiatry* 44(7), 634–41.

23 O'Rourke, D. H., Gottesman, I. I., Suarez, B. K., Rice, J., and Reich, T. (1982). Refutation of the single locus model in the aetiology of schizophrenia. *American Journal of Human Genetics* 33, 630–49.

24 Alzheimer, A. (1897). Beitrage zur pathologischen Anatomie der Himrinde und zur anatomischen Grundlage einiger Psychosen. *Monatsschrift für Psychiatrie und Neurologie* 2, 82–120.

25 Haug, J. O. (1962). Pneumoencephalographic studies in mental disease. *Acta Psychiatrica Scandinavica* 38(Suppl. 165), 1–104.

26 Johnstone, E. C, Crow, T. J., Frith, C. D., Husband, J., and Kreel, L. (1976). Cerebral ventricular size and cognitive impairment in chronic schizophrenia. *Lancet* 2, 924–6.

27 Reveley, A. M., Reveley, M. A., Clifford, C. A., and Murray, R. M. (1982). Cerebral ventricular size in twins discordant for schizophrenia. Lancet 1(8271), 540–1.

28 Rose, S., Karnin, L. J., and Lewontin, R. C. (1984). *Not in our genes*. Harmondsworth: Penguin.

29 Lewis, S. W. and Murray, R. M. (1987). Obstetric complications, neurodevelopmental deviance, and risk of schizophrenia. *Journal of Psychiatric Research* 21(4), 413–21.

30 Weinberger, D. R. (1987). Implication of normal brain development for the pathogenesis of schizophrenia. *Archives of General Psychiatry* 44, 660–9.

31 Lewis, S. W. and Murray, R. M. (1987). Is schizophrenia a neurodevelopmental disorder? *British Medical Journal (Clinical Research Edition)* 295, 681–2.

32 Keshavan, M. S. (1999). Development, disease and degeneration in schizophrenia: a unitary pathophysiological model. *Journal of Psychiatric Research* 33(6), 513–21.

33 Broome M. R., Woolley J. B., Tabraham, P. et al. (2005). What causes the onset of psychosis? *Schizophrenia Research* 79(1), 23–34.

34 Sakoğlu, U., Upadhyay, J., Chin, C. L. et al. (2011). Paradigm shift in translational neuroimaging of CNS disorders. *Biochemical Pharmacology* 81(12), 1374–87.

35 Friston, K. J. and Frith, C. D. (1995). Schizophrenia: a disconnection syndrome? *Clinical Neuroscience* 3(2), 89–97.

36 Fearon, P., Kirkbride, J. B., Morgan, C. et al. (2006). AESOP Study Group. Incidence of schizophrenia and other psychoses in ethnic minority groups: results from the MRC AESOP Study. *Psychological Medicine* **36**(11), 1541–50.

37 van Os, J., Hanssen, M., Bijl, R. V., and Ravelli, A. (2000). Strauss (1969) revisited: a psychosis continuum in the general population? *Schizophrenia Research* **45**(1–2), 11–20.

38 Johns, L. C., Cannon, M., Singleton, N. et al. (2004). Prevalence and correlates of self-reported psychotic symptoms in the British population. *British Journal of Psychiatry* **185**, 298–305.

39 Berrios, G. (2003). Schizophrenia: a conceptual history. *International Journal of Psychology and Psychological Therapy* **3**(2), 111–40.

40 Brockington, I. F. (1992). Schizophrenia: Yesterday's concept. *European Psychiatry* **7**(5), 203–7.

41 van Os, J. and Kapur, S. (2009). Schizophrenia. Lancet **374**(9690), 635–45.

Social science and psychiatry, and the causes of mental disorders

Dana March and Ezra Susser

We look forward to the day when enough will be known about sociocultural factors to allow prevention in a public health sense through deliberate change in the human environment (1).
—*Alexander Leighton*

Introduction

Social science has played a critical role in conceptualizing and investigating the causes of mental illness. Nowhere is this more apparent than in the history of the epidemiology of psychiatric disorders. In contemporary psychiatry, the emphasis on biological and genetic determinants of, and pharmaceutical interventions for, mental illness has often eclipsed a focus on social determinants and the social contexts in which mental illness develops. Addressing such issues is taken up by social psychiatry. The influence of social science on psychiatry generally has been both penetrating and profound, meriting reflection at a time in which the dominant paradigm of the discipline could be greatly enhanced by a creative relationship with social science. Towards this end, we will draw out several strands of research exemplifying the contribution of social science in our understanding of the causes of mental illness. We will also note the welcome signs of its rejuvenation since the 1990s.

Early antecedents

The importance attached to social factors in the context of mental illness has fluctuated for over a century and a half. During the second half of the 19th century and the first half of the 20th, many influential figures in public health thought that the causes of mental disorders were partly or even largely sociocultural in nature, a perspective that may have reflected a wider concern with the corrosive effects of large-scale social developments—primarily industrialization, urbanization, and migration (2,3).

Perhaps the best-known seed for the subsequent blossoming role of social science in psychiatry was that planted by the father of sociology, Émile Durkheim, in *Suicide*, published in 1897 (4). In his classic study Durkheim sought to explain variation in the rate of suicide. He explored the influence of social isolation and a sense of control in various groups such as those with different religious affiliations and marital status; he concluded that the rate was higher among Protestants compared to Catholics and Jews, and among single than married people. He attributed this to the result of social isolation and deficits in social control, in turn associated with unsavoury effects of industrialization and the fraying of the societal fabric emblematic of modernity.

Against the backdrop of Durkheim's pioneering work, scores of studies in the early 20th century addressed social phenomena as possible causes of mental disorders, primarily severe forms. Of particular interest during this period were migration and its role in illnesses such as schizophrenia and other psychoses. These concerns were fuelled by a broader preoccupation with social dependency in migrants. Studies like those conducted by Ödegaard (5) in Minnesota and Norway and Malzberg (6) in New York State reflected demographic shifts in the United States and the fear of the potential needs of newly arrived groups, their possible burden on American society, and the potential impact of psychological disability on the country's social, economic, and political progress (2,3).

Striking differences were found between social groups and across social contexts in the prevalence of schizophrenia and related psychoses. In order to test theories that social arrangements might be of aetiological significance, sociologists and social psychiatrists attempted to capture and study markers of the dynamic social processes of industrialization, urbanization, and migration. Various social constructs, among them stratification, disorganization, and isolation, crystallized from sociological theories and informed the identification of social variables that were examined quantitatively to deepen our understanding of the causes of mental disorders (7). Studies addressing these social phenomena were aligned along two axes: urban ecology and social causation-selection.

Mental disorders in urban areas

The urban scape and its social architecture became a special locus of study for social scientists interested in mental health. In this context, a pioneering study was carried out by Robert Faris and Warren Dunham, members of the Chicago school of sociology, in the 1930s. They examined the relationship between what was then called 'functional psychoses' and social organization. They theorized that social isolation and poor interpersonal communication were associated with mental disorders. Applying the concentric zone model of urban organization, developed a decade earlier by their mentor, the sociologist Ernest Burgess, Faris and Dunham tested their theories empirically in a cross-sectional ecological study. In this model inner urban zones consisted of the most disorganized communities, and were characterized by isolation and poor communication. Social organization improved as circles radiated from the epicentre, with outer zones containing the most organized communities.

They conceived of social organization as a function of interaction within a given context, captured by administrative data covering type of residence (e.g. rooming-house, rental), characteristics of the populations, both fixed (e.g. race and country of birth) and dynamic (e.g. mobility and government assistance status), framed in terms of the community (e.g. percentage of minority residents in a particular neighbourhood). Consistent with their hypothesis, a distinct social pattern of schizophrenia (though not bipolar disorder), emerged with the highest rates in the most socially disorganized areas (8).

As many have pointed out, these findings do not confirm the role of social disorganization as a cause of schizophrenia. Given the limitations of a cross-sectional design and the use of administrative data, the results might have reflected a downward drift of those with schizophrenia, but the researchers concluded that this could not fully account for their results.

The work of Faris and Dunham helped to cement the role of social science in psychiatry, especially their theory-driven attempt to conceptualize and measure aspects of the social environment (7), and to apply these measures quantitatively within an ecological approach. Moreover, they appreciated that social factors operate in tandem with other factors—psychological and constitutional—in causing mental illness and are not mutually exclusive. At the time that Faris and Dunham were carrying out their research, causality was conceptutalized in terms of three primary domains: constitutional, psychological, and sociological, which accounted for both individual and population-level variation in the prevalence of mental illness.

Social class and mental illness

The growing interest in social determinants of mental illness during the interwar and post-World War II years, particularly in the United States, was tethered to historical concerns about social dependence. A related strand of research addressed the issue of whether an individual's social class position was a cause or consequence of mental illness. This subject has deep historical roots, with studies of insanity and social class conducted by Edward Jarvis in the 1850s (9). Perhaps the most rigorous early work was done by a notable pairing of August Hollingshead, a sociologist, and Frederick Redlich, a psychiatrist. They brought their joint interests to bear in a study in the early 1950s, examining the relation between mental illness and social class in New Haven, Connecticut (10). They demonstrated that each social class manifested specific patterns of illness and presented in distinct clinical ways, including pathways to treatment. They also examined the socio-historical context of the New Haven community, the cultures of the social classes, and the institutions in which psychiatrists practiced. Striking inequalities in care were identified, a pattern that has endured to the present in the United States (11). Mentally ill people from lower social classes often come to psychiatric care through compulsory and other coercive means and receive poorer quality and continuity of treatment compared to their higher-class counterparts.

The study also gave rise to methodological advances, especially the Hollingshead Index of Social Position, which blended weighted categories of occupation and education. While the index had limitations, and was subsequently revised (12), it represented a noteworthy contribution to this area of research. Whether social class is a cause or consequence of mental illness continued to be keenly debated for decades.

The ecology of mental illness

On the heels of the work of Hollingshead and Redlich, social science and psychiatry were interwoven in two landmark epidemiology studies, the Midtown Manhattan Study and the Stirling County Study. Both studies were conducted at a time of critical policy shifts and expanding psychiatric research, stimulated by the postwar boom (13). The purpose of the Midtown Manhattan Study was to examine sociocultural determinants of mental health and to establish the need for community psychiatric services.

Thomas Rennie, the progenitor of the multidisciplinary approach in this investigation, called for 'a working relationship between the social scientist and the psychiatrist' (14). He and his collaborator Alexander Leighton, both influenced by the celebrated psychiatrist Adolf Meyer, recognized that psychiatric disorders, like somatic disorders, occurred in a particular context with its own conflicts, history, and dynamic changes. Their aims were to capture the prevalence of mental disorders in the community, and not only in people presenting for treatment ('treated rates' were criticized as underestimating the true burden of mental illness), within a social environment perceived as either 'benign' or 'noxious', and to establish a scientific basis for preventing mental illness and promoting mental health. Indeed, the integration of social factors into their investigations was so profound that the conceptualization of psychiatric outcomes was defined in terms of a continuum of from health to ill-health. An additional composite rating of mental health was devised (the Global Judgment of Mental Health). The components were not only focused on 'disorder' *per se*, but also on health, well-being, and overall functioning.

The high rate of mental health problems, especially anxiety, generated controversy, but was plausible to the investigators, given the New York City-based community under study with its population density, degree of crowding in public places, and pace of life.

A similar study in a less urbanized area in Nova Scotia (the Stirling County Study, led by Leighton) also found a comparably high rate, which was interpreted as reflecting economic decline and limited opportunities, with people suffering a sense of loss of control over their lives (1).

The holistic approach that typified the above three major studies gave way to a narrower conceptual framework during the second half of the 20th century: primacy was given (and still is today) to 'constitutional factors'—essentially biological and genetic—in psychiatric disorders, in keeping with shifts in science and medicine. Far less attention was paid to social factors, especially social contexts. Moreover, a dimensional conception of mental illness was supplanted by a categorical one. Although a bias towards discrete disorders contributed to major advances in psychiatric epidemiology as well as to the public's acceptance of mental ill-health as warranting investment in services and research, limitations became apparent, generating vigorous debate.

Social science as background in US studies of burden and need

From the 1970s onwards, psychiatric epidemiology in the United States largely moved away from community studies and the integration of social science therein (mostly to try and establish causality) because it was not sustainable to collect such rich information, and did not serve the needs of the federal government, or states that increasingly administered services.

Following the Midtown Manhattan Study, the next ambitious attempt to examine the burden of mental illness in the United States, and related service requirements, was the Epidemiologic Catchment Area (ECA) Study(15). This study represented a shift away from the rich social science foundation of its epidemiological predecessors. The ECA served the needs of the State by establishing the burden of psychiatric disorders, in five US communities. The data could be weighted back to the general population.

The National Comorbidity Surveys (NCS) (16,17) were nationally representative studies conducted in the 1990s and 2000s, following the ECA and its indication that psychiatric comorbidity was an understudied burden. The NCS drilled further into the complexities of burden and service use than the ECA could and did not. This was necessary to understand what kind of problem psychiatric illnesses posed for the US health care system, and whether the services available—both public and private—were adequate and used effectively. While the State could not address social causes, it could address what services could be provided, given an established burden.

Both the ECA and the NCS examined prevalence and correlates, and included social variables only as correlates. Their purposes and affiliated designs had little to do with social causes or social science, and as such, they were a type of technology, from which social science was absent almost entirely, that shifted the emphasis to burden and need.

International studies and the course of social science in psychiatry

As the role of social science began to diminish in the United States, an international project launched in the late 1970s by the World Health Organization (WHO) proved a landmark in the history of the role of social science in shedding light on aspects of psychiatry. The Ten Country Study was designed to compare the incidence and course of schizophrenia and related psychoses in diverse sociocultural settings. Examining sociocultural context and adopting discrete categories for diagnosis (18), the research team found compelling evidence of different kinds of psychosis (19), and a more favourable course of illness, as indicated by five of six best outcome measures, in developing countries compared to developed ones. The data on incidence were more ambiguous, partly due to small samples of subjects, a limited number of research sites in developing countries where it proved feasible to measure incidence (only urban and rural Chandigarh in India), and a variety of methods to determine diagnosis.

One of the present authors (ES) used the data from the WHO study to show that acute and transient psychoses were as much as tenfold more common in developing than developed countries. Much previous research had suggested this, as well as anecdotal evidence, but it could not be confirmed without being able to compare sociocultural environments (as facilitated by an internationally based study). We also found that the classification of acute and transient psychoses in widely used manuals was derived from small studies in only 10% of the globe (where almost all psychiatric research has been conducted for generations), and did not correspond well with their actual manifestations and clinical course. In a long-term follow-up study, we found that in both long- and short-term psychoses, course was on average more favourable in developing countries; although there was more variance, with poor as well as good outcomes more common in the developing countries. The explanation may lie partly at the level of family support, as proposed by Leff and his colleagues (see this volume, pp. 96–116), and confirmed by work at Columbia.

The broader social ecology also may have played an important role. People with psychoses in developing countries were less likely to be segregated in institutions (mainly due to limited resources). Remaining in their community, they could participate in its informal economy and have a place in the extended family household, and had the opportunity to achieve a measure of social integration. The current patient-led 'recovery' movement in developed countries that has become a potent force in rehabilitation would surely endorse this hypothesis as warranting serious consideration.

The findings of the Ten Country Study on clinical course have been challenged by other investigators; this is legitimate, given that massive urbanization in the developing world, with its associated profound social changes, had not occurred when the WHO investigation was under way. Historical time, as well as place, is an essential context in any psychiatric research, especially within the social psychiatry paradigm.

Reviving social science in psychiatry

While social science was dormant in psychiatry in the United States beyond the 1970s, a couple of research strands provided a strong foundation for the revival of social science in psychiatry on the international stage. Bruce Dohrenwend, a sociologist and psychiatric epidemiologist, and his team sought definitive answers to the social selection-social causation issue in an Israeli cohort, finding that lower social class was the *result* of schizophrenia and that social causation might be relevant to other psychiatric disorders (especially depression in women and antisocial personality disorder in men) (20).

Perhaps most notably, studies of migrants in the United Kingdom and Western Europe (see Leff, this volume, pp. 96–116) served as a foundation for new work from which emerged a pattern of high rates of psychosis in migrant groups belonging to certain ethnic minorities (21). Two key studies have generated continuing curiosity about these questions. The Aetiology and Ethnicity of Schizophrenia and Other Psychoses (ÆSOP) investigation reported markedly increased rates of schizophrenia in specific ethnic groups compared to the white population (22) in three British cities. These ethnic groups were largely comprised of former immigrants and two generations of their descendants. The Hague Incidence Study yielded a similar pattern (23).

The features of the social environment itself that might be contributing to the differential rates have been examined closely. For example, rates of schizophrenia are lower in ethnic minority and migrant groups living in neighbourhoods where they constitute a sizable proportion of the local residents—the so-called ethnic density effect (24). This effect was first reported by Faris and Dunham in *Mental Disorders in Urban Areas* (8). They observed that rates of hospital admissions for schizophrenia among black Americans residing in areas of Chicago where they constituted a majority were lower than for those living among other migrant and ethnic groups. Nearly 70 years later, fuelled by research addressing elevated rates of psychosis among ethnic minority immigrants in western Europe, this effect was investigated in south-east London. Again, rates of schizophrenia were lowest among non-whites (e.g. black Africans and Afro-Caribbeans) living in areas in which they were the majority (25). Another investigation in the same area of London, this time using the ÆSOP data (see above), yielded similar findings but the lowest rates of schizophrenia were in neighbourhoods in which the black population had 'medium' ethnic density (26).

Limitations of the studies addressing ethnic density effect warrant attention. First, all have been cross-sectional, precluding the determination of a cause–effect relationship. If the effect does operate, then we might expect it to do so over time or at a critical period in development but not at the point of illness onset. Second, only in The Hague study were particular groups with elevated schizophrenia rates examined (Surinamese, Moroccan, and Turkish). Third, the neighbourhoods under study did not include ones in which ethnic minorities constituted all of the residents or only very few of them. As a result, whether ethnic density has an effect on rates of schizophrenia cannot be determined fully.

In an attempt to surmount these difficulties, our team undertook a study of urbanicity and ethnic density at birth in the United States (27). When controlling for family socio-economic status (SES) at birth, black people were three times more likely to be diagnosed with schizophrenia than their white neighbours (28). A high population density at birth was associated with being black and with increased schizophrenia, but after adjusting for this factor, a substantial black–white difference in the odds ratio for schizophrenia remained (2.96). When we restricted our sample to Blacks, there was a marked protective effect of birth in racially mixed neighbourhood, not explained by family SES at birth. Compared to Blacks born into majority black neighbourhoods (72–96% black), those born in racially mixed neighbourhoods (17–42% black) had a lower risk of schizophrenia (0.11). Similar results obtained when majority white neighbourhoods (0–16% black) were used as the referent.

These findings demonstrate the need for social science research to take into account the full range of potential factors when investigating the risk of schizophrenia or indeed any other mental illness in a particular racial or ethnic minority. An approach is called for that blends historical and epidemiological investigations to understand the complex web of social, economic, and political determinants, both deleterious and protective. The influence of age at the time of migration and the experience of discrimination reinforces this point. For example, in the above-mentioned Dutch study (29), migrants who arrived in Holland under the age of five had the highest rate of schizophrenia in adult life, suggesting that social stress has long-term effects on the developing brain which in turn may render them more susceptible to psychiatric illness as they grow up. According to the Dutch research work (30), the prevalence of schizophrenia in migrant minorities may also be associated with the experience of discrimination.

Future prospects

In the current era of investigating social causes of mental disorders, community-based phenomena and the mechanisms by which they operate (e.g. gene–environment interactions, epigenetics) have proved appealing. 'Upstream' social factors such as poverty and discrimination are insufficient on their own to lead to disorders but they can contribute to causation in conjunction with 'downstream' risk factors (i.e. more proximal to the person). It is essential therefore that the entire range of social factors (with their multilevel effects) is granted systematic attention.

The recent emergence of epigenetics in psychiatric research provides a golden opportunity for social factors to be considered in concert with biological and genetic ones. Many investigators who previously gave short shrift to the social dimension have been drawn to study it in order to understand how social experience can shape the expression of genes. At present, this is most evident in research on the early origins of psychiatric disorders (34). However, the same trend is taking shape in other fields as the dynamic nature of epigenetic changes over the lifespan is increasingly recognized.

Research regarding migration, urbanization, and schizophrenia, with notable historical roots, may prove in the immediate future the most amenable to the contemporary integration of social science and psychiatry in using novel approaches. For example, although there is evidence regarding the role of discrimination (as we mentioned earlier), it is still poorly understood why migrants have elevated rates of psychosis. Similarly, the mechanisms of the ethnic density effect remain unclear. In addition, the mechanisms by which urban areas elevate rates of schizophrenia are elusive. However, both areas are ripe for rigorous social psychiatric investigations. For example, systematic research addressing how social causes get under the skin to produce illness in individuals and in populations is necessary in order to identify targets for intervention at multiple levels (e.g. individual, community).

Psychiatric epidemiology is deeply connected to social psychiatry and is well poised to bring together the requisite elements to understand the many roles social factors play in the causes, course, and consequences of psychiatric illness. The integration of descriptive and analytic psychiatric epidemiology in order to both document risk and protective factors and subsequently explain how they affect illness, using integrative social and biological investigations over the lifespan, is needed. By building on the rich history of research in the social sciences regarding the causation of mental illness, psychiatry can leverage the knowledge gained thus far and even set the laudable aim of preventing mental disorders by, as Alexander Leighton put it, 'deliberate change in the human environment.' To this, psychiatry can look forward.

References

1 Leighton, A. (1959). *My name is legion: foundations for a theory of man in relation to culture.* New York: Basic Books.

2 Grob, G. N. (1983). *Mental illness and American society, 1875–1940.* Princeton: Princeton University Press.

3 Grob, G. (1985). The origins of American psychiatric epidemiology. *American Journal of Public Health* **75**(3), 229–36.

4 Susser, E., Schwartz, S., Morabia, A., and Bromet, E. (2006). *Psychiatric epidemiology: searching for the causes of mental disorders.* New York: Oxford University Press.

5 Ödegaard, Ö. (1932). Emigration and insanity. *Acta Psychiatrica Neurologica Scandinavica Suppl* **4**, 1–206.

6 Malzberg, B. (1940). *Social and biological aspects of mental disease.* Utica, NY: New York State Hospitals Press.

7 March, D., Hatch, S., Morgan, C., et al. (2008). Psychosis and place. *Epidemiologic Reviews* **30**(1), 84–100.

8 Faris, R. and Dunham, H. (1939). *Mental disorders in urban areas.* Chicago: University of Chicago Press.

9 Jarvis, E. (1855/1971). *Insanity and idiocy in Massachusetts: report of the Commission in Lunacy.* Cambridge, MA: Harvard University Press.

10 Hollingshead, A. and Redlich, F. (1958). *Social class and mental illness.* New York: John Wiley and Sons.

11 Miranda, J., McGuire, T. G., Williams, D. R., and Wang P. (2008). Mental health in the context of health disparities. *American Journal of Psychiatry* **165**(9), 1102–8.

12 Liberatos, P., Link, B. G., and Kelsey, J. L. (1988). The measurement of social class in epidemiology. *Epidemiologic Reviews* **10**, 87–121.

13 Srole, L., Langner, T. S., Opler, M. K., Michael, S. T., and Rennie, T. A. C. (1962). *Mental health in the metropolis: the Midtown Manhattan study.* New York: McGraw-Hill.

14 Rennie, T. A. C. (1978). Introduction. In: Srole, L., Langner, T. S., Michael, S. T., Opler, M. K., Rennie, T. A. C (eds.) *Mental health in the metropolis: the Midtown Manhattan Study (revised edition).* New York: New York University Press.

15 Robins, L. N. and Regier, D. A. (eds.) (1991). *Psychiatric disorders in America: The Epidemiologic Catchment Area study.* New York: Free Press.

16 Kessler, R. C., McGonagle, K. A., Zhao, S. et al. (1994). Lifetime and 12-month prevalence of DSM-III-R psychiatric disorders in the United States: results from the National Comorbidity Survey. *Archives of General Psychiatry* **51**(1), 8–19.

17 Kessler, R., Birnbaum, H., Demler, O. et al. (2005). The prevalence and correlates of non-affective psychosis in the National Comorbidity Survey Replication (NCS-R). *Biological Psychiatry* **58**, 668–76.

18 Jablensky, A., Sartorius, N., Ernberg, G. et al. (1992). Schizophrenia: manifestations, incidence, and course in different cultures. A World Health Organization ten-country study. *Psychological Medicine Monograph Supplement* **20**, 1–97.

19 Susser, E. and Wanderling, J. (1994). Epidemiology of nonaffective remitting psychosis vs. schizophrenia: sex and sociocultural setting. *Archives of General Psychiatry* **51**, 294–301.

20 Dohrenwend, B. P., Levav, I., Shrout, P. E. et al. (1992). Socioeconomic status and psychiatric disorders: The causation-selection issue. *Science* **255**(5047), 946–52.

21 Cantor-Graae, E. and Selten, J. (2005). Schizophrenia and migration: meta-analysis and review. *American Journal of Psychiatry* **162**(1), 12–24.

22 Fearon, P., Kirkbride, J. B., Morgan, C. et al. (2006). Incidence of schizophrenia and other psychoses in ethnic minority groups: results from the MRC ÆSOP Study. *Psychological Medicine* **36**(11), 1541–50.

23 Veling, W., Selten, J. P., Veen, N. et al. (2006). Incidence of schizophrenia among ethnic minorities in the Netherlands: a four-year first-contact study. *Schizophrenia Research* **86**(1–3), 189–93.

24 Veling, W., Susser, E., van Os, J. et al. (2008). Ethnic density of neighborhoods and incidence of psychotic disorders among immigrants. *American Journal of Psychiatry* **165**, 66–73.

25 Boydell, J., van Os, J., McKenzie, K. et al. (2001). Incidence of schizophrenia in ethnic minorities in London: ecological study into interactions with environment. *BMJ* **323**, 1–4.

26 Kirkbride, J. B., Morgan, C., Fearon, P. et al. (2007). Neighbourhood-level effects on psychoses: re-examining the role of context. *Psychological Medicine* **37**(10), 1413–25.

27 March, D., Susser, E., Bresnahan, M., and Schaefer, C. (2013). Race, schizophrenia, and neighborhood context in the U.S.: Evidence from a California birth cohort. *International Congress on Schizophrenia Research*. Orlando, FL.

28 Bresnahan, M., Begg, M., Brown, A. et al. (2007). Race and risk of schizophrenia in a US birth cohort: another example of health disparity? *International Journal of Epidemiology* **36**, 751 8.

29 Veling, W., Hoek, H. W., Selten, J. P., and Susser, E. (2011) age at migration and future risk of psychotic disorders among immigrants in the Netherlands: a 7-year incidence study. *American Journal of Psychiatry* **168**, 1278–85.

30 Veling, W., Selten, J. P., Susser, E. et al. (2007) Discrimination and the incidence of psychotic disorders among ethnic minorities in The Netherlands. *International Journal of Epidemiology* **36**(4), 761–8.

Essay 5

The history of cultural psychiatry in the last half-century

Anne E. Becker and Arthur Kleinman

Introduction

Cultural psychiatry is a transdisciplinary field, principally drawing from interpretive social sciences (e.g. medical anthropology), social and psychiatric epidemiology, clinical psychiatry and psychology, and the concerns of mental health professionals from non-Western ethnic, diasporic, and national groups.

Plural agendas set forth over the past half-century can be discerned. The dominant narrative of change for cultural psychiatry in the last half-century is migration from description to action and from Eurocentric preoccupations to global concerns. However, there is a recursive quality in this history, and some major preoccupations persist throughout this period: What are the commonalities and differences in mental illness across diverse cultural contexts? What are their implications for aetiological understanding and therapeutic interventions? What are the social structural determinants of risk and distribution of mental disorders? Moreover, the declared intention to eradicate the most vexing methodological limitations undermining previously held valid cross-cultural assessment resonates with the same machinations on the threshold of publishing the newest iteration of the American Psychiatric Association's *Diagnostic and Statistical Manual for Mental Disorders* (DSM) (1).

Cultural psychiatry has a heterogeneous constituency comprising academic disciplines that remain somewhat insular and compartmentalized, despite many attempts to bridge them. Preoccupation with excavating presumed 'core' and universal underpinnings of mental illness persists. Further, the impact of social structural adversity and rapid social change on mental health continue to be central questions inhering in epidemiological studies.

For 50 years the intricate interface of social, psychological, cultural, and biological dimensions of the mental disorders has persisted, additionally complicated by such contingencies as the possibility of epigenetic impacts, an expanding inventory of physiologically and socially hazardous exposures, and large-scale transnational migration that has reconfigured the social realities of ethnic and national identity and cultural diversity. We continue to wrestle with the validity of universalizing diagnostic classification, while recognizing its pragmatic utility for policy-making and constructing globally useful and locally effective mental health services. The polemics of both extreme cultural relativism and biopsychological reductionism have given way to appreciation of the integration of biological, social, and psychological factors, as well as of social theory with clinical practice. This recognition is necessary given the staggering burden of global mental illness, and obstacles that continue to thwart the delivery of mental health services.

The recent history of cultural psychiatry dwells in multiple historical and social currents. Its unselfconsciously ethnocentric approach in the mid-20th century emerged from a colonial-era legacy, just as its present globally oriented agenda reflects the advantages of scientific and communications technologies, heightened visibility, a social justice discourse committed to championing health as a human right, and expanding economic opportunities for the pharmaceutical industry.

Cultural psychiatry has emerged from a fundamentally Eurocentric interest in prevalence and phenomena of mental disorders to focus on redressing the inequities of global shortfalls in research, resources, and treatment. In the past half-century, discerning universal core psychopathology among culturally diverse phenotypes was broadly motivated by aetiological questions, producing endless debates about cultural plasticity, risk mediators, and modifiers. The century ended with a broader global agenda. Cultural diversity, the realities of social mediation, and moderation of risk were firmly established in the scientific record. However, the *clinical* salience of cultural diversity engendered marginal interest until incontrovertible evidence of ethnic disparities in mental health outcomes came to light.

Cultural psychiatry's ignoble colonial legacy

The dominant preoccupations of cultural psychiatry mid-20th century, emerging from the motives and practices characterizing tropical medicine during the colonial era, were largely devoted to safeguarding and optimizing imperialist economic and political ambitions (2). Notwithstanding earlier interest in African studies as a means of discerning universal psychological processes (3), the latter half of the century witnessed a preoccupation with racial and cultural difference (4) that constructed and emphasized qualities of racial 'otherness' (5).

The inordinate impact of a few expatriate men practicing psychiatry in remote settings buttressed a colonial ideology (6). For example, in 1953, the World Health Organization published *The African Mind in Health and Disease: A Study in Ethnopsychiatry*, by John Carothers, a psychiatrist who administered the Mathari Mental Hospital in Nairobi from 1938 to 1951. A sequel monograph, *The Mind of Man in Africa*, concurred with Prince's formulation of 'brain fag', a syndrome of Africans acquiring literacy, positing 'expression of a subconscious antagonism to the written word' (7). Carothers supported this position elsewhere (8), seemingly unaware of social factors and inequities that confounded the presentation of mental illness.

Contrast this with Fanon's formulation of madness, based on his experiences as an Afro-Caribbean psychiatrist practicing in North Africa during the Algerian war for independence: 'We believe that in the cases [of psychotic reaction] presented here the triggering factor is principally the bloody, pitiless atmosphere, the generalization of inhuman practices, of people's lasting impression that they are witnessing a veritable apocalypse' (9, p. 153).

Thomas Lambo, a Nigerian psychiatrist, wrote about the profound psychological impact of social structural changes imposed by colonialism. He also impugned 'the moral arrogance of nineteenth- and twentieth-century Europe in setting up its civilizations as the standard by which all other civilizations are to be measured' (10, p. 345). In their repudiation of stereotypes of a 'primitive mind', Lambo and Fanon laid a foundation for a discourse on the social determinants of mental illness and poor health—the macrosocial structures overlaid on the microsocial—later described and elaborated as 'structural violence'.

Novel therapeutics and interventional paradigms at mid-century

Several major events laid the foundation for the increasingly medicalized approach to classifying, understanding, and treating mental illness during the mid-20th century. The first double-blind randomized clinical trial in 1949, conducted by the US National Institute of Mental Health, established the standard for psychotropic clinical research. Several psychopharmacological agents (e.g. reserpine, chlorpromazine, imipramine, and lithium) subsequently revolutionized care of patients with psychotic disorders. In 1952, the American Psychiatric Association published the first edition of the DSM, which promulgated assumptions about the discrete and universal nature of diagnostic categories. These and other events catalysed a shift from the mind to the brain as a dominant paradigm for understanding and responding to mental illness. Subsequent editions of the DSM further overhauled psychiatric classification introducing standardized criteria for psychiatric diagnosis (DSM-III, 11) that promoted an atomistic emphasis on disease categories. Such work facilitated assessment of the global burden of mental health, by ascertaining the prevalence of mental disorders in non-Western contexts.

A persistent dialectic of commonalities and diversities: epidemiological approaches and contributions to cultural psychiatry

In contrast to the influential conceptual frame of mental illness as culturally particular and relative in the first half of the 20th century, many cultural psychiatrists and epidemiologists subsequently favoured a universalist frame. Cultural diversity in the presentation of mental disorders, well-recognized by mid-20th century, became an intellectual springboard for discerning universal core psychopathology, and a platform for informing aetiological models of mental illness. Approaches to cultural variation in expression and risk for mental illness responded to scientific and social contexts that located pathogenesis at an individual level as opposed to a societal level. This profoundly shifted the radical theoretical stance of cultural relativism of Margaret Mead, Ruth Benedict, and others in the 1930s and 1940s, that had advanced the theory of mental illness as entirely socially constructed.

By the second half of the 20th century, pathoplasticity (the idea that symptoms are malleable even if aetiology is not) of mental disorders was acknowledged as a *de minimis* influence of the cultural milieu, but interpretation of culturally distinctive phenomenological presentations lacked consensus. Among those who posited universals in psychopathology, cultural variation was viewed as a methodological vexation—as reflected in Leighton's assertion that 'the content of symptomatic expressions may interfere with our recognizing a syndrome, and so lead to misidentification'–but not necessarily as counter-evidence of core commonalities (12, p. 162). This view was opposed by some, reflected in Eric Wittkower's query whether it is 'possible or permissible (though it may be desirable) to press mental disorders observed in African natives into the Procrustean bed of American nosology?' (13). The premise was widely shared that certain major mental disorders were universal, even if 'masked' by distinctive cultural forms.

Culturally distinctive phenotypes of mental illness observed and reported in the scientific literature raised questions not just about their relation to clinically observed forms of mental illness in Europe and North America, but also what they signalled about their etiological pathways. Although proponents of a greater quantitative understanding of psychopathology placed explicit emphasis on the need for greater methodological rigour through more systematic sampling and careful attention to valid assessment, the agenda was curiously focused on matters with relevance to European and North American populations.

However, in writing about the impact of colonial domination and rapid economic change on mental health, Lambo noted that societies in African nations 'constitute the most rewarding and extraordinary laboratory of human and social interactions' (10). And Leighton, in comments from the panel discussion on Transcultural Studies at the Third World Congress of Psychiatry in 1961, included the 'importance of the comparative analysis of nature's experiment as a means of extending knowledge of causes' of mental disorders (12, p. 180). The clinical relevance of cultural diversity was poorly appreciated and of marginal interest—at least in the United States—whereas the scientific value of comparative studies both in detecting universal core pathology and in informing aetiological models rationalized several large epidemiological studies. Most surprising here is that much cultural psychiatry in this period lacked any sustained interest in building mental healthcare systems in poor countries or among the poor in the West. Whereas comparative studies of like cases undeniably yielded useful data, they failed to address how differences might be reconciled with aetiological theories premised on commonalities.

Global standardization of psychiatric diagnosis

Over the past half-century, a number of large epidemiological studies set the stage for rigorous systematic comparisons across diverse cultural contexts using standardized assessments. Prior to this, lack of standardization of both methods (14) and clinical nosological categories drew sharp criticism as major impediments to cross-cultural comparisons that could inform therapeutic and health policy.

The perceived scientific and clinical utility of standardization mobilized an international collaborative effort, and in the early 1960s the World Health Organization (WHO) initiated attempts to standardize diagnostic classification of the mental disorders. The unprecedented and Herculean nature of this task was evident and Norman Sartorius observed that 'Reaching such agreement signal[led] something of a revolution and a major international effort was necessary to approach this goal' (15). Although the programme produced both 'an internationally workable classification' and 'an internationally acceptable glossary, which was developed in collaboration with psychiatrists from 62 countries,' notwithstanding the honest effort and ambitious and laudable goals, the classification represented something of a 'compromise' that 'appeared theoretically conservative and unenterprising' (15, p. 80). Fifteen years later, the 'definition of mental disorders in different cultures' was still cited as a major barrier to overcome (15), even though WHO had by then sponsored a nine-country International Pilot Study of Schizophrenia and was preparing for an analogue international study on depressive disorders (15).

The increasing operationalization of diagnostic criteria in general psychiatry eventually led to standardized assessments deployed in the service of cross-national studies. These included the Stirling County Study, launched in Canada in 1955 (16), the WHO Collaborative Study on the Assessment of Depressive Disorders (SADD), launched in 1972 (17), the WHO International Pilot Study of Schizophrenia (IPSS) launched in the 1960s (18), the Determinants of Outcome of Severe Mental Disorder (DOSMeD) launched in 1978 (19), and the International Study of Schizophrenia (ISoS), launched in the 1990s (20).

Notwithstanding large studies that advanced understanding of the global prevalence of major mental disorders, uncertainties about cross-national and cross-cultural prevalence persist, in part because we have not yet overcome challenges to diagnostic validity in cross-cultural assessment (21). The Lancet's 2011 series update on their 2007 launch for global mental health observed the wide range of prevalence estimates of mental illness in children and adolescents globally, citing heterogeneity of assessments, risk exposures, and cultural contexts as possible explanations (22).

Complementary to the influential work of the culture and personality school that preceded them, these epidemiological studies undeniably raised the scientific standards for cross-cultural psychiatry. The systematic assessments required to address comparative questions of interest were necessarily reductionistic, however, and focused attention on universal phenotypes rather than pursuing other interesting questions about cultural diversity. For example, the IPSS criteria for inclusion in the study cohort were narrow in order to exclude outliers that might confound the relationships between caseness and outcomes. Although this was a reasonable methodological strategy, it also perpetuated the Western biomedical nosological hegemony, and thereby systematically excluded cases with greatest diversity.

The inherent bias was acknowledged in the early comparative work on schizophrenia (23). While acknowledging commonalities in the expression of psychopathology across cultures, Yap underscored the cultural bias in the 'the grammar and language of psychiatry' as well as 'the danger of an ethnocentric reduction of psychiatric manifestations everywhere to an arbitrary uniformity based on the Kraeplin–Bleuler schema, accompanied by misconception of or even blindness to culture-bound reactions' (24, p. 836).

Critics of these multinational studies have pointed out that they may have simply identified symptom profiles most familiar in European and North American populations and excluded outliers more salient in their local contexts. Cultural critics have subsequently argued that selective publication of clinical trials representing European and North American populations has contributed to reification of mental illness phenotypes typifying these populations to the relative exclusion of populations representing over 90% of the world (25). Likewise, the subsequent widespread distribution and global use of the DSM foregrounds clinical presentations based on diagnostic criteria developed for these populations. Cultural variation in the DSM-1V was relegated to the appendices, reflecting perceived marginal relevance to American psychiatrists, even as they practice in increasingly multicultural clinical settings (26).

The interest in a parsimonious nosological framework that could encompass cultural diversity was also reflected in a paper by Blashfield and colleagues in anticipation of the release of the DSM-IV. They commented on the steady increase in the number of diagnostic categories: from 106 in the first edition of the DSM in 1952 to 285 in the third edition in 1980. They argued that proliferation of categories would undermine their clinical utility, and observed the risk that 'diagnostic categories in an official classificatory system tend to be reified'. They also enumerated inclusion and exclusion criteria as a standard to consider when endorsing a new diagnostic category (27). They proposed that 50 scientific papers be published (at least half based on empirical data) as a minimum eligibility standard for diagnosis, and that assessment tools and inter-rater reliability studies be available for the disorder.

The formalization of diagnostic categories in the DSM tended both to reify the presentations described and to exclude culturally diverse clinical presentations—both because the latter may not have come to the attention of the DSM Task Force, and also because they could not meet the high standards for inclusion as a diagnostic category. In this respect, the steep gradient in economic and scientific resources between high- and low-resource regions arguably continues to have profound impact on how psychiatric diagnosis is conceptualized, recognized, and treated.

Notwithstanding their considerable methodological limitations, these large-scale attempts to standardize psychiatric diagnostic assessment established the imperative of including investigators in low-resource countries as participants in collective efforts to examine comparative epidemiology (15). They may be viewed as a major departure from the predominantly Eurocentric agenda that motivated cultural comparative psychiatry at the outset of the half-century. This departure appeared in the recognition that findings from cross-cultural comparative studies would be essential to adapting therapeutic strategies to local contexts of mental health services (12,28–30).

The studies organized by WHO confirmed not just the scientific uses and local clinical utility of the data, but rationalized in-country capacity building as a prelude to the Movement for Global Mental Health that emerged over the ensuing decades. This work promoted the 'training of psychiatrists and other mental health workers from various cultures in the use of such [assessment] instruments' (23, p. 484). The relevance of cultural psychiatry to supporting local, in-country needs beyond the Western scientific agenda that had previously primarily motivated comparative research became increasingly evident.

Comparative psychiatry was eventually appreciated for its contributions to understanding the mediation and moderation of social environmental factors on mental disorders to enhance aetiological understandings that could, in turn, inform thera-peutic interventions and public policy. Leighton and colleagues were particularly influential proponents of enshrining rigorous standards of systematic comparative epidemiological research and can be credited with building its sound methodologi-cal foundation. They succeeded in elevating the perceived relevance of cultural differ-ence in mental disorders in contrast to anecdotal and poorly-informed accounts that perceived cultural forms of mental disorders as having little relevance to mainstream psychiatry.

Contributions of cultural psychiatry to understanding social structural determinants of mental illness

Although initially perceived as a means of advancing aetiological understanding of mental disorders, the standardization of diagnostic criteria and assessments and en-hanced methodological rigour in data collection concerning prevalence and risk correlates documented the burden of mental illness in regions where such data were previously scarce. The resulting quantitative empirical base also highlighted the rela-tionship of mental disorders to macrosocial factors. Possibly the least contested ideas of the last half-century were assertions that confrontations with change and difference begat psychological turbulence. Although the mediators between acculturation and psychopathology are far from agreed upon, the evidence of deterioration in the face of rapid cultural change has been robust and incontrovertible.

In tandem with findings from the large-scale multinational social epidemiological studies, scientific articles stated and restated the apparent adverse impact of rapid so-cial change on mental health. The mediators of psychopathology in the context of social change have been theorized as due to 'social disintegration' (31), or acculturative stress in a 'stress-diathesis' model (32) among other hypotheses. Subsequent formulation has posited that cultural reservoirs of resilience may be eroded in the setting of urban or transnational migration. Even if the mediators and moderators were incompletely de-scribed and agreed upon, the observed effects were indisputable. As Lambo wrote in 1966 'the task of telescoping the period of social and economic progress of advanced countries to bring about almost a phenomenal transition from subsistence to market economy in developing countries [. . .] is more than an immense task' (28, p. 80). In aggregate, numerous studies have demonstrated the health hazards of social change, whether in the context of colonization, migration, urbanization, or globalization. The salience of cultural change as a risk and maintaining factor for mental illness has sur-vived across the last half-century as an aetiological accomplice.

Decade after decade, the velocity of change has been declared unprecedented. While this claim may be warranted, it does not recognize that cultural change is a relatively fixed, and therefore chronic, exposure. Cumulatively, what can be gleaned is the dy-namic interaction between social and cultural currents and physical and mental health. It was not until relatively late in the 20th century that the processual dimension of culture—as contrasted with its content dimension alone—was appreciated (33,34): that is to say, culture is not a variable that can be summarized by a single metric like income or education, but influences through meanings and values the very procedures of classifying, perceiving, expressing, interpreting, experiencing, and evaluating symptoms and treatments. In this respect, earlier descriptions of 'culture-bound syndromes' appear naive in their assumption about the stability or insularity of their cultural contexts and influence.

If the epidemiologists were focused on commonalities across culturally distinct populations, medical anthropologists and cultural psychiatrists trained their intellectual focus on understanding the great diversity in expression and distribution of mental illness. This focus countered the prevailing universalizing and clinical frames imposed on mental illness, emphasizing instead the importance of meaning-centred approaches to mental illness. Several key critiques emerged from this work.

Arriving at a biosocial perspective

The first major summary of this deeper cultural perspective is found in Kleinman's article on the 'new cross-cultural psychiatry' which, he argued, required an anthropological grounding in ethnographic studies that examined particular contexts and their influence on the lived experience of symptoms, the interpretation of their cause and significance, the study of how they affected course and outcome; and that reciprocally showed how the culture of psychiatry and bioscience more generally imbued categories and experiences of the practitioners and the researchers with social values (35). Kleinman cited works from anthropology, social psychology, sociology, history of medicine and science, and primary care that psychiatric epidemiologists and self-identified ethnopsychiatrists failed to examine. These works showed that disease interpretations and illness experiences were inseparable from cultural processes that provided symptom clusters with a social course that was constructed as much by the local worlds of the patient and the clinician as by presumed output of genetic programmes. For example, more favourable prognosis of schizophrenia identified and reported in developing societies in the IPSS had potential clinical and social implications that suggested resilience factors could be unearthed and applied in the service of better patient care.

Theoretical assertions that illness experience is profoundly socially constructed had a second act in the late 1970s in the form of labelling theory, which underscores the impact of social labels not just on how illness is framed, but also on its course (36). During that period, cultural psychiatrists challenged the universality of mental illness upon which cross-cultural epidemiological studies were premised, and exposed professional ethnocentrism and its contribution to scientific bias.

The 'new cross-cultural psychiatry' (35) was transdisciplinary and integrative. While accepting the utility of a standardizing comparative framework for mental illness, it challenged the assumption that it had got the core psychopathology right. For example, there was an inattention to engagement of local knowledge in favour of imposition of nosological categories. Kleinman critiqued the entrenched preoccupation with universals, an approach wherein cultural difference was trivialized as epiphenomenal, consistent with the view that culture had a pathoplastic (shaping of symptoms), but not pathogenic (causing the disease) impact on mental disorders (35). This disregard of how culture shaped mental illness outside of familiar European and North American social contexts, and how the culture of psychiatry understood mental disorders in relation to their socio-cultural context, resulted in a pseudo-naturalized, distorted perception of mental illness as primarily biologically based. The assumption that symptoms had fixed physiological referents was critiqued for failing to recognize the professional construction of psychiatric nosology as inherently a cultural interpretation of lived experience that was different in a patient's local world (37). Kleinman drew attention to biases based on exclusion of non-Western local worlds where most people worldwide lived, but whose experience of symptoms was absent from much psychiatric research (38). The medicalization of emotional distress as illness was also critiqued, as reflected in iterations of the DSM; disorders appeared or were removed as the social, political, and economic contexts shifted professional understandings of their clinical salience. Such professional transformation of collective suffering was dangerous in obscuring social determinants that could not be satisfactorily addressed when relocated into a clinical domain (37).

Failing to engage and incorporate patient experience, indigenous categories, and local knowledge into models for mental illness was a serious threat to validity (37). Manifestations and expressions of distress could be attended to as idioms of distress (39), rhetorical devices for communication with local cultural salience promoted or constrained by local political and economic realities. In this respect, cross-cultural psychiatric assessment requires a detailed and nuanced understanding of the context in which the illness is disclosed or manifested. Cross-cultural psychiatry also rejected the relegation of cultural factors as merely pathoplastic, and posited 'the role of culture in shaping vulnerability and precipitating factors' while maintaining the need to understand illness in both micro- (cultural) and macro- (social) contexts, conceptualizing it as culturally constructed and socially produced (40).

In this respect, '[c]ultural norms reciprocally interact with biological processes to pattern these body/self experiences so that different archetypes of distress are predominant in different social groups' (37). The benefits of the epidemiological frame of analysis were acknowledged as valuable but insufficient; however, epidemiologists were criticized for an overly reductionistic approach, and anthropologists were critiqued for overlooking the biological and personal contributions to mental illness, and exigency of developing treatment interventions (37).

The pragmatic benefits of clinically informed medical anthropology to advancing a culturally sophisticated understanding of mental disorders were increasingly recognized in the 1970s and 1980s among medical anthropologists and cultural psychiatrists alike. Kleinman's ideas were supported by his research in Taiwan in the 1970s and in China in the 1980s and 1990s. In 1980, he studied 100 psychiatric outpatients with the diagnosis of neurasthenia at one of the major teaching hospitals of the Hunan Medical School (formerly the Yale in China Medical School). Kleinman showed that 87% could be rediagnosed, using DSM-III criteria, as suffering from depressive disorder. But he also demonstrated that their depressive disorders were primarily experienced as somatic conditions in which the leading symptoms—dizziness, fatigue, and pain—were understood by family members, clinicians, and other neurasthenia patients as culturally meaningful and socially acceptable complaints. Their metaphorical meaning of exhaustion and alienation indirectly criticized radical Maoist policies. These policies culminated in the Cultural Revolution, which had roiled Chinese society and injured enormous numbers of intellectuals and political cadres, including patients Kleinman studied. He demonstrated that the illness experience of Chinese patients was distinctive (most lived depression without sadness as a major symptom), and that the understanding of the pathophysiology of depression for Chinese psychiatrists was so different from that of American psychiatrists that only 1% of psychiatric outpatients were diagnosed with depression. Moreover, a follow-up study showed that these same depressed patients with neurasthenia responded clinically to antidepressant therapy with improvement of their vegetative complaints, yet did not cease complaining of somatic symptoms until their political or social conditions improved.

Over the next decades, Kleinman's research showed how Chinese psychiatry globalized to fall in line increasingly with Euro-American classification, such that the diagnosis of neurasthenia disappeared while that of depression became as common as in the West. At the same time, the urban and younger Chinese population became more globalized, and increasingly comfortable using psychological terminology; consequently, their experiences of depression came to resemble those in America and Europe. Not surprisingly, epidemiological surveys counted higher and higher numbers of patients with depression, so that a once uncommon disease became roughly as common as in the West.

To understand these changes in cultural terms, Kleinman reasoned that since there was no biological test to diagnose psychiatric disorders, those diseases needed to be understood as the clinician's interpretation (based on his/her classification) of the family's interpretation of symptoms. In turn these represented culturally patterned bodily experiences that patients had been socialized to express in particular ways. The findings of cultural psychiatry and medical anthropology thereby challenged the idea of what constitutes a psychiatric disorder. All psychiatric disorders (and even medical disorders for which there was a clear biological basis) bore the imprint of the particular cultural worlds of patients and the historical transformations of the profession and its cultural productions. And culture did not work alone, but in conjunction with political, economic and institutional realities, as the Chinese case illustrates, to shape health behaviour, illness experiences, and disease pathology.

The research of Kleinman and other medical anthropologists indicated that it is more useful for global health research and clinical practice to understand culture in terms of socially differentiating conditions of the individual—for example, economic status, age, gender, religious orientation, than as uniformly shared beliefs and stereotypical behaviour of entire groups. The latter approach has the unintended negative clinical consequence of obscuring personal needs and rights. Kleinman increasingly argued that culture was most deeply understood as central to moral–emotional orientations and practices that defined what was most at stake for individuals in health, sickness, and care. Stated in terms that related biology and culture together to medical conditions and clinical practices, cultural psychiatry and medical anthropology showed that the bodily, the subjective, the moral, and the medical aspects of illness are inseparable—and not just for exotic conditions, but for everyday routine diseases, professional practices and institutional policies.

Clinically applied medical anthropology: from the 1980s through the 1990s

The journal *Culture, Medicine and Psychiatry* (CMP), a major hub for scholarly cross-disciplinary exchange among clinicians, medical anthropologists, and other social scientists, was launched in 1977. It has been instrumental in locating, articulating, and developing a discourse discerning the social determinants of health and the cultural patterning of the lived experience of illness, and in deconstructing the social complexity of healthcare access and delivery. Still, cultural psychiatry's 'main messages were not reaching larger audiences' until the late 1980s (33).

Subsequent to the development of this journal, new opportunities for anthropologists and clinicians to examine cultural issues influencing mental disorders arose. A Training Program in Clinically Relevant Medical Anthropology—which later became the Training Program in Culture and Mental Health Services Research—was funded by the U.S. National Institute of Mental Health at Harvard and supported nearly 70 postdoctoral and predoctoral trainees from 1984 to 2008. Other funding sources—Carnegie Corporation, Freeman Foundation, Rockefeller Foundation, MacArthur Foundation—created and sustained training and research programmes at Harvard in anthropology and psychiatry, culminating in the World Mental Health report of 1995—that combined anthropology, epidemiology, social medicine, and clinical psychiatry in the first overview of global mental health. This report built upon two decades of relevant publications, including *Culture and Depression* (41), a 'cross-disciplinary colloquy' for anthropologists, psychologists, and psychiatrists that promoted ethnographic and historical accounts more central to the field.

In addition to critiquing perceived ethnocentric assumptions inherent in mainstream psychiatric nosology, medical anthropologists produced ethnographic studies that related symptoms of emotional distress not just to mental disorders but to large-scale social processes as well as to local cultural realities in dynamic interplay within a community. For example, an important body of work on the cultural syndrome *ataque de nervios* demonstrated that, notwithstanding its phenomenological similarities to panic episodes, it is a 'more inclusive construct than panic disorder' (42) and an indicator of both psychiatric vulnerability and social vulnerability or disharmonies.

Medical anthropologists presented a compelling rationale for augmenting the study of mental disorders with research methods that could better capture the full phenomenological range of their expression across diverse cultures. For example, the inclusion of culture-specific terms and questions (43) and use of continuous measures as well as categorical measures (44) in survey assessments would record information potentially omitted by criteria designed for diagnostic assessment in Western populations. The importance of partnerships with communities of study in developing research agendas and interventions was also highlighted (43,45).

Ethnographic and qualitative in-depth interviews were endorsed as means of highlighting socially complex moorings of mental disorders in individual lives in their local context, as well as the lived experience of symptoms and chronicity (44,46,47). This was not just a matter of enhancing validity and relevance, but also of humanizing clinical encounters such that clinicians would 'see not a broken brain, but a social history' (47).

A central theme in this reconstruction of the human side of mental illness was the emphasis on stigma as a moral problem that required advocacy and political action for human rights, similar to that seen in the HIV/AIDS movement (48). For example, Yang and Kleinman (49) and Guo and Kleinman (50) showed that in Chinese culture, the stigma of psychosis nullified the personhood and even the humanity of the sufferer, resulting in a non-person who could be abused with impunity.

Within the shared intellectual space for psychiatrists and social scientists created by specialist journals and other publications, as well as joint training opportunities, there was a growing interest in clinical relevance. In their historic retrospective from 1988 through 2000, Lopez and Guarnaccia pronounced cultural psychopathology research as finally 'on the map' (33). They also declared that its 'ultimate goal' was 'to alleviate suffering and improve people's lives.'

In addition to advocating approaches that integrated qualitative and quantitative methods (33), there was an acknowledged need for anthropologists to present their work as relevant for clinical application. Chrisman and Maretzki described 'the need to build bridges between clinical and academic emphases' (51), and the 'new cross-cultural psychiatry' (35). Journals such as *CMP*, the medical anthropology section of *Social Science and Medicine*, *Anthropology and Medicine*, and *Transcultural Psychiatry*, are venues for psychiatrists and social scientists to continue a scientific dialogue about cultural and mental disorders. Several professional organizations (e.g. the World Federation of Mental Health, the World Psychiatric Association, the Group for Advancement of Psychiatry, the American Psychiatric Association) provide the infrastructure for collaborative interdisciplinary work concerning the understanding and relevance of cultural factors in the pathogenesis, maintenance, and presentation of mental disorders. One example of a concrete contribution was Kleinman's development of the Explanatory Model method of eliciting relevant cultural orientations to specific disease and treatment episodes around eight questions for any diagnostic evaluation (52). The Cultural Formulation developed by a taskforce of psychiatrists and anthropologists for DSM-IV also provides a clinical method to specifically assess culture in psychiatric evaluations (53).

As the American Psychiatric Association prepared to revise the DSM-III, cultural psychiatrists drew attention to its inadequacies in addressing cultural diversity (54). In 1991, a major conference on Culture and Diagnosis was convened with support from the U.S. National Institute of Mental Health and the American Psychiatric Association. Multidisciplinary expertise in cultural psychiatry was well represented and the conference resulted in detailed recommendations for modifying standing diagnostic criteria and text guidance so as to create a more culturally informed and broadly relevant diagnostic manual. However, these recommendations were incorporated only minimally and regarded largely as disappointingly insufficient by the cultural experts (55).

With the release of the APA's DSM-IV, new attention was focused on integrating social and cultural dimensions within diagnostic assessment. The Cultural Formulation approach incorporated a patient-centred assessment of the meanings, experience, and preferences related to mental illness with the rationale that 'clinicians need a method that systematically allows them to take culture into account when conducting a clinical evaluation' (56). The outline itself is allocated less than 2 of 943 pages in the latest iteration of the DSM-IV-TR (53). Although the Cultural Formulation has become a primary component of psychiatric residency training in cultural issues, it is underutilized in clinical practice (57). While largely syntonic with patient-centred approaches to clinical work, ubiquitous institutional pressures and financial incentives to increase clinical efficiency militate against an approach that requires more time and may not yield tangible, immediate benefits.

Twin trajectories towards improved healthcare equity for mental illness trace kinship to cultural psychiatry as it developed from the mid-20th century and onward. These are: (1) the robust portfolio of scholarly and advocacy efforts to improve mental healthcare training, services access, and quality in low- and middle-income regions of the world best capsulated by the present term, 'global mental health'; and (2) the steady progress towards identifying and redressing ethnic-based disparities in mental healthcare treatment access and outcomes. Both sets of activities have drawn from the scholarly foundation comprising cultural psychiatry and have crossed disciplinary boundaries towards policy and advocacy. The scholarly and advocacy activities have become well organized within several professional and other organizations where scientific and clinical expertise reside.

World mental health: from a local agenda to a global agenda

A watershed event for articulating the scientific, clinical, and resource needs for global mental health was the publication of *World Mental Health: Problems and Priorities in Low-Income Countries* (58). This report leveraged the metrics of Disability Adjusted Life-Years (DALYs) and Quality Adjusted Life-Years (QALYs) to illustrate the high global burden of neuropsychiatric disease previously not fully appreciated by conventional metrics of mortality data alone. It integrated ethnographic narratives with epidemiological data to provide a compelling agenda for policies and programmes of the future.

This tally of the considerable global burden of neuropsychiatric disease also drew attention to disproportionately low allocation of public-sector healthcare resources towards interventions for mental disorders (59) which could be articulated within a rights-based argument for improving health services and access to care. Several other major achievements built upon this platform by marshalling scientific, clinical, and social justice evidence to advocate for a concerted effort to remedy the considerable gaps that characterize clinical resources for mental disorders around the globe. The trajectory of these collective efforts reached another inflection point in 2007 when the *Lancet* published a special series devoted to global mental health, giving high visibility to the powerful credo, 'No health without mental health' (60), and calling for scientific, policy, and collective action to scale up high-quality treatments for mental disorders. The launch of the Movement for Global Mental Health followed a year later as a strategy for mobilization of resources and stimulation of action to address profound global shortfalls in mental health treatment (61). Inspired by the success of the movements for the care of people living with HIV/AIDs in low- and middle-income countries, this approach facilitated collective action (61). In 2010, WHO unveiled its signature mental health Global Action Plan (mhGAP) elaborating guidelines for treatment of major mental disorders (61,62). In July 2011, *Nature* published the results of the Grand Challenges in Mental Health Initiative (63) that articulated priorities for a global research agenda. This initiative, led by the U.S. National Institute of Mental Health and the Global Alliance for Chronic Disease, utilized a Delphi method with over 400 panellists articulating a research agenda for global health. Interestingly, several of the priorities resonate with the call for high-quality prevalence and risk data across global regions, presaged a half-century earlier. In October 2011 the *Lancet* published a follow-up series on global mental health to coincide with World Mental Health Day and the World Mental Health Federation alliance with the Movement for Global Mental Health—the most recent effort by cultural psychiatrists to mobilize political will in the service of promoting global mental healthcare.

The intellectual infrastructure engendered by the medical anthropological approach to cultural psychiatry over the past half-century is arguably the core of consensus priorities for global mental health. These encompass culturally informed and valid modes of diagnostic assessment and an evidence base that interrogates the social and cultural disparities of mental illness, as well as a call for methods to eliminate the stigma and discrimination that continue to diminish the lives and opportunities of the mentally ill and their families.

The intellectual products of cultural psychiatry have provided a foundation and purpose for the present coalescence of scientific, clinical, and patient/carer advocacy to redress the vast economic, human resource, research, policy, and clinical services deficits in mental healthcare in underserved populations. The social and clinical achievement and advances in the broader field of global health also provided a template for the social change strategies and cultivation of political will that are integral to mobilizing support for advancing the treatment of both non-communicable diseases and mental disorders.

Cultural psychiatry and its impact on response to the global burden of mental illness and paradigms for in-country capacity building

If the social epidemiological studies on comparative prevalence and socio-demographic risk factors for mental disorders were atheoretical, they ultimately served a utilitarian purpose in evaluating and critiquing the appropriateness of exporting and implementing Western treatment paradigms for other populations. In the 1970s and 1980s the question of how the large-scale comparative studies could inform cultural relevance and potential culture-specific effectiveness for psychiatric treatment emerged among psychiatric epidemiologists (64,65). The dubious relevance of Western psychiatric treatment models had been identified much earlier by the indigenous psychiatrists Lambo (66) and Neki. Lambo rejected the wholesale importation of unsuitable Western models of care and described the locally perceived poor acceptability of these approaches. In this respect, he was a pioneer in incorporating local knowledge in adaptation of treatments for a culturally rational strategy. Lambo had proposed an alternative to the asylum model of care just as the census of patients managed within that model peaked (10), a model therapeutic community in Aro (Nigeria) that by contrast managed patients within their social milieu (66).

Resonating with this, and writing from his south-east Asian perspective, Neki advocated for culturally syntonic therapeutic approaches that tapped indigenous treatment models (67). Likewise, he criticized the deployment of clinicians without sensitivity and informed local cultural engagement, and advocated instead psychiatric training with skills development that would foster communication (68).

Even if the radically cultural relativist paradigm was ultimately overshadowed by the emergence of operationalized diagnostic criteria, it did begin a critical dialogue about the incontrovertible relevance of culture to diagnosis, help-seeking, treatment adherence, and therapeutic engagement. This relevance, moreover, became not just an intellectual exercise but fundamental to the feasibility, social acceptability, and effectiveness of mental healthcare delivery. Arguably, the work done in the 1930s and 1940s, and subsequently amplified by influential in-country psychiatrists, laid the foundation for training not just specific to biological aspects of disease, but also to social and cultural dimensions of the patient's world and the community. Lambo's critique in 1966 was, in that respect, long overdue but foreshadowed a central component of a global mental health research agenda in 2011. With it, the debate about universal versus culturally relative psychopathology was rendered somewhat moot; cultural diversity in clinical presentation now warranted attention, regardless of its interpretation.

Wittkower and Warms called for attention to cultural differences and impact on therapy, adaptation of Western treatments to local contexts, integration of indigenous concepts with Western therapeutic strategies, and developing local capacity in order to deliver care by indigenous psychiatrists (69). The call for integration of indigenous models notably contrasted with previous colonial laws restricting the activities of local healers (3). Further it was 'increasingly recognized that skills and resources from the developing countries can be important inputs for the developed' (70, p. 65), and that psychiatry trainees must acquire training that could be applied in local contexts (68, p. 264). Although local adaptation of empirically supported therapeutic approaches for the treatment of depression to low- and middle-income settings is seen as essential to their effectiveness (71), cultural psychiatry has not had a large intellectual footprint on mental health services in resource-constrained regions. The desirability of community-based models and resources for mental healthcare has been well-recognized, but empirical data evaluating the effectiveness and feasibility of mental health service models and human resources are still urgently needed to respond to the vast health burden imposed by mental disorders in those locations (72).

Social justice and clinical utility

Cultural psychiatrists since the 1960s have lobbied for more robust mental health community services and have generated models of how such services might function. The Aro village model developed by Lambo aimed to strengthen traditional village-based relations as a means of providing social support and treatment. Henri Collomb's approach in Senegal drew on traditional healers and emphasized cultural processes that can make psychiatric treatments better understood and more acceptable. Joop de Jong showed how community service in Burkina Faso could make it feasible to empty beds at warehouse-like psychiatric hospitals and provide the same therapeutic services with the assistance of community health workers. Thara and Phillips, working in India and China respectively, have demonstrated the value of family support groups as a means of extending rehabilitation of psychiatric patients from the clinic into the home. There are literally dozens of such innovative programmes but only a few have been robustly evaluated and almost none have been generalized. There must be a continuing tale here; the limits on resources has the effect of driving psychiatry into the community, yet progress in developing community services as generalizable programmes is stymied by lack of resources. Perhaps the highly successful model of the non-governmental organization, Partners In Health, that promotes accompaniment of patients by community health workers will be one of the first examples of a task-sharing model that can be successfully implemented for mental healthcare delivery as well.

The US Surgeon-General's report on mental health marked another watershed for cultural psychiatry when highlighting ethnic and social disparities in access to mental health services (73). This document, and the subsequent *Mental Health: Culture, Race, and Ethnicity: A Supplement to Mental Health*, became a lever for policy changes that required attention to race and ethnicity in federally supported research and demonstration of core competencies related to culturally informed care (74). For example, the Accreditation Council for Graduate Medical Education and the American Board of Psychiatry and Neurology established requirements for psychiatry residents' formal training in cultural dimensions of care. Two studies were conducted in the United States alongside the National Comorbidity Study Replication to investigate the prevalence of mental disorders and associated impairment and service utilization among specific underserved ethnic groups of African Americans and Afro-Caribbeans (75) and Latinos and Asians (76). Both Jackson and colleagues and Alegria and colleagues heralded these studies as a strategic means of discerning and responding to the specific needs of ethnic minority populations in the United States, including evidence of poorer access to mental health services. Subsequent research documented ethnic disparities not just for access, but also for outcomes (77). The sources of these disparities remain poorly understood and suffer from a lack of empirical data evaluating interventions such as culturally focused clinics, but support the need for better professional education about ethnic and cultural variation in presentation of mental illness. Francis Lu developed culturally relevant mental health services for Asian Americans at San Francisco General Hospital and Roberto Fernandez for Latinos at Columbia University; there are many other examples of cultural approaches being applied in the United States. For example, Bell and colleagues have elaborated strategies that utilize community- and school-based human resources to promote mental health among impoverished urban youth (45,78). Although the research literature on such services is still limited, the practices have become widespread and involve thousands of mental health professionals. Yet, there can be little question today that in North America, Europe, Australia, and elsewhere the movement to make 'culture' central to clinical care has taken off to an extent no one could have predicted 40 years ago with both important mainline effects and certain unintended consequences, such as ethnic politics and social marketing effects of the 'cultural competence' as both a political and a business enterprise.

Summary

The professional ethnocentrism that characterized cultural psychiatry in the mid-20th century has gradually transitioned from a local to a global agenda for research and implementation. Within this trajectory, the scholarly products of cultural psychiatry—descriptive, empirical, and theoretical—have been increasingly applied in healthcare and policy domains, in the service of mitigating the substantial global burden of mental illness and persisting inequities in mental healthcare access. As described in this essay, cultural psychiatry has also been characterized by an unremitting preoccupation with the universality versus cultural particularities of mental disorders. The keen interest in understanding phenomenological differences, as well as relative prevalence, in psychopathology was initially rationalized as an opportunity to discern the aetiological contributions of social and cultural exposures. Although this rationale can be seen to have emerged from a relatively self-serving position, it ultimately laid the foundation for an essential critique of methodological limitations in cross-cultural psychiatry. Several large-scale epidemiological studies were designed and launched in the 1970s with the intention of collecting data on course and prevalence of major mental illnesses with improved systematic rigour of sampling and diagnostic assessment. While striving to hone methodological quality, however, these studies were themselves inherently flawed. Their design reflected a bias for discerning core commonalities of the major mental disorders while, in aggregate and inadvertently or not, they have elided and trivialized cultural variation. One could argue, on the other hand, that earlier anthropological emphasis on intellectually intriguing 'exotic' and culture-bound syndromes did a parallel disservice in its distraction from exigent on-the-ground clinical realities and their attendant suffering.

In the 1970s an emergent medical anthropology discourse within the 'new cross-cultural psychiatry' critiqued the failure to engage local knowledge in cross-cultural clinical and research encounters. This approach instead promoted a fundamentally integrative framework for understanding the nexus of culture and mental health and made a compelling argument for the necessity of interpreting patterns of mental illness against their contexts of structural violence, local historical legacies, and cultural semiotics and rhetoric. This biosocial perspective was not just theoretically sound, it reoriented clinical and public health approaches to seriously engage local knowledge and experience in delivery of care.

Engagement of local knowledge and moral worlds, an understanding of the social determinants of mental health—both at a macro-level and micro-level—and an attunement to the ways in which culture includes the trajectory of affective and embodied experience have resulted in meaningful intellectual and pragmatic traction in the application of research data to mental health care. These are favourable signs of progress—good for patients, clinicians, and scholars of medicine and the social sciences alike. At the same time the field has not entirely escaped its polemic tendencies, and a still more integrative frame—which manages complexity, navigates among the advantages of reductionism and vivid thick description, properly interrogates the exclusive attribution of illness to just biology, society, or psychology—is not yet within reach. This deficit leaves too much at stake for cultural psychiatry's translational promise. Yet the new emphasis on mental healthcare delivery in the context of a global psychiatry is evidence that psychiatry is steadily defining a new era of cross-cultural and transnational work in medicine around access to quality treatment. In this regard, it might be argued that the shipwreck of ethnopsychiatry in the early and mid-20th century on the rocks of racism, colonialism, and ethnocentrism set the stage for the entrance of a new medical anthropology into the very heart of the subject. This transition has had the consequential, though still uncertain, impact of making a deeper and more complexly human understanding of culture central to the mental health field—an understanding that culture is a perceptual, relational, classificatory, interpretative, and ultimately moral process that is inherent to illness experience and disease pathology, as it is to communities and the profession of psychiatry itself. As there is no health without mental health, there can be no psychiatry (or medicine) without culture.

References

1 Jackson, J. S., Abelson, J. M., Berglund, P. A. et al. (2011). The intersection of race, ethnicity, immigration, and cultural influences on the nature and distribution of mental disorders. In: Regier, D. A., Narrow, W. E., Kuhl, E. A., and Kupfer D. J. (eds.) *The conceptual evolution of DSM-5*. Arlington, VA: American Psychiatric Publishing, pp. 267–85.

2 Worboys, M. (1976). The emergence of tropical medicine: a study in the establishment of a scientific specialty. In: Lemaine, G., Macleod, R., Mulkay, M., and Weingart P. (eds.) *Perspectives on the emergence of scientific disciplines*. The Hague: Mouton, pp. 75–98.

3 Bullard, A. (2011). Denial, la crypte, and magic. In: Anderson, W., Jenson, D., and Keller R. C. (eds.) *Unconscious dominions: psychoanalysis, colonial trauma, and global sovereignties*. Durham, NC: Duke University Press, pp. 43–74.

4 Vaughan, M. (1991). *Curing their ills: colonial power and African illness*. Palo Alto, CA: Stanford University Press.

5 Fanon, F. (1967). *Black skin, white masks*. New York: Grove Press.

6 Nasser, L. (2011). *The great divide, or how an obscure diagnosis from colonial Africa ended up in Playboy magazine*. Doctoral dissertation. Unpublished.

7 Carothers, J. C. (1972). *The mind of man in Africa*. London: Tom Stacey Ltd.

8 Carothers, C. (1960). Further thoughts on the African mind. *East African Medical Journal* 37, 457–63.

9 Fanon, F. (2004). *The wretched of the Earth*. New York: Grove Press.

10 Lambo, T. A. (1971). The African mind in contemporary conflict. The Jacques Parisot Foundation Lecture, 1971. *WHO Chronicle*, 25, 343–53.

11 Eisenberg, L. and Guttmacher, L. B. (2010). Were we all asleep at the switch? A personal reminiscence of psychiatry from 1940 to 2010. *Acta Psychiatrica Scandinavica* 122, 89–102.

12 Leighton, A. H., Lin, T. Y., Yap, P. M., Kline, N. S., and Lambo, T. A. (1962). Transcultural Studies: Panel discussion at the Third World Congress of Psychiatry. *Acta Psychiatrica Scandinavica* 38, 157–82.

13 Wittkower, E. D. (1963). Discussion in: Psychiatric Disorder in West Africa. *American Journal of Psychiatry* 120, 525–7.

14 Jablensky, A. and Sartorius, N. (1975). Culture and schizophrenia. *Psychological Medicine*, 5, 113–24.

15 Sartorius, N. (1978). Diagnosis and classification: cross cultural and international perspectives. *Mental Health and Society* 5, 79–85.

16 Leighton, D. C., Harding, J. S., Macklin, D. B., Hughes, C. C., and Leighton, A. H. (1963). Psychiatric findings of the Stirling County Study. *American Journal of Psychiatry* 119, 1021–6.

17 Thornicroft, G. and Sartorius, N. (1993). The course and outcome of depression in different cultures: 10-year follow-up of the WHO Collaborative Study on the Assessment of Depressive Disorders. *Psychological Medicine* **23**, 1023–32.

18 Sartorius, N., Jablensky, A., Korten, A., et al. (1986). Early manifestations and first-contact incidence of schizophrenia in different cultures. A preliminary report on the initial evaluation phase of the WHO Collaborative Study on determinants of outcome of severe mental disorders. *Psychological Medicine* **16**, 909–28.

19 Jablensky, A., Sartorius, N., Ernberg, G., et al. (1992). Schizophrenia: manifestations, incidence and course in different cultures. A World Health Organization ten-country study. *Psychological Medicine Monograph Supplement* **20**, 1–97.

20 Harrison, G., Hopper, K., Craig, T., et al. (2001). Recovery from psychotic illness: a 15- and 25-year international follow-up study. *British Journal of Psychiatry* **178**, 506–17.

21 Kessler, R. C., Wang, P. S., and Wittchen, H. (2010). The Social Epidemiology of Mental Disorder. In: Morgan, C. and Bhugra, D. (eds.) *Principles of social psychiatry* (2nd edn). Chichester: John Wiley and Sons, pp. 91–101.

22 Kieling, C., Baker-Henningham, H., Belfer, M., et al. (2011). Child and adolescent mental health worldwide: evidence for action. *Lancet* **378**(9801), 1515–25.

23 Sartorius, N. and Jablensky, A. (1976). Transcultural studies of schizophrenia. *WHO Chronicle* **30**, 481–5.

24 Yap, P. M. (1969). Perspectives of transcultural psychiatry. A search for order in diversity. *International Journal of Psychiatry* **8**, 834–9.

25 Patel, V. and Sumathipala, A. (2001). International representation in psychiatric literature: survey of six leading journals. *British Journal of Psychiatry* **178**, 406–9.

26 Alarcon, R. D., Becker, A. E., Lewis-Fernandez, R., et al. (2009). Issues for DSM-V: the role of culture in psychiatric diagnosis. *Journal of Nervous and Mental Disease* **197**, 559–660.

27 Blashfield, R. K., Sprock, J., and Fuller, A. K. (1990). Suggested guidelines for including or excluding categories in the DSM-IV. *Comprehensive Psychiatry* **31**, 15–19.

28 Lambo, T. A. (1966). Socioeconomic change, population explosion and the changing phases of mental health programs in developing countries. *American Journal of Orthopsychiatry* **36**, 77–83.

29 Yap, P. M. (1967). Classification of the culture-bound reactive syndromes. *Australian and New Zealand Journal of Psychiatry* **1**, 172–9.

30 Neki, J. S. (1976). An examination of the cultural relativism of dependence as a dynamic of social and therapeutic relationships. I. Socio-developmental. *British Journal of Medical Psychology* **49**, 1–10.

31 Leighton, A. H. (1974). The erosion of norms. *Australian and New Zealand Journal of Psychiatry* **8**, 223–7.

32 Fabrega, H. (1969). Social psychiatric aspects of acculturation and migration: a general statement. *Comprehensive Psychiatry* **10**, 314–26.

33 Lopez, S. R. and Guarnaccia, P. J. (2000). Cultural psychopathology: uncovering the social world of mental illness. *Annual Review of Psychology* **51**, 571–98.

34 Kleinman, A. and Benson, P. (2006). Anthropology in the clinic: the problem of cultural competency and how to fix it. *PLoS Medicine* **3**, e294.

35 Kleinman, A. (1977). Depression, somatization and the 'new cross–cultural psychiatry'. *Social Science and Medicine*, **11**, 3–10.

36 Waxler, N. (1981). The social labeling perspective on illness and medical practice. In: Eisenberg, L. and Kleinman, A. (eds.) *The relevance of social science for medicine*. Dordrecht: D. Reidel, pp. 283–306.

37 Kleinman, A. (1988). *Rethinking psychiatry*. New York: Free Press.

38 Lin, K. M., Kleinman, A., and Lin, T. Y. (1980). Psychiatric epidemiology in Chinese cultures: An overview. In: Kleinman, A., Lin, T. Y. (eds.) *Normal and abnormal behavior in Chinese culture*, Dordrecht, Holland: D. Reidel, pp. 237–71.

39 Nichter, M. (1981). Idioms of distress: alternatives in the expression of psychosocial distress: a case study from South India. *Culture, Medicine and Psychiatry* 5, 379–408.

40 Weiss, M. G. and Kleinman, A. (1988). Depression in cross-cultural perspective. In: Dasen P. R., Berry J. W., Sartorius N., World Health Organization (eds.) *Health and cross-cultural psychology: toward applications*. Newbury Park, CA: Sage, pp. 179–205.

41 Kleinman, A. and Good, B. (eds.) (1985). *Culture and depression: studies in the anthropology and cross-cultural psychiatry of affect and disorder*. Berkeley, CA: University of California Press.

42 Lewis-Fernandez, R., Guarnaccia, P. J., Martinez, I. E. et al. (2002). Comparative phenomenology of ataques de nervios, panic attacks, and panic disorder. *Culture, Medicine and Psychiatry* 26, 199–223.

43 Beals, J., Manson, S. M., Mitchell, C. M., Spicer, P., and AI-SUPERPFP Team. (2003). Cultural specificity and comparison in psychiatric epidemiology: walking the tightrope in American Indian research. *Culture, Medicine and Psychiatry* 27, 259–89.

44 Phillips, M. R. (2010). Rethinking the role of mental illness in suicide. *American Journal of Psychiatry* 167, 731–3.

45 Bell, C. C. and McKay, M. M. (2004). Constructing a children's mental health infrastructure using community psychiatry principles. *Journal of Legal Medicine* 25, 5–22.

46 Kleinman, A. (1988). *The illness narratives*. New York: Basic Books.

47 Luhrmann, T. M. (2007). Social defeat and the culture of chronicity: or, why schizophrenia does so well over there and so badly here. *Culture, Medicine and Psychiatry* 31, 135–72.

48 Kleinman, A. (2009). Global mental health: a failure of humanity. *Lancet* 374 (9690), 603–4.

49 Yang, L. H. and Kleinman, A. (2008). 'Face' and the embodiment of stigma in China: the cases of schizophrenia and AIDS. *Social Science and Medicine* 67, 398–408.

50 Guo, J. and Kleinman, A. (2011). Stigma: HIV/AIDS, mental illness, and China's nonpersons. In: *Deep China: the moral life of the person. What anthropology and psychiatry tell us about China today*. Berkeley, CA: University of California Press, pp. 237–62.

51 Chrisman, N. J. and Maretzki, T. W. (1982). Anthropology in health science settings. In: Chrisman, N. J. and Maretzki, T. W. (eds.) *Clinically applied anthropology: anthropologists in health science settings*. Dordrecht: D. Reide, pp. 1–31.

52 Kleinman, A. (1980). *Patients and healers in the context of culture*. Berkeley, CA: University of California Press.

53 American Psychiatric Association. (2000). *Diagnostic and statistical manual of mental disorders* (4th edn), Text Revision. Arlington, VA: American Psychiatric Association.

54 Westermeyer, J. (1987). Cultural factors in clinical assessment. *Journal of Consulting and Clinical Psychology* 55, 471–8.

55 Mezzich, J. E., Kirmayer, L. J., Kleinman, A., et al. (1999). The place of culture in DSM-IV. *Journal of Nervous and Mental Disease* 187, 457–64.

56 Lewis-Fernandez, R. and Diaz, N. (2002). The cultural formulation: a method for assessing cultural factors affecting the clinical encounter. *Psychiatric Quarterly* 73, 271–95.

57 Lewis-Fernandez, R. (2009). The cultural formulation. *Transcultural Psychiatry*, 46, 379–82.

58 Desjarlais, R., Eisenberg, L., Good, B., and Kleinman, A. (1995). *World mental health: Problems and priorities in low-income countries*. Oxford: Oxford University Press.

59 Saxena, S., Thornicroft, G., Knapp, M., and Whiteford, H. (2007). Resources for mental health: scarcity, inequity, and inefficiency. *Lancet* 370(9590), 878–89.

60 Prince, M., Patel, V., Saxena, S., et al. (2007). No health without mental health. *Lancet* 370(9590), 859–77.

61 Patel, V., Collins, P. Y., Copeland, J., et al. (2011). The movement for global mental health. *British Journal of Psychiatry* 198, 88–90.

62 World Health Organization (2011). *WHO Mental Health Gap Action Programme (mhGAP)*. Available at: http://www.who.int/mental_health/mhgap/en/[Accessed November 2011].

63 Collins, P. Y., Patel, V., Joestl, S. S., et al. (2011). Grand challenges in global mental health. *Nature* 475(7354), 27–30.

64 Sartorius, N. (1986). Cross-cultural research on depression. *Psychopathology* 19(Suppl 2), 6–11.

65 Sartorius, N., Jablensky, A., and Shapiro, R. (1978). Cross-cultural differences in the short-term prognosis of schizophrenic psychoses. *Schizophrenia Bulletin* 4, 102–13.

66 Lambo, T. A. (1956). Neuropsychiatric observations in the western region of Nigeria. *British Medical Journal* 2(5006), 1388–94.

67 Neki, J. S. (1979). An examination of the extent of responsibility of mental health services from the standpoint of developing communities. *International Journal of Social Psychiatry* 25, 203–8.

68 Neki, J. S. (1973). Psychiatry in South-East Asia. *British Journal of Psychiatry* 123, 257–69.

69 Wittkower, E. D. and Warms, H. (1974). Cultural aspects of psychotherapy. *Psychotherapy and Psychosomatics* 24, 303–10.

70 Orley, J. (1990). International collaboration for postgraduate psychiatric education. *Social Psychiatry and Psychiatric Epidemiology* 25, 65–6.

71 Patel, V., Simon, G., Chowdhary, N., Kaaya, S., and Araya, R. (2009). Packages of care for depression in low- and middle-income countries. *PLoS Medicine*, 6, e1000159.

72 Kakuma, R., Minas, H., van Ginneken, N., et al. (2011). Human resources for mental health care: current situation and strategies for action. *Lancet* 378(9803), 1654–63.

73 US Department of Health and Human Services (1999). *Mental health: a report of the Surgeon General*. Rockville, MD: US Department of Health and Human Services, Substance Abuse and Mental Health Services Administration, Center for Mental Health Services.

74 U.S. Department of Health and Human Services (2001). *Mental health: culture, race, and ethnicity—a supplement to Mental health: a report of the Surgeon General*. Rockville, MD: US Department of Health and Human Services, Substance Abuse and Mental Health Services Administration, Center for Mental Health Services.

75 Jackson, J. S., Torres, M., Caldwell, C. H., et al. (2004). The National Survey of American Life: a study of racial, ethnic and cultural influences on mental disorders and mental health. *International Journal of Methods in Psychiatric Research* 13, 196–207.

76 Alegria, M., Takeuchi, D., Canino, G., et al. (2004). Considering context, place and culture: the National Latino and Asian American Study. *International Journal of Methods in Psychiatric Research* **13**, 208–20.

77 Good, M. D., James, C., Good, B. J., and Becker, A. E. (2005). The culture of medicine and racial, ethnic and class disparities in health care. In: Romero, M. and Margolis, E. (eds.) *The Blackwell companion to social inequalities*. Malden, MA: Blackwell, pp. 396–423.

78 Atkins, M. S., Frazier, S. L., Birman, D., et al. (2006) School-based mental health services for children living in high poverty urban communities. *Administration and Policy in Mental Health* **33**, 146–59.

History and development of social psychiatry

Julian Leff

Introduction

I should start by defining social psychiatry, but this is not easy. I am tempted to resort to a tautology and state that social psychiatry is what is practised by social psychiatrists. But who are they? After completing my training at the Maudsley Hospital in London I was soon offered a position in John Wing's Social Psychiatry Unit, and from then on I considered myself to be a social psychiatrist. But I also have a background and a history, which together impelled me to accept the position that defined the kind of psychiatry I was to practice. My father was a general practitioner before World War II: in fact I was born above his surgery. He was a Marxist and believed that improving the conditions in which people lived would eliminate many diseases. After the war he became active in the Socialist Medical Association, which worked towards the establishment of the National Health Service (NHS) in 1948 by the Labour government. My father then gave up being a GP and was appointed as Medical Officer of Health for a London borough. This position enabled him to practise the preventive measures that he believed would alleviate the burden of disease that fell disproportionately on the poorer sections of society. He did not conduct any research himself, but he used epidemiological data collected by others to strengthen his arguments with the Conservative council that employed him. These arguments were always about his insistence that more facilities should be made available to local working people.

Defining social psychiatry

Is social psychiatry, then, a younger sibling of social medicine? In contrast to my father I spent most of my years in the health service as a full-time scientist, designing and conducting research. Throughout that time I continued to care for patients, running half an admission ward and a busy outpatient clinic. My research could not exclusively be classified as social psychiatric, because I utilized biological measures in some of the studies. For instance, the first study I was directed by John Wing to design and conduct was an evaluation of the effectiveness of antipsychotic medication for prevention of relapse of schizophrenia (1). I was surprised by the fundamentally biological nature of this undertaking and decided to include an element of social significance, so incorporated the Life Events and Difficulties Schedule developed by Brown and Harris (2). Life events clearly fall under the simple definition of social psychiatry I proposed in a previous publication: 'Social psychiatry is concerned with the effect of the social environment on the mental health of the individual, and with the effects of the mentally ill person on her/his social environment.'

Altering the social environment

With hindsight, this definition implies only half of the activity of social psychiatrists, namely research. It omits remedial actions taken with the intention of changing the social environment of the patient to reduce their psychiatric morbidity. This interventionist approach brings social psychiatry much closer to social medicine and my father's brand of social engineering. It also brings into the compass of social psychiatry attempts to alter the environment of institutions for those with psychiatric illnesses to improve their outcome. In this historical perspective, probably the first pioneer to forbid chaining psychiatric patients was Vincenzo Chiarugi, director of Santa Dorotea Hospital in Florence, who issued this edict in 1788. In Britain the Quaker founders of the York Retreat can be viewed as some of the earliest social psychiatrists, before the term psychiatry was introduced. William Tuke opened the Retreat in 1796 and instituted a supportive and healing environment based on Quaker principles. The main tenet was that every person, regardless of their mental disturbance, has an element of God within them.

It is surely more than a coincidence that just a year after the Retreat was opened, Jean-Baptiste Pussin, Pinel's mentor, replaced the shackles on the psychiatric patients at the Bicêtre in Paris with cloth straitjackets. Pinel, who had left for the Salpêtrière earlier, sympathized with the French Revolution and applied its banner slogan of individual liberty to the treatment of the mentally ill in the Salpêtrière, removing their chains 3 years after Pussin's innovatory act. The anti-authoritarian movement, epitomized by the French Revolution, was affecting the whole of Europe, creating great anxiety among autocratic rulers, as does the unrest in the Arab world today. Sadly the example of the York Retreat was not followed by the great majority of institutions for the mentally ill in Britain. The Bethlem Hospital as depicted by Hogarth in 1735 not only confined patients in chains, but charged the curious one penny to come and stare at the lunatics.

The asylum era

The building of asylums in England and Wales was the largest and most expensive public works programme in the history of the country. When Queen Victoria ascended the throne there were nine such institutions. By the end of her reign there were 77. Building did not cease with her death: by 1975 the number had grown to 130. This massive expansion was partly fuelled by the overcrowding that developed in psychiatric institutions. Very few discharges occurred and there was an apparently unstoppable tendency for the indications for admission to become increasingly broader. When patients began to be discharged, among them were women who had never suffered from a psychiatric disorder, but had given birth to an illegitimate baby. The overcrowding led to beds being set up in what had been originally designed as recreational spaces. Not only were the planned uses of the spaces lost, depriving the patients of healthy activities, but the sheer number of patients became unmanageable by the staff, who resorted to brutal practices. The ensuing public scandals gave impetus to the movement to retreat from the asylums. But there were larger social forces at work, without which the asylums would probably have continued with minor cosmetic changes. These forces were generated by World War II.

Influences from World War II

Psychiatrists working in military hospitals saw that healthy young men, sent back from the front with serious psychiatric disorders, recovered with treatment in a safe environment in Britain. This convinced the psychiatrists that recovery from psychiatric illnesses induced by major stresses was a reality. In addition, through lack of personnel, they had to treat the disturbed soldiers in groups. Tom Main, a psychoanalyst as well as a psychiatrist, who was an advisor to a section training military psychiatrists, recognized the value of group treatment. At the end of the war he was posted to a large military psychiatric hospital where he developed his ideas on the therapeutic value of groups. In 1946 he became director of the Cassel Hospital in Carshalton, Surrey, which he transformed into a therapeutic community. Another military psychiatrist, Maxwell Jones, on returning to civilian life, founded a unique treatment centre, the Henderson Hospital in London, which was also run as a therapeutic community. Treatment was based on large group meetings in which patients were given the same rights to voice their opinions and to be treated with respect as the staff. Even the rules for running the community were put to the vote. The general effect of the entry of these military psychiatrists into asylums was a modification of the custodial atmosphere and a new-found optimism, leading to the discharge of patients formerly considered incurable.

The stimulus to discharging patients in the United States stemmed from a different source. Young men who refused to fight on the grounds of conscience were offered a variety of alternative ways of serving their country, one of which was working as attendants in psychiatric hospitals. This was in contrast to the situation in the United Kingdom where conscientious objectors were put to work in the coal mines. It is estimated that 3000 of these young men with high moral values entered the US asylums and brought humane attitudes to the care of the patients. They felt it was their mission to improve standards and find non-violent methods of managing the patients. One of these young men, a Quaker named Steve Cary, is quoted in the *Friends' Journal* of December 2006 as saying, 'There is no doubt in my mind that the greatest contribution which we made in that era was in the whole field of mental health'. Their influence stemmed from the same Quaker ethos which motivated William Tuke to found the Retreat. Discharges from US psychiatric hospitals became increasingly frequent, allowing beds to be reduced, but closure of psychiatric hospitals has not been as dramatic as in the United Kingdom.

The first moves out of the asylums

Even before the peak occupancy of psychiatric beds in England and Wales was reached in 1954, a few pioneering psychiatrists began to introduce innovatory conditions in the hospitals and extramural services. The psychiatrist Duncan Macmillan, who was appointed superintendent of Mapperley Hospital, Nottingham, in 1942, opened outpatient clinics, increased the proportion of voluntary admissions, and in 1952 arranged for all wards to be unlocked. Mapperley became the first fully open psychiatric hospital in England. Douglas Bennett, who had worked with Maxwell Jones, developed rehabilitation in Netherne Hospital (at Hooley, Surrey) and then came to the Maudsley where he opened a day hospital, which became the fulcrum for the development of community services.

The importance of the hospital environment in shaping patients' behaviour was brought home to me in a project I initiated in Warley Hospital (Brentwood, Essex) in the 1990s. In studying the process of closing two Victorian psychiatric hospitals in North London, Friern and Claybury, it emerged that there was a group of long-stay patients who were considered too dangerous, too vulnerable, or too disturbing to be discharged to community residences. Seventy-two patients who were the responsibility of Friern Hospital fell into this category of difficult-to-place (DTP) patients. They were transferred to four different facilities with high staffing levels. They were followed up by the Team for the Assessment of Psychiatric Patients (TAPS), which I directed with the remit of evaluating the government's policy on community care. My assistant director, Noam Trieman, constructed an assessment schedule to identify DTP patients in a hospital undergoing closure. This was known as the Special Problems Rating Scale (SPRS) (3). A follow-up of the DTP patients after 5 years showed that only 40% had been discharged. I considered that this proportion could be considerably increased with a more active and focused regime. Consequently I negotiated with the management of Warley, another Victorian hospital that was in the process of closing, and was authorized and funded to create an intensive rehabilitation unit in the hospital grounds. I was given the use of a separate villa, a pleasant domestic-style building in the grounds, which contained 16 male and 6 female beds. Before this unit was developmed, Trieman conducted a survey of the remaining hospital population with the SPRS. The SPRS data were used to select 22 patients for the new unit. For administrative reasons, the men were moved in first and then the women after a delay of 1 year. During this period, no active rehabilitation was instituted, the men were maintained on their previous medication regimes, and were looked after by the same staff that had moved with them from their wards in the main building, which had been declared unfit for human habitation. At the end of the first year the active rehabilitation programme was due to start, but first the SPRS was completed again for the 16 men to update the baseline. A third assessment was made of all 22 patients after a further year.

The mean number of special problems among the 16 men was 3.0 before their move into the villa. The nursing staff who opted to work in the villa, with the exception of the nurse manager, were themselves institutionalized, and continued in a custodial role. After 1 year in the new environment, with no alteration to the medical and nursing care, the mean number of special problems exhibited by the men dropped to 1.8. This serendipitous experiment demonstrated the major impact on disturbed behaviour of a move from a vast crumbling building to a pleasant residence built to a human scale. It is worth recording that 36% of the Warley DTP patients moved to the community after 2 years.

The accumulation of knowledge about social factors

Early studies of the influence of the social environment on the incidence of psychiatric illness were conducted in the United States by Faris and Dunham (4) and in the United Kingdom by Hare (5) and by Goldberg and Morrison (6). A large corpus of research in social psychiatry did not begin to accumulate until the 1960s. Probably the most influential figure in this sphere was Sir Aubrey Lewis, not so much on account of his own research, which was highly erudite, although not directly clinical, but due to his assembling a critical mass of outstanding social scientists, and facilitating their collaboration. He was appointed the first director of the Medical Research Council (MTC) Social Psychiatry Research Unit at the Institute of Psychiatry in London in 1948. Members of this unit in its early years included Eliot Slater, who established the Maudsley Twin Register, and Morris Carstairs, Norman Kreitman, Michael Shepherd, Michael Rutter, George Brown, and John Wing, all of whom became directors of their own research units, which made major contributions to the understanding of social influences on psychiatric disorders. These merit consideration in some detail.

The UK Medical Research Council units

The Medical Research Council (MRC) established six units in the general area of social psychiatry across the United Kingdom. Michael Shepherd directed the General Practice Research Unit at the Institute of Psychiatry from the late 1950s. His interest was in the role of GPs in the treatment of neuroses. He conducted epidemiological studies in general practices and was appointed to the first chair in epidemiological psychiatry. Epidemiology was to prove a fundamental tool in social psychiatry research. David Goldberg joined the unit and developed the General Health Questionnaire to detect the presence of neuroses in attenders at general practices. This instrument has subsequently proved its value in many countries worldwide. With Peter Huxley, David Goldberg identified the filter process whereby GPs select patients for referral to secondary and tertiary psychiatric services, and went on to train GPs to improve their clinical skills in recognizing their patients' psychiatric symptoms.

Morris Carstairs directed a unit in Edinburgh for Epidemiological Studies in Psychiatry, investigating parasuicide and alcoholism. Norman Kreitman moved from the Institute of Psychiatry to the MRC unit in Chichester directed by Peter Sainsbury, and assisted with the research on suicide. After 6 years in Chichester he moved again to join Morris Carstairs in Edinburgh, where he continued the ongoing lines of research and added studies on depression in women, an interest stimulated by his previous association with George Brown. Michael Rutter established the Child Psychiatry Unit at the Institute of Psychiatry in 1984 and engaged in epidemiological studies on autism, and the deleterious effects of institutional care on children. George Brown, a medical sociologist, was a seminal influence in John Wing's Social Psychiatry Unit, and together with Morris Carstairs and Elizabeth Monck they studied the outcome for a group of men with schizophrenia discharged from psychiatric institutions to the community (7). It emerged that the best predictor of readmission to hospital was the kind of home to which the men were discharged. Those discharged to live with close relatives fared worse than men who went to live with more distant relatives or with private landlords.

Brown's hunch was that the emotional relationship between the patients and their close relatives was responsible for the deterioration in their mental state. In order to test this hypothesis, he needed to develop a method of measuring the emotional response of the family members to their sick relative. He accomplished this over a number of years in collaboration with Michael Rutter (8). The instrument they created is based on an interview with the relative about the patient's symptoms and behaviour over the previous 3 months, and is called the Camberwell Family Interview (CFI). The interview is audiotaped and the tape is rated later. The ratings are used to define relatives as either high or low on Expressed Emotion (EE). High-EE relatives are characterized by making many critical remarks about the patient, expressing hostility towards him or her, or behaving in an overinvolved manner towards the patient. Relatives' EE was found to have a strong association with the outcome of schizophrenia, as Brown had hypothesized (9). This finding was replicated by Christine Vaughn and myself, and extended by including a group of patients with depression who lived with a partner. Critical remarks made by the relative were also found to predict the outcome of a depressive illness (10). Subsequent research by many other groups has shown that relatives' EE is a potent predictor of outcome for most psychiatric conditions and for a number of non-psychiatric illnesses such as diabetes and myocardial infarction.

Research in social psychiatry has developed in other countries, particularly in Australia where Scott Henderson directed the unit in Sydney and was concerned with social aspects of old-age psychiatry. In South Africa the local MRC unit in Cape Town under the direction of Lynn Gillis conducted epidemiological surveys of the general population, and studied the impact of life events on the different ethnic groups living there, using the schedule developed by George Brown. In the United States Michael Goldstein made major contributions to the literature on relatives' EE, as did Gerry Hogarty in Pittsburgh. Arthur Kleinman, psychiatrist and social anthropologist, worked in China and studied the relationship between clients and traditional healers. He also examined the concept of neurasthenia, which is commonly used in China for neuroses, and found that most people given this diagnosis satisfied the US diagnosis of major depression. He treated a group of these people with antidepressants and assessed them as recovered. However many of them complained that their situation had not improved as they were still suffering from the effects of the Cultural Revolution. Kleinman concluded that it was important to alter the patients' social environment if they were to gain relief from their symptoms.

When Aubrey Lewis retired from directing the Social Psychiatry Research Unit in 1965, John Wing was appointed as director and pursued his interests, which were both local, centring on the epidemiology of mental illness and the service needs in Camberwell, and international, working with the mental health unit of the World Health Organization (WHO) on their ambitious studies of schizophrenia. The director of the WHO unit at this time was Tsung-Yi Lin, a psychiatrist from Taiwan. The first major research project undertaken was the International Pilot Study of Schizophrenia (IPSS), which was designed to investigate whether it was possible to train psychiatrists from nine different countries to apply standardized assessment procedures to patients with psychotic illnesses. The participating centres were situated in high-, middle-, and low-income countries, to render the study as representative as possible. The standard assessment of patients' mental state used in this study, the Present State

Examination (PSE), was developed by John Wing in collaboration with John Cooper from Nottingham, and Norman Sartorius, who later became director of the WHO mental health unit. The IPSS was very successful, largely due to Sartorius's (see this volume, pp. 117–32) genius for coordinating a disparate group of people from different cultural backgrounds. Each centre was expected to interview at least 100 patients with a diagnosis of schizophrenia or another psychosis, using the same set of instruments in which the psychiatrists had been trained, often in joint sessions during site visits.

The US/UK study was being conducted at about the same time as the IPSS and was designed to identify the causes of major discrepancies between American and British prevalence figures for schizophrenia, mania, and personality disorder. John Cooper was one of the principal investigators and the central assessment instrument was the PSE, as in the IPSS. Both international studies concurred in finding that the US psychiatrists involved held a much broader concept of schizophrenia than British psychiatrists, and in the IPSS, than psychiatrists from the other centres, with the exception of Moscow. While these two studies had no direct bearing on social influences, they established the methodological basis for the successor to the IPSS, the Determinants of the Outcome of Severe Mental Disorders (DOSMeD), and this made a major contribution to social psychiatry (11).

The strength of this study lay in the training of the participating psychiatrists to use the PSE reliably; the use of a computer program, CATEGO, to act as a standard against which local diagnoses could be compared; and the epidemiological nature of the study population. Only patients making a first contact with the psychiatric services for a psychotic illness were eligible to be included.

Does the social environment influence the incidence of schizophrenia?

The epidemiological basis of the DOSMeD study enabled the incidence of schizophrenia to be calculated in the participating centres. The findings are often quoted as showing that the incidence is uniform across countries widely differing in their cultural and social conditions, hence pointing to a predominantly biological aetiology. However, the uniformity of incidence rates is only evident in schizophrenia defined by Schneider's first-rank symptoms. These are a group of delusions and hallucinations identified by Kurt Schneider as delineating a central syndrome of schizophrenia. While they occasionally occur in other psychoses, they are much more frequently found in schizophrenia. When non-Schneiderian schizophrenia is separated out and the incidence calculated, a very different picture emerges. The variation in incidence between countries for Schneiderian schizophrenia is no more than would be expected by chance, while the variation for schizophrenia without Schneiderian symptoms has a negligible possibility of occurring by chance. This clearly indicates that there are two types of schizophrenia, one with an invariant incidence, which is mainly determined by biological factors, while in the other, the incidence of which varies dramatically across cultures, social factors play a substantial role in aetiology. I will address this issue below in discussing migrants, but first I will consider the influence of social factors on the outcome of schizophrenia.

The emotional impact of the family on the mentally ill person

The research on this issue began in the MRC Social Psychiatry Unit in the 1950s with the collaboration between Brown and Rutter, mentioned above. There have been well over 20 studies of the relationship between EE and the outcome of schizophrenia, spanning many different cultures and languages. The results are remarkably consistent, with an average of 56% of patients relapsing over 9 months after returning to a high-EE home compared with 18% of those returning to a low-EE home. In other words, a patient with schizophrenia in a high-EE home has a three times greater risk of relapse than one in a low-EE home. These findings led several groups to develop and evaluate ways of working with families in order to produce a less stressful, more supportive environment. Common to these different groups was educating families about the illness of their relative, teaching them how to tackle daily problems, improving communication in the family, modifying high-EE attitudes, and reducing contact between high-EE relatives and the patient. Where this was achieved, the relapse rate in high-EE homes was reduced from around 50% to 10% over 9 months. The key studies took place in the United States, the United Kingdom, China, and Japan, indicating a similarity in families' response to the interventions despite very different family structures and functions. The accumulation of these results plus cost-benefit analyses persuaded the UK National Institute of Clinical Excellence (NICE) to recommend that family members caring for a relative with schizophrenia should receive this kind of family work.

As already mentioned, the association between relatives' EE and other psychiatric conditions has been established. These conditions are bipolar disorder, major depression, eating disorders, alcoholism, and post-traumatic stress disorder (PTSD). With the exception of PTSD, family interventions have been developed and evaluated, and have proved capable of ameliorating the family environment and improving the patient's outcome. As an example, a randomized controlled trial was conducted of antidepressants versus couple therapy for depressed people with a critical partner as determined by the CFI. The results were that couple therapy was more effective than antidepressants in treating depression during the first year of the trial, and during the second year in maintaining the patients after all treatment was discontinued. Furthermore, couple therapy was no more expensive than antidepressants (12). Couple therapy is not the only social treatment that is effective in depression. Cognitive behaviour therapy and interpersonal therapy are also evidence- based, as is befriending patients who lack a supportive partner.

Family influences on the course of schizophrenia

Over the years several studies in low-income countries have suggested that, despite the paucity of community services, and often the unavailability of antipsychotic medication, the outcome for patients with schizophrenia was better than in high-income countries. These results met with scepticism, which was one of the spurs to the initiation of the DOSMeD study. Elizabeth Kuipers and I hypothesized that if the WHO study confirmed this surprising finding, it might well be explained by a lower prevalence of high-EE carers. Therefore we tacked on to DOSMeD a study of EE which would be conducted in Chandigarh, North India. We received full cooperation from Narendra Wig, the director of the centre, who seconded two of his researchers to this sub-study: a psychologist, Keerti Menon, and a social anthropologist, Harminder Bedi. We took great care over the training of these two researchers, and included a third Hindi speaker to check the transferability across cultures of the technique of measuring EE. The results were striking: whereas just over half of British relatives were rated as high-EE, the proportion for urban Chandigarh was 30%, and for the peasant farmers in the surrounding rural areas only 8%. Comparison of the DOSMeD first-contact sample of patients with schizophrenia in Chandigarh with a comparable sample in London revealed that twice as many of the Indian patients had a good outcome. Twice the whole Chandigarh sample of relatives were rated as low-EE compared with the London relatives, and this difference completely accounted for the better outcome of the Indian patients (13).

Migrants and ethnic minorities

Migration of human populations has become a dramatic feature of the past 100 years. In 2003 the Office of the United Nations High Commissioner for Refugees estimated that 38 million people were displaced worldwide, and that figure must have increased substantially since then. A migrant community living side by side with an ethnic majority offers the opportunity to compare rates of psychiatric illness and to explore possible cultural and social factors that might account for any differences in rates found. Both pull factors, the promise of economic betterment, and push factors, escape from persecution and civil war, exert a pressure to migrate. The flow is almost always from low-income countries to middle- and high-income countries. Research on social and cultural factors has been concentrated in just a few high-income countries: the United States, Canada, Australia, the Netherlands, the United Kingdom, and Sweden. One of the first pieces of psychiatric research to include a specific focus on an ethnic minority was the epidemiological study of the admission rates for schizophrenia in the city of Chicago. Faris and Dunham examined the admission rates for African Americans living in areas with high-density black population with those for African Americans living in low-density black areas, and found that the latter had higher admission rates than the former (4). This phenomenon has become known as the ethnic density effect.

Some of the largest ethnic minority populations are to be found in the United States, where Mexican Americans constituted over 10% of the population in 2009, and Spanish is now the second language. The United Kingdom was the destination for large numbers of Afro-Caribbeans who were recruited to staff the transport system and the NHS after nationalization in 1948 by the Labour government. During the same period there was an influx of people from South Asia in search of economic betterment or escaping from the sectarian violence that followed the partition of India. When the Dutch granted independence to their Caribbean colonies in 1975, one-third of the populations of Surinam and the Dutch Antilles emigrated to the Netherlands. Research on the Mexican Americans in the United States mainly focused on their relationship with the majority white population, and the effects of assimilation. In the Netherlands a high incidence of schizophrenia was found in the immigrants from the Caribbean, which increased in the second generation, while a study in Sweden found higher rates in im- migrants from a wide variety of countries than in native whites. In the United Kingdom a series of studies recording a very high incidence of schizophrenia in Afro-Caribbeans and an excess of involuntary admissions provoked accusations from the black commu- nity of racism in the psychiatric services and the judicial system. It became essential to investigate these accusations thoroughly, particularly in light of the well-documented Soviet abuse of psychiatry. Three studies of the incidence of schizophrenia using the PSE were conducted in Trinidad, Barbados, and Jamaica. All three found that the inci- dence of schizophrenia in the islanders was no higher than that in the white population of Britain. This result focused research on possible causal factors in the social environ- ment in the United Kingdom.

Social factors in three ethnic groups in the United Kingdom

A comparison was made between Afro-Caribbeans, South Asians, and white British, who acted as the reference group. The South Asians showed no excess of schizophrenia compared with the whites, while the Afro-Caribbeans had double the incidence rate of the whites. A range of social factors was measured in the three groups, including a meas- ure of ethnic identity developed for this study. The patients with schizophrenia were compared with matched individuals randomly selected from the general population. The South Asian patients were found to be deeply integrated in their ethnic community, whereas the Afro-Caribbean patients aspired to assimilate with the white community, which rejected them. At the same time the Afro-Caribbean patients had less contact with their families, leaving them in a marginal position. Other factors that distinguished the Afro-Caribbean patients from their healthy controls were: living alone, being un- employed, and having experienced separation from their parents in childhood. Each of these would lead to social isolation, which was therefore identified as a candidate causal factor for the high incidence of schizophrenia in this ethnic group (14). This finding substantiates the pioneering studies of schizophrenia and the social environment (4–6). It also suggests the possibility of remedial action on a social level to attempt to halt the escalating incidence of schizophrenia in UK Afro-Caribbeans, which has reached an alarming level in the third generation of migrants, as shown in the AESOP study in three British cities (15). This large-scale epidemiological study has also replicated the ethnic density effect in the area of London in which the Maudsley Hospital is sited.

Are cities pathogenic?

A series of studies in Sweden and the Netherlands, using the linkage of records kept by their governments, has established that being born or brought up in cities is a risk factor for the development of schizophrenia. The incidence is up to twice as high for those born in cities as for those born in small towns or the countryside. These observa- tions from northern Europe are substantiated by a study in China which found that the prevalence of schizophrenia in cities was double that in rural areas. It cannot be as- sumed that the social environment in cities is responsible for this disparity. It is possible that population density favours the spread of infections during pregnancy, that pollutants in the atmosphere affect the child's developing brain, or that many other physical factors in the city environment exert an adverse influence. Identifying the root causes will require a series of detailed studies comparable to those conducted on the different ethnic groups.

From psychiatric hospital to the community

So far I have focused on the attempts to humanize care within the asylums and to begin the development of psychiatric services in the community. It is true to state that England and Wales were at the forefront of these efforts. It has been claimed that the introduction of chlorpromazine to psychiatry in the early 1950s initiated the process of deinstitutionalization, but as we have seen, some pioneers began to develop extramural services some years earlier. The so-called Italian Experience began with a political activist, Franco Basaglia, who with the support of the Communist members of parliament passed Law 180 in 1978. This effectively closed the front doors of the psychiatric hospitals in Italy and forced the development of alternative services. By its nature this could not be a slow evolution and resulted in an uneven distribution of facilities in the community, with the south of the country lagging far behind the north.

In the United States the Senate passed the Community Mental Health Centres Act in 1963 in response to President Kennedy's call for a new approach to the provision of services to people with psychiatric illness. For this purpose the sum of $2.9 billion was appropriated from the federal budget. This invigorated the community mental health movement, which was based on the principles of social psychiatry: the humane treatment of people with mental illness, equality of access to healthcare, and the right of all citizens to full participation in society. I will deal with the issues raised by social inclusion later in the essay.

Many idealistic young people took posts in the community mental health centres (CMHCs) and attempted to provide a high quality of care to the long-term patients being discharged from the psychiatric hospitals. However, many of these patients had been subjected to custodial care and needed prolonged rehabilitation, which was not available in the CMHCs. The youthful workers found themselves facing opposition from the public who held stigmatizing attitudes, and were also blocked by entrenched financial interests which they lacked the political experience to combat effectively. A system of 'board and care' was established which in effect paid landlords to house the discharged patients, but gave no guidance on management of the many daily living problems of long-term psychotic patients, so that the care element was missing. Many discharged patients were living in conditions that were no better than the hospitals from which they had come. A considerable number became homeless or ended up in prison, giving rise to the term 'transinstitutionalization'. The financial provision for the CMHCs was undermined by President Nixon's misappropriation of the federal funds in 1973. The accumulation of these problems dealt a severe blow to the community mental health movement which largely failed to achieve its aims. Nevertheless, the psychiatric hospitals continued to reduce their beds, and some enthusiasts managed to develop innovative and cost-effective community services.

In England and Wales the closure of the psychiatric hospitals has been dramatic. Of the 130 hospitals functioning in 1975, no more than a dozen are still open today. Unlike in Italy, this was an evolution rather than a revolution. A steady stream of discharges was maintained at a pace determined by the provision of adequate replacement services in the community. Most of the residences provided for the long-term patients were converted domestic houses, not new buildings. This was an advantage, since these homes were indistinguishable from the neighbouring houses. This did not mean that ex-patients were easily integrated into their neighbourhoods. The comprehensive series of studies of this process by TAPS found that the discharged patients' social networks did not increase in size. Their quality was somewhat enhanced by the addition of two new friends and one confidant over 5 years after discharge, but the networks were dominated by other patients and mental health personnel (16).

The main problem besetting the process of deinstitutionalization in England and Wales has been the admission wards in general hospitals. The planners assumed that once patients were discharged from long-term care they would no longer require admission, so they reduced the number of beds. Their assumption turned out to be false. In the TAPS 5-year follow-up it was found that, at any one time, one in ten of the discharged patients occupied an admission bed (17). Furthermore, a considerable number of patients admitted to hospital wards stayed for long periods, occupying beds that were intended for acutely ill people. This became evident early on in the TAPS study of Friern Hospital in North London, where there was a steady accumulation on the admission wards of patients who stayed over 1 year. The number of these new long-stay patients admitted varied considerably across the different districts in the catchment area; the districts with the greatest degree of socio-economic deprivation generated the highest number of these patients. This observation should help planners to estimate the resources required for admission wards and, hopefully, make more realistic decisions.

Back doors and front doors

The British programme became known as a 'back door' policy because patients continued to enter the front door while the long-stay patients left through the back door. By contrast, the Italian programme was known as a 'front door' policy because the front door was closed to new patients, while the existing patients remained in the institutions in conditions which were often far from ideal. The most balanced programme was developed in Finland, where long-stay patients were returned to well-planned facilities in their communities, while patients referred for admission were carefully assessed over several days, including an interview with their family members.

While community psychiatric services have been established in North America and in much of western Europe, there are still many countries in the world where mentally ill people are kept in inhumane conditions, often being chained, sometimes beaten to drive out evil spirits, and separated from their families for years. In low-income countries psychiatric illnesses are given low priority by governments, which are unwilling to provide funds to shift the site of care from the old hospitals to the community. One solution, promoted vigorously by WHO, is to train community health workers to deal with psychiatric illnesses. There are some successful schemes of this kind. In Kerala

State, India, not only were primary healthcare staff trained in the detection and management of psychiatric disorders, but training was extended to police, prison warders, and schoolteachers. In Iran a national programme of the training of primary healthcare staff included local community health workers. These were recruited from *behvarzes*, who have a general education up to secondary school level and 2 years training in healthcare, including 1 week of formal training in mental health. Ntete in Uganda has developed the most comprehensive and impressive service integrating psychiatry into primary care. Village health teams, made up of volunteers, have been formed to help identify, refer, and follow up people with mental disorders. The volunteers were trained in basic community mental health, identification of mental disorders, and referral of cases to local health centres. They were able to identify and refer many people who previously would have been left untreated. In addition, a consumer organization was formed in the district with the aim of providing patient support and advocacy functions. This organization started income-generating projects, which not only provided economic assistance, but also gave consumers a sense of purpose and dignity. These innovative examples show what can be achieved in low-income countries with little or no financial input from the government.

Social inclusion

It is one thing to transfer people from outmoded long-stay institutions to sheltered residences in the community. It is another to ensure that they are integrated into the community in which they live. As we saw from the TAPS study of the discharged patients' networks, they often have very little social contact with people who were not part of the mental health services as either users or providers. I have deliberately introduced the term 'user' here because the rise of the User Movement, accompanied by the Recovery Movement, has brought the issue of social inclusion into prominence. Since the 1980s, user organizations have been established in a number of high-income countries, and some have achieved national status. In the United Kingdom, Mind is a national users' organization which receives a sizable annual grant from the government. In the United States the two most prominent organizations for users are the National Mental Health Consumers Association and the National Alliance for Mental Patients, but there are many others. The increasing power of users has occurred in the context of major societal changes affecting the relationship between professionals and their clients. The flattening of the hierarchy came about partly as a result of World War II, following which there was greater upward social mobility in high-income countries. An additional factor in Europe was European Union legislation granting patients the right of full access to their medical notes. This legitimizes the claim that information about the patient's body (and mind) belongs to the patient, not to their medical attendants.

The development of community mental health teams also contributed to this shift in power. There is much greater equality between the different professionals in these teams than existed on the hospital wards. Even the psychiatrist's previously unique right to prescribe medication has now been eroded in the United Kingdom by granting psychiatric nurses limited prescribing rights. The same privilege has been given to psychologists in the United States. The combination of all these influences has nar-rowed the status gap between professionals and users. In both the United Kingdom and the United States, users have taken up roles previously denied to them. In the United Kingdom, users serve on ethical committees, and collaborate with scientists in the de-sign and conduct of research studies. In my research on people who hear persecutory voices, the follow-up interviews have been conducted by a user who heard such voices himself some years ago but then became free of them. In the United States, users are often members of the governing and advisory boards of their service organizations and also serve on their executive and quality-improvement committees. Although these positive changes have boosted users' self-confidence and self-esteem, their integration into society requires a reciprocal response from the general public, many of whom hold stigmatizing attitudes towards people with psychiatric illness.

Reducing stigma

The stigma of mental illness has attracted increasing interest from the psychiatric com-munity in recent years, which has resulted in attempts to tackle it at many levels, using a variety of interventions. The Royal College of Psychiatrists' first effort was the Defeat Depression Campaign, launched in January 1992 in association with the Royal College of General Practitioners. The method of informing the public was through a media campaign and the distribution of leaflets, books, and audiotapes. An educational pro-gramme aimed at GPs was also mounted, and included consensus conferences and statements, guidelines for the recognition and management of depression, and training videotapes. Three polls of the general population were conducted before the campaign, in the middle of it, and 1 year after it ended. They showed changes of attitude of the order of 5–10%. However, the public continued to view antidepressants as addictive. The impact on GPs was much greater: 40% had definitely or probably made changes to their practice as a result of the campaign.

In 1997, a year after the Defeat Depression Campaign ended, the Royal College of Psychiatrists initiated a new campaign, Changing Minds, this time against the stigma of a broad range of psychiatric illnesses. Fact sheets, videos, and downloads were made available, and in 2000 a 2-minute film on mental illness was shown in all Odeon cin-emas before the main feature. Fact sheets produced for the campaign were largely in-effective in changing stigmatizing attitudes towards schizophrenia and alcoholism. Before-and-after surveys revealed only small reductions in stigmatizing attitudes.

The results of both these campaigns were disappointingly small, which was hardly surprising when the resources of the Royal Colleges are compared with those dedi-cated by international marketing companies to sell their products. Repeated exposure of a product for long periods on all possible media—television, cinemas, newspapers, radio, hoardings, T-shirts—costs huge sums of money, way beyond the reach of profes-sional organizations. I was involved in the planning of the Changing Minds Campaign and believed from the start that a scattergun approach to a broad range of psychiatric illnesses was a tactical error. A much more focused effort was planned by the World Psychiatric Association (WPA), led by its president, Norman Sartorius. His view was that a long-term effort was more likely to succeed than a brief campaign and this was accepted by a meeting in Geneva of 38 psychiatrists from more than 20 countries, and representatives of consumer groups. The participation of such an international assembly of psychiatrists and consumers indicated how social thinking about psychiatric illnesses had spread around the world.

The global programme of the World Psychiatric Association

The purpose of this programme was to combat the stigma of schizophrenia worldwide. It was launched in 1996 and was still active 10 years later, fulfilling the aim of its originators. Many different activities were pursued by the participants, one of the earliest being studies of public attitudes towards schizophrenia in the member countries. Comparison of the findings showed that the most positive attitudes were expressed by people in Canada and Germany, while the most negative were found in a cluster of eastern Mediterranean countries: Greece, Macedonia, and Turkey. The treatment of mentally ill people on the Greek island of Leros became an international scandal. I visited one of the four psychiatric hospitals in Macedonia and found patients living in appalling conditions. I have not been inside a Turkish psychiatric hospital, but have been informed by colleagues that the treatment of psychiatric patients has been far from enlightened. There is a strong link between hospital-centred care of a poor standard, and repressive public attitudes towards the mentally ill. It is likely that the high visibility of closed institutions from which few patients return to their families feeds the public stereotype of madness as dangerous and incurable. On the other hand, the persistence of such institutions is an indication of general societal attitudes towards psychiatric illness.

The Canadian city of Calgary was the pilot site for the WPA programme. An intensive educational campaign was run using local radio, and was evaluated with telephone surveys of a random sample of the general population, and by scanning local newspapers for items featuring mental illness. Once again a large-scale media campaign failed to make an appreciable impact. Rogers pointed out that the effectiveness of social marketing campaigns is increased by 'audience segmentation': partitioning a mass audience into relatively homogeneous sub-audiences and devising appropriately targeted promotional strategies and messages (18). This is what the Calgary group did next. They targeted high-school students and used a variety of methods of communicating anti-stigma messages. A teaching guide was prepared for the school staff, an art competition was held for the students to create anti-stigma messages, and people with psychiatric illness were recruited and coached to speak to students and answer their questions. Many studies have shown that personal contact with people who have a psychiatric illness modifies negative stereotypes. This component of the Calgary programme was very effective in altering the students' attitudes towards and knowledge about schizophrenia. The proportion of students with a perfect knowledge score increased from 12% to 28%, and the proportion expressing no social distance between themselves and people with schizophrenia increased from 16% to 30%. The success of this approach to high-school students led to replications in several other countries participating in the WPA programme.

Targeting neighbours

As reported above, when we measured the social networks of the discharged patients in the TAPS project, we found that few ordinary citizens were included. The policy of the resettlement teams was to slip the patients into the community as quietly as possible to avoid hostile responses from neighbours. Two surveys of public attitudes to deinstitutionalization in the localities chosen to resettle the patients revealed that a majority of people expressed a high level of goodwill towards patients discharged from the old psychiatric hospitals. It became apparent that the hostile groups of residents who campaigned against patients being moved into their neighbourhoods constituted a small but vocal minority. I concluded that the policy of secrecy was an error because it failed to mobilize the goodwill of the silent majority. Therefore we decided to mount an educational campaign in advance of moving patients into a specific neighbourhood, and to do so in the context of a randomized trial in which the control neighbourhood, in which long-stay patients from the same hospital were being placed, would receive no intervention. The materials for the education programme consisted of a video about the process of deinstitutionalization and the rationale for it, and interviews with professional carers, shopkeepers in an area in which patients had already been resettled, and users. This was supplemented with leaflets on community care and psychiatric illnesses. A meeting for neighbours was held in a local church hall at which the video was shown, and staff and a user were available for questioning. The meeting was attended by about 30 people, and was catered by a Caribbean chef. After the presentations, I joined the group of neighbours around the food table, who were talking animatedly. Several of them said that were very pleased to be at this meeting in that it gave them an opportunity to meet their neighbours. So much for the concept of community! Neighbours who had not attended the meeting were offered copies of the video and leaflets by knocking on doors. Social events such as bring-and-buy sales and barbecues were held in the patients' residence, to which all neighbours were invited.

Analysis of the data from the before-and-after assessments showed that, compared with neighbours in the control street, those in the experimental street showed a small gain in knowledge and a significant reduction in fear of mentally ill people and the wish to exclude them from society. Neighbours in the experimental street were much more likely to know the names of users, and to visit them, invite them to their homes, and count them as friends. This was confirmed by charting the users' social networks (19). As in the Calgary programme, targeting a specific group proved to be an effective method of reducing stigmatizing attitudes, and in this case led to a demonstrable improvement in the social inclusion of users. Before beginning this study I considered that since TAPS was evaluating government policy on phasing out the old asylums, we had to maintain a strictly independent position. Consequently I resisted pleas from the planning groups for TAPS to provide an input. When we completed the evaluation and sent a final report to the Department of Health (20), I felt that my hands were no longer tied. That is when I initiated the trial of educating local neighbours, based firmly on what we had learned from TAPS surveys of public attitudes. It was extremely gratifying to find that the knowledge we gained through our research enabled us to improve the social integration of users discharged from psychiatric hospitals.

Employment

Employment has numerous advantages for people with psychiatric illness, but unfortunately it is difficult for many of them to find a job and to keep it, particularly in tough economic climates. Many decades ago, Douglas Bennett observed that when the economy was booming, his day hospital at the Maudsley Hospital emptied, and vice versa. A paid job gives workers a sense of achievement and enhances their self-esteem. It offers them the possibility of supporting themselves and/or contributing to their family's income. It structures their weekday, and offers the possibility of leisure activities, which are unaffordable for most patients on benefits. It also enlarges their social network with people from the general population, rather than users and providers of psychiatric services.

Many of the old asylums put patients to work in the hospital farms, laundries, and gardens. Of course their work was unpaid, although they contributed to the economy of the asylum. After the trade unions put a stop to this exploitation, there was an eventual development of sheltered workshops in the asylums. The work was repetitive and boring, and patients' earnings were very small. As more humane practices were introduced, the available tasks became more complex. For example, Netherne Hospital in South London developed a graded programme of work, starting with the folding of cardboard light-bulb sleeves, and progressing to the winding of armatures for rocket motors in guided missiles. Friern Hospital maintained an industrial therapy workshop which employed 120 patients daily and included horticulture, wooden furniture assembly, and metal work. The most skilled worker was a patient of mine who drilled precision holes in metal blocks and was the highest earner.

During the period of development of community services, sheltered workshops were set up in the community, but they rarely, if ever, acted as a stepping stone to open employment. Attempts to remedy this deficiency include supported or transitional employment schemes, such as Fountain House in New York. In a further development, clients have been supervised and trained on site, and meetings arranged with employers. However, even with this degree of professional input and care no more than 50% of clients progress to open employment. The answer to this problem may lie in the development of social enterprises.

Social firms

Social enterprises first began in Italy, based on the existing worker cooperatives. In English they are referred to as social firms or affirmative businesses. Franco Basaglia and his team in Trieste set up the first worker cooperative for discharged patients in 1973. It provided employment in cleaning and maintaining public buildings, and by 1985 was employing 130 workers. The success of this model led to expansion into other enterprises, including a hotel, a café, a restaurant, a transportation business, and a building renovation business. By 1997 there were about 1600 social cooperatives in Italy employing around 40,000 workers, 40% of whom were disabled. From their origins in Italy, social firms have spread to other European countries. Germany has probably been at the forefront of this development: in 1999 it had 300 social firms employing 6000 workers, of whom one-half are disabled. The United Kingdom has over 70 social firms with more than 400 workers, one-third of whom are of whom disabled. In 1999 a survey estimated that there were about 2000 social firms in Europe as a whole, with about 47,000 employees, about one-half being disabled. Recently I stayed in a 12-bedded hotel in Cracow, Poland, run almost entirely by users. The rooms were impeccable and the service friendly and efficient.

The shift from unpaid work in the asylums to social firms run entirely by users has occurred in the course of 50 years, and is an index of a dramatic change in professional attitudes to people with psychiatric illness, and a marker of the burgeoning power of the user movement. The largest employer of labour in Europe is the UK NHS. It can be argued that the NHS has an obligation to employ people with psychiatric illness, and some NHS Trusts have already done this. In the Pathfinder Trust in south-west London 10% of employees suffer from psychiatric illness, mostly psychoses. In Denver, Colorado, people with psychiatric illness are trained to become case-manager aides, staff members in sheltered homes, and job coaches in mental health centres. Over 100 people have been placed in these positions, and two-thirds are still in post after 2 years. In Boulder, Colorado, the mental health centre run by Richard Warner employs people with psychiatric illness as case-manager aides, residential counsellors, job coaches, clubhouse staff, office workers, and research interviewers.

The responsibilities in running businesses, working in health facilities alongside professional staff, and participating as researchers, which are currently borne by users, would have been unimaginable even 30 years ago. This would not have been achieved without the pioneering work of social psychiatrists in many countries, and the efforts of professionals and users to modify the negative stereotypes that existed for centuries and were maintained by the custodial ethos of the old asylums. I never cease to be amazed by the fact that there are young psychiatrists today who not only have never worked in a mental hospital, but have never even seen one.

The future of social psychiatry

A spectre is haunting social psychiatry: biological determinism. During the second half of the 20th century new techniques of imaging the human brain at rest and in action, and the unravelling of the human genome gave rise to optimism that a biological approach to psychiatric disorders would yield a breakthrough in discovering their causes, and hence the development of new and effective physical treatments. The brave new world of psychiatric research was heralded in the United States by designating the last 10 years of the century 'the Decade of the Brain'. The United Kingdom was not untouched by these developments, but was not swept along on this tide of enthusiasm for biological explanations that dominated the United States. However, it did have an impact on one sector, the MRC units dedicated to social psychiatry research. By 1995 five units, including my own, which I took over from John Wing, had been closed. Only Michael Rutter's unit remained. At the time of the closure of my unit, the MRC explicitly stated that in future they would not support a unit that focused on social psychiatry without its being integrated with biological research. Michael Rutter, always a canny politician, had anticipated this policy and was successful in establishing a Social, Genetic and Developmental Psychiatry Centre at the Institute of Psychiatry.

This was not of course the death-knell of social psychiatry research, which continued in many centres in the United Kingdom and Europe outside the MRC unit structure. However, it did become sparse in the United States, as evidenced by a study I did of the papers published in the *British Journal of Psychiatry* (*BJP*) and the *American Journal of Psychiatry* (*AJP*) over the years 1951–2005 (20). Between 1961 and 1966 there was a steep rise in the proportion of psychosocial articles in both journals, which maintained the high level reached over the next decade, during which community psychiatry developed in the United Kingdom and the United States. As the US community mental health movement began to fail, the proportion of psychosocial articles in the *AJP* diminished. This fall continued in an almost linear fashion over the next two decades, reaching its lowest level in 50 years in 2001. At this point the *AJP* featured almost twice as many articles of a biological nature as psychosocial articles. By contrast, the proportion of psychosocial articles in the *BJP*, after a moderate fall from 1966 to 1981, rose slowly but steadily to 59% in 2005, the highest level in the 55 years of the survey. This indicates that despite the closure of the MRC units, research in social psychiatry in the United Kingdom continued to flourish. It is noteworthy that while the Decade of the Brain produced no novel biological treatment for psychiatric illnesses, during that period UK psychiatrists and psychologists established the effectiveness of family work for schizophrenia and depression, developed cognitive behaviour therapy for psychoses, and introduced cognitive remediation for schizophrenia. At the heart of social psychiatry, both in research and practice, lies a concern with relationships, and this will never be eclipsed by advances in the biology of the brain.

Possible future developments

What direction is social psychiatry likely to take during the next decade? One obvious problem to be solved is the difficulty in making psychosocial interventions of proven efficacy available to all those who could benefit from them. Unlike new drugs, psychosocial treatments do not generate big profits, so no commercial organization is interested in marketing them. Even when a government recommends the use of a specific intervention, as has the UK Department of Health for working with family carers of people with schizophrenia, its availability countrywide is patchy. The situation is even worse for cognitive behaviour therapy for psychosis. There is now ample evidence that involving family carers in the treatment of a wide variety of psychiatric illnesses improves the outcome for the patients, but few clinicians take heed of this. A high priority needs to be given to studies of the failure of psychiatrists and managers to implement evidence-based psychosocial treatments. The eradication of stigma will continue to concern psychiatric professionals, users, and their family carers. Given the relatively small impact of national campaigns, future efforts will probably be targeted on specific groups. There have been no advances in the pharmacological treatment of psychoses in the past two decades, yet the lives of a high proportion of patients are still devastated by these illnesses. Innovative psychosocial therapies are needed to ameliorate this situation (21). These suggestions are more of a wish list than an informed guess about the future of social psychiatry. I hope my wishes are fulfilled.

Coda

Since I wrote this, one of my wishes has been fulfilled. I have developed a computer-assisted therapy for patients who continue to be harassed by persecutory voices despite adequate antipsychotic medication. This novel psychological therapy has succeeded in abolishing the hallucinations in three patients and in reducing the frequency and intensity of the voices in many others.

References

1 Leff, J. P. and Wing, J. K. (1971). Trial of maintenance therapy in schizophrenia. *British Medical Journal* 3, 599–604.

2 Brown, G. W. and Harris, T. (1978). *The social origins of depression*. Tavistock: London.

3 Trieman, N., Hughes, J., and Leff, J. (1998). The TAPS Project 42: The last to leave hospital—a profile of residual long-stay populations and plans for their resettlement. *Acta Psychiatrica Scandinavica* 98, 354–9.

4 Faris, R. E. L. and Dunham, H. W. (1939). *Mental disorders in urban areas*. Chicago University Press: Chicago.

5 Hare, E. H. (1956). Mental illness and social conditions in Bristol. *Journal of Mental Science* 102, 349–57.

6 Goldberg, E. M. and Morrison, S. L. (1963). Schizophrenia and social class. *British Journal of Psychiatry* 109, 785–802.

7 Brown, G. W., Monck, E. M., Carstairs, G. M., and Wing J. K. (1962). Influence of family life on the course of schizophrenic illness. *British Journal of Preventive and Social Medicine* 16, 55–68.

8 Brown, G. W. and Rutter, M. L. (1966). The measurement of family activities and relationships. *Human Relations* 19, 241–63.

9 Brown, G. W., Birley, J. L.T., and Wing, J. K. (1972). The influence of family life on the course of schizophrenic disorders: A replication. *British Journal of Psychiatry* 121, 241–58.

10 Vaughn, C. E. and Leff, J. P. (1976). The influence of family and social factors on the course of psychiatric illness: a comparison of schizophrenic and depressed neurotic patients. *British Journal of Psychiatry* 129, 125–37.

11 Jablensky, A., Sartorius, N., Ernberg, G. et al. (1992). Schizophrenia: manifestations, incidence and course in different cultures: A World Health Organization ten-country study. *Psychological Medicine Monograph Supplement 20*. Cambridge: Cambridge University Press.

12 Leff, J., Vearnals, S., Brewin, C. R. et al. (2000). The London Depression Intervention Trial: Randomised controlled trial of antidepressants versus couple therapy in the treatment and maintenance of people with depression living with a partner: clinical outcome and costs. *British Journal of Psychiatry* 177, 95–100.

13 Leff, J., Wig, N. N., Ghosh, A. et al. (1987). Expressed emotion and schizophrenia in North India. III. Influence of relatives' expressed emotion on the course of schizophrenia in Chandigarh. *British Journal of Psychiatry* 151, 166–73.

14 Bhugra, D., Leff, J., Mallett, R., Morgan, C. and Jing-Hua, Z. (2010). The Culture and Identity Schedule a measure of cultural affiliation: Acculturation, marginalization and schizophrenia. *International Journal of Social Psychiatry* 56, 540–56.

15 Fearon, P., Kirkbride, J. K., Morgan, C. et al. (2006). Incidence of schizophrenia and other psychoses in ethnic minority groups: results from the AESOP study. *Psychological Medicine* **36**, 1541–50.

16 Leff, J. and Trieman, N. (2000). Long-stay patients discharged from psychiatric hospitals. Social and clinical outcomes after five years in the community. The TAPS Project 46. *British Journal of Psychiatry* **176**, 217–23.

17 Gooch, C. and Leff, J. (1996). The TAPS Project 26: Factors affecting the success of community placement. *Psychological Medicine* **26**, 511–20.

18 Rogers, E. M. (1996). The field of health communication today: an up-to-date report. *Journal of Health Communication* **1**, 15–23.

19 Wolff, G., Pathare, S., Craig, T., and Leff, J. (1996). Public education for community care. A new approach. *British Journal of Psychiatry* **168**, 441–7.

20 Leff, J., Trieman, N., Knapp, M. and Hallam, A. (2000) The TAPS Project: A report on 13 years of research, 1985–98. *Psychiatric Bulletin* **24**, 165–8.

21 Leff, J. (2007). Climate change in psychiatry: periodic fluctuations or terminal trend? In: Morgan C., McKenzie, K., and Fearon P. (eds.) *Society and psychosis*. Cambridge: Cambridge University Press, pp. 11–22.

Psychiatry in developed and developing countries

Norman Sartorius

Introduction

When the editors suggested that I should write about psychiatry in developed and developing countries in the past 50 years I thought that they might have made the title shorter, say, call it 'Psychiatry worldwide', or 'Psychiatry, its development and perspectives': yet when thinking about it some more I felt that the title should be left as it is because it reminds us that many of the developing countries have parts that are highly developed and most of the countries that consider themselves highly developed have parts which are similar to the poorest of developing countries. The distinction between the two types of countries is not categorical but dimensional. Countries differ in the proportion of their populations that is poor because there are poor people everywhere. It makes no sense to propose solutions for developed and other solutions for the developing countries: solutions should refer to specific problems, not to countries in which the problems are to be solved. Clearly, the application of the solution will depend on the local circumstances and on the environment in which the problem exist; however, that does not imply that the solutions to problems should be different from one another. Once this principle is accepted it will be easier to learn from each other and to use the experience of others in building one's health services or other parts of societies' structures. This also makes it easier to collaborate in searching ways that can improve the lot of people with mental illness and their families worldwide.

The acceptance of this point of view means that it is not, for example, justified to propose the use of different medications (or other health interventions) for one set of countries but not for the other. It might well be that a medication that is most effective in dealing with a disease and causes least side effects is of such a price that the person who needs it cannot buy it: this should launch us on a campaign that will make the drug cheaper or reimbursable by the government or insurance companies, rather than proposing that the patient should receive a cheaper yet less effective medication or a medication with serious side effects because his country is classified as being poor. The example of the fight for affordable medication to treat AIDS showed the former course is possible and better than the decision to select less appropriate treatments.

Most of the recommendations for mental health policies and programmes in the 'developing' countries have been based on the latter strategy. The logics is that 'developing' countries have few resources and that therefore mental health services should use the cheapest medications or other interventions regardless of whether they are also the best for the diseases for which they are prescribed. This is not regarded as a temporary solution, but a reasonable and acceptable approach often embedded into the policies governing health care. A related message was that solutions lie in a better use of available resources rather than in the search for additional resources. This might well be true in some instances, but not in many others. What is worse is that in the field of mental health such a strategy contains the meta-message that mentally ill people are of little or no value to society or to themselves, thereby justifying second-best solutions—as long as they are cheaper. This meta-message is a strong confirmation of the content of the stigma that is attached to mental illness, suggesting that persons with a mental illness are of no value, incurable and in addition difficult, dangerous, and lazy. It also confirms the stigma attached to people in the developing countries implying they are less educated, less intelligent, less able to create or live in a civic society, unaware or dismissive of ethical principles—in short, less valuable or worthy of investment. It is of course true that in precarious situations it is better to use less effective interventions than none, and that lives can often be saved with second- or third-best interventions, even though they may have a high cost in terms of significant side effects. However, the use of less than best interventions and strategies should at all times be seen as a temporary surrogate of what is needed and understood as the best practice.

Recent years have seen major socioeconomic changes with considerable potential impact on mental health and the treatment of mental illness (1). Globalization, for example, can impose significant change in the value systems of countries participating in the global exchange. In part this is due to the fact that the flow of information between countries is not balanced; richer countries with highly developed technology send more information than they receive, influence more than they are influenced. Value systems prevalent in some European countries and the United States are being promoted (and imposed) in developing countries with the argument that they are more likely to make societies better, although the evidence for this statement is lacking. The striving for independence and autonomy of the individual, for example, is often presented as being preferable to accepting the interdependence of individuals living as a group. Clearly neither independence nor interdependence alone can make societies a safer and better place to live. A judicious mix of the two would be ethically and practically the best: unfortunately the defenders of the two stances are entrenched in their opinion and use extreme examples of the application of the opponent's' views to promote their ideas.

Another change relevant to psychiatry and the provision of mental health care is the trend of 'commodification' promoted by, among others, the World Bank and many governments. Commodification describes the tendency to handle all of the services and transactions in societies in economic and financial terms as if they were a commodity. Health care, for example, should be organized in a manner that will ensure a profit to the agency or government that is providing it. The position is rejected that helping feeble members of one's society—children, elderly people, those with disabilities—is an ethical imperative of civilized societies. The economic imperative requires that help should be provided in a manner that will bring measurable and immediate economic benefits to society, particularly in terms of increased productivity. A reflection of this trend is also the abandonment of the terms 'least developed', 'developing', and 'developed' countries which are now referred to as 'low income', 'middle income' and 'high income' countries.

Changes in sociodemographic structure over the past several decades have also greatly influenced psychiatry. For example, the change of age distribution in many societies has increased the prevalence of geriatric mental disorders, and the diminution of the size of the family in most countries has reduced their capacity to look after chronically ill members.

Most societies are also experiencing changes of the size of their middle class. In developing countries it has grown exponentially, thus creating a large market for health and related industries; the growing middle class already attracted a strong private health care sector, developed within the country or imported from abroad. The urgency to strengthen primary health care has diminished in parallel with this development, although the governments continue to emphasize the need to build it up The upward-striving members of the middle class want to be treated by the most qualified and famous specialists (and now can afford this); they do not want nurses and general practitioners as their main care providers; they do not want the kind of care that they see as being for the poor who cannot afford better.

In many settings policies and recommendations about primary health care are not supported by a commensurate increase in the budget. The emergence of 'specialized' primary health care—i.e. the placement of specialists' services as the first point of contact—also belies the original intentions of the primary health care agreement embodied in the Alma Ata declaration (and report) on primary health care (2,3). Other changes of the social structure, such as those caused by diminishing natality and increased rates of divorce, are not universal but exert a powerful impact on health care in the countries where they exist.

Finally, another massive social change derives from migration—economic, voluntary, or forced—from rural to urban areas and from country to country. The impact of migration on mental health varies with the manner in which it took place. In some instances candidates for migration are screened by medical authorities to exclude those with an illness. The consequence of this procedure, currently in place in a variety of countries, is that the migrants generally have fewer diseases than the host population while the prevalence of diseases in the donor country increases. Refugees, on the other hand, often have higher rates of mental disorders than the host population—a finding that is particularly striking in instances in which the rules forbid repatriation if the refugees are mentally or physically ill.

Paradigms of psychiatry and their change

This volume contains fine descriptions of developments that have had a significant impact on psychiatry and its application over the past 60 years. These include the rise of psychopharmacology, the development of powerful neuroimaging methods, the production of a multitude of standardized diagnostic procedures, the revolutionary advances of genetics, and the discoveries of other basic sciences. Most of these discoveries have opened the door to further research and scientific advances; however, the stark reality is that they have not significantly affected the provision of services to the mentally ill. Other developments—such as those mentioned in the introduction—had an impact on the practice of psychiatry and eroded several of the paradigms on which its practice is based. The formulation of new paradigms that are more harmonious with the environment in which mental illness occurs, and in which treatment takes place, is not likely to be difficult. What will represent a major challenge will be to demonstrate to all who hold current or past paradigms sacred that they must abandon them and accept their change or substitution. The following pages will examine six such paradigms and propose components that could be used in reformulating them.

The paradigm of community care

The first of these paradigms concerns the site of psychiatric treatment. In the late 19th and early 20th century most of the industrially developed countries erected large mental hospitals. Those that had colonies did the same in many of these locations. Psychiatric treatment at that time included a variety of interventions, most of them based on the opinion of the leading psychiatrists rather than on evidence about their effectiveness. Some of these treatments were based on the notion that severe stress might bring the patients to their senses—a rationale resembling that used with crackling old radios which, when hit, sometimes had an improved sound. Patients were immersed in cold water, exposed to conditions of sensory deprivation, placed in turning cages (4,5). Less drastic treatments were also employed—patients were taken for walks in the parks, made to listen to gentle and harmonious music. Treatments which involved infection with malaria, search for sources of 'focal sepsis' with a consequent surgical removal of those sources (6), insulin coma treatment, leucotomies and lobotomies, treatment with special diets, and various convulsive therapies all had their time; a common denominator to all these efforts was that they were usually performed in mental hospitals. Some of these were huge, like the Pilgrim State Hospital in the state of New York, USA (with more than 13,000 patients and several thousand staff), some small, some private, some managed by the government. The smaller private hospitals were often run by a psychiatrist who employed members of his family as key personnel in the institution.

The mental hospitals built in colonial times in developing countries resembled those in the industrialized world. Practically all of the funds that the government was providing for mental health care had to be used to maintain the hospitals. The funds provided to the hospitals were, however, insufficient to maintain the buildings, to ensure regular clean water supply and the elimination of waste, to maintain the parks that often surrounded them, and to pay decent salaries to hospital staff. Even when the funds given to the hospital were substantial, their use frequently lacked any form of effective control and tended to be left in the hands of the hospital directors who were not necessarily skilled managers. The result of underfunding and poor management of institutions—which were usually far away from the public eye—was the physical deterioration of the facilities, loss of staff, and a continuously lessening quality of care. The abuse of hospitalized patients was a frequent occurrence, often not reported. There were no systems in place to ensure that patients would get appropriate treatment or be protected against abuses of their human rights.

In the middle of the 20th century the idea of providing treatment to patients living in the community gained ground. Communities were to accept people with mental illness as their members and support their families or other carers. Mental hospital beds were to be reduced to a minimum. Inpatient and outpatient services were to be placed in the institutions providing general health care. Governments were easily persuaded by the advocates of community psychiatry who often claimed that the reform of mental health care arrangements would reduce the cost of care as well as improve the quality of life of the mentally ill. In some countries the reduction of beds was drastic—in the United States, for example, several hundred thousand beds were eliminated and in Italy the parliament passed a law by which all state mental hospitals had to be abruptly closed, without delay. In other countries the reduction of the numbers of beds was slower but the goal of reducing the size of mental health institutions was accepted by most professionals and by the governments.

As time went by and the experience of closing inpatient facilities grew, several facts emerged. First, the transition of inpatient facilities to a community mental health care system did not reduce the cost of care; in fact, while the transition was under way the cost of care was increased because it was also necessary to maintain the hospital in operation during the period of transfer. Subsequently, well-run community services seemed to be just as expensive as hospital care (and sometimes more so). When settled in the community patients reported an improvement of their quality of life, but the symptoms of chronic mental illness did not change very much (7).

In other settings, where the transition from hospital care to community care was more abrupt, and where the investment into the development of appropriate mental health services in the community did not occur, patients' conditions often deteriorated and many of them—now that the treatment facilities were reduced in size—ended up in prison (8,9). Thus, deinstitutionalization, the goal of the reformers, turned into transinstitutionalization—from hospital to prison—offering a considerably less appropriate environment for the many incarcerated mentally ill.

Another fact that emerged was that the capacity of the family to look after the mentally ill was constantly diminishing. This was due to the gradual disappearance of the multilayer extended family that could cope with the burden of care for a chronically ill member. Nuclear one-tier families could not provide care for a person with mental illness without external help, particularly in settings in which women also accepted or sought work outside the house.

In addition, there was the difficulty of transferring staff from the hospital to the community, problematic because of the reluctance of personnel to work in a community setting and the need to retrain many who were trained for work in hospital and only had experience of care provided to inpatients—a retraining that required considerable additional resources. These problems were present in developed countries which were introducing community care. In developing countries that also made attempts to introduce community care it was not easy to overcome prejudice and tradition or to find funds to support change. Islands of such care were sometimes created by gifted leaders: but what they built usually did not survive their departure.

For all these reasons the paradigm of community care will have to be reformulated. If community care is to be successful it will be necessary to invest additional resources into the development of health services in the community; staff recruited to work in the mental health services will have to be aware that their place of work will be in the community; a certain number of beds will have to be maintained to provide care to patients who require hospital care, and the facilities in which they will be placed will have to be covered by arrangements for quality assurance; families and other carers will require substantial help in terms of appropriate financial aid, additional education, and moral support; outreach qualified services, which have demonstrated their value in various settings, will have to be added to the community mental health services; and collaborative arrangements will have to be developed with institutions caring for people with mental illness who also have physical illnesses, and those living in institutions such as care homes and prisons. In addition it will be necessary to have inpatient and outpatient facilities that can provide emergency services to people with mental illness and deal with acute and incipient mental disorders.

The realization of such an array of services will take time and at present might not be feasible in many places. Nevertheless, in terms of quality and components of mental health services it is a model of this kind that has to be seen as the necessary goal for both developing and developed countries. The original paradigm of total or nearly total transfer of responsibility for the mentally ill to the community has to be significantly reformulated. Recent publications seem to indicate that these changes of community care paradigms are beginning to be recognized (10).

The paradigm of 'task shifting'

Some 40 years ago an Expert Committee of the World Health Organization (WHO) considered strategies that could be employed to extend mental health care to those in need of it (11). It recommended that personnel employed in primary health care services should be given additional training that would enable them to recognize the most severe forms of mental disorders and provide appropriate treatment. The Expert Committee's recommendation was not a total novelty; the idea that tasks related to mental health should be undertaken at general and primary health care level had been voiced by experts on previous occasions and as early as in 1871 by Isaac Ray (12), but it was felt that a report by a prestigious WHO Expert Committee would give that notion additional weight and facilitate its promotion. In the years that followed, WHO carried out a multicentre study to explore whether the recommendation could be realized. Investigators in Senegal, Colombia, India, and the Philippines participated in the study, which demonstrated that short training courses can teach primary care staff how to recognize and treat 'priority conditions'—including serious mental and neurological disorders such as schizophrenia and epilepsy (11,13). Publication of data obtained in this study was then used to promote the idea of shifting the tasks related to the recognition and treatment of mental health problems from psychiatrists and mental health services to simply trained staff and general health care services. The paradigm of task shifting seemed well-formulated and the hope was that health services would provide care to people with serious mental illness.

The formulation of the paradigm did not lead to significant changes of practice. While the usefulness of the strategy could be demonstrated in well-selected areas, with strong leaders, national recognition, and external support (such as recognition and support by WHO) the work in pilot study areas could not be generalized and implanted in other areas without additional resources or outstanding leaders keen to see the project work (14). When external support ceases, the new community care model withers away—an experience reported from many countries over the years. In the first decade of the 21st century WHO had to state, regretfully, that the gap between needs for mental health care and its actual provision has grown, and that a vast number of people with serious mental illness in developing countries do not receive necessary treatment. A new WHO programme, 'Mental Health Gap Action Programme', has been launched to reduce this gap (15) and it is to be hoped that it will be successful.

Nevertheless, there are good reasons to reconsider the value of the 'task shifting' paradigm. Doctors and other staff working in general health care services are often reluctant to accept tasks related to the care of mental disorders. Sometimes this can be overcome by adding an incentive, for example the financial incentives offered to general practitioners (GPs) in the United Kingdom who are regularly using depression screening questionnaires. But often the willingness to deal with mental disorders stops once they are recognized, resulting in referral to a mental health service. Courses given to GPs and other health care staff in developed and developing countries often show no effect in terms of practice change (16). A vast majority of general health care personnel have received only rudimentary training about mental health in their basic education and often share the negative and discriminatory opinion of the general public about the mentally ill.

A reformulation of the task shifting paradigm might include the following elements. First, training about the recognition and management of mental disorders should only be offered to general health care personnel who are interested in such learning. Second, the training should not be a systematic education about all psychiatric disorders, but address specific frequently encountered problems giving their solution (e.g. on the recognition and treatment of depression). The modules should be deliverable in a short course (possibly one half-day duration) because GPs often find it impossible to stay away from their practice for very long. Third, the courses should not be given by mental health specialists but by well-informed general health workers of the same level (e.g. a nurse trainer for nurses, a GP teacher for GPs) with a mental health specialist as a resource person present and willing to give advice and guidance when asked to do so. Fourth, teaching should not focus exclusively on the recognition of conditions, but rather the provision of skills necessary for the delivery of interventions by the trainees. The above-listed elements might help to shift the responsibility for some of the mental health tasks to non-mental-health personnel, though much of the responsibility of the management of severe and complex mental disorders is likely to remain with specialized personnel and a well-organized care system. This in turn means that the training and employment of mental health personnel remains important and cannot be circumvented by shifting tasks to other categories of personnel.

The paradigm of primacy of primary health care

The notion of task shifting is closely related to the paradigm of primacy of primary health care, which states that emphasis of health service development should be on strengthening primary health care even if this means relative neglect of specialized services and a decreased priority for basic or applied scientific work. The origin of that paradigm can probably be traced back to the years after World War II during which simple interventions—such as spraying with insecticides which could be done by untrained workers—saved lives of millions of people from malaria, typhus, and other insect-borne diseases. In remote regions of the Soviet Union, for example, simply trained staff known as *feldschers* proved their worth in the years that followed World War I and subsequently did very well dealing with the prevention of communicable diseases, introducing hygienic measures and health education, and providing first aid to the wounded. In some other countries similarly trained personnel (e.g. the 'barefoot doctors' of China) helped decrease morbidity and mortality from illness. Similar schemes were put into operation in various other countries and reports of these successes in China, Cuba, Guatemala, India, Indonesia, Niger, Tanzania, and Venezuela published in 1975 (17) prepared the ground for a meeting of Ministers of Health and numerous experts in Alma Ata in 1978. The Alma Ata conference produced a report and a declaration listing the 10 essential ingredients of primary health care. The declaration and the report stated a number of principles that should govern the organization of primary health care (2). Most of these were ethical desiderata which could be used to strengthen the case for the introduction of mental health programmes and could serve as a boost for psychiatrists (18). The definition of primary health care, however, contained also the phrase that primary health care should include elements which '. . . the countries can afford', allowing countries to do little about primary health care if they decided that they 'could not afford' to introduce it.

At this point WHO and governments in most countries viewed primary health care as the answer to the world's health problems. Many drafted health policies based on primary health care principles, and made significant efforts to reform the health care system so as to be congruous with the principles of the Alma Ata declaration. As could be expected, it was easier to draft policies than to implement them, and the follow-up of the Alma Ata declaration was in many places reduced to lip service to the principles it announced.

While the notion of strengthening primary health care has significant merit it also has a dark side, namely reducing support to the development of specialized health care. This was particularly harmful for disciplines that were largely ignored previously and because of this policy became even more retarded in their development. Pediatrics, despite its obvious importance in a world in which half the population consists of children and adolescents, was one of the neglected disciplines. Psychiatry was in a similar situation. In both instances neglect of the specialty reduced the possibility of enhancing knowledge and translating it into tools for use in primary and general health care.

The paradigm of spontaneous destigmatization

The changes of opinions and attitudes relating to leprosy, tuberculosis, and sexually transmitted diseases are examples of the destigmatization of diseases that occurs when an effective treatment has been discovered and applied. It was the hope of many decision-makers, social scientists, and mental health specialists that the same would happen with mental disorders. Good treatment would lead to a reconstitution of mental functions (and thus the disappearance of reasons for the stigma) and make people with mental disorders acceptable by society.

This paradigm continues to have defenders, although stigma of mental illness persists despite the range of effective, or partially effective, treatments that have emerged in the past six decades. While cognitive therapy and pharmacotherapy may not be perfect, they are now available as routine treatment options in developed countries. Medications prescribed to the mentally ill are better (in terms of reduction of symptoms and prevention of relapses) than medications for the treatment of various physical illnesses that are not stigmatized (19). Nevertheless, the stigma of mental disorders has not diminished, and may even be more pronounced. Recent reports indicate that people with mental illness experience stigmatization in all walks of life and are additionally burdened with self-stigmatization (20,21). The reasons for failure of this expectation and of the paradigm based on it are not well understood, but seem to include a number of factors. Psychiatrists have still not arrived at a consensus about the best ways of treating mental illness. Schools of psychiatry argue publicly against treatments whose effectiveness they question and, consequently, diminish the credibility of the specialty of psychiatry and its armamentarium. Some treatments appropriate for specific psychiatric disorders have been used too widely. Their inappropriate use not only failed to help patients and harmed some of them but also reduced faith that the treatment offered by psychiatrists was effective. Another reason for the persistence of stigma despite effective treatments is the reluctance of patients with mental illness to disclose information about their illness or to talk about its treatments, regardless of whether it was effective or not. The good news about the effective treatment of mental illness is thus not spread by people who experienced it, a situation very different from that in the field of physical illness and its treatment. While a surgical intervention leading to recovery from a potentially lethal illness is usually widely praised by fortunate patients, a parallel scenario has only recently become a reality in psychiatry. At last, there is an increasing number of testimonies from well-known people—such as the prime minister of Norway—who now discuss their mental illness and its successful treatment. Unfortunately, on the other hand, the failures of mental health treatments—confirming a previously widespread prejudice—seem to be of far more interest to the media than their successes.

Among reasons for the failure of the paradigm could also be the well-organized antipsychiatric propaganda by groups such as the Church of Scientology and the recent actions of producers of psychotropic medications. The latter have, in recent years, adopted the strategy of pointing out the weaknesses or side effects of the competitors' drugs in order to sell their own. As a result, the credibility of all medications used in psychiatry has been diminished and the prevailing opinion about them in the mind of the general public, and health workers in the fields other than psychiatry, is that they are unlikely to help and are often harmful. A further consequence of the image of dangerousness of psychotropic mediations is that GPs and specialists in other branches prescribe psychotropic drugs in doses far too low to achieve an effect, which contributes to their poor opinion about these drugs. An institutionalized example of this tendency is the recommendation of a nursing association about the treatment of depression—to treat it by giving patients a non-therapeutic dose of an antidepressant.

The paradigm of destigmatization by the demonstration that psychiatric disorders can be successfully treated could still be saved if all those involved—patients, their families, psychiatrists, and other health care workers—were to place more emphasis on presenting the positive outcomes of psychiatric treatment in a realistic manner. While admitting weaknesses, they should highlight and assemble evidence as a basis for a consensus about the best treatment for specific mental disorders. This will not remove all stigma, but is likely to diminish it.

The paradigm of single-disease morbidity

The 1960s were marked by a growth of interest in public health aspects of psychiatry— a development that seems to have stemmed from vestiges of military medicine which was successfully using mass approaches to the promotion of health during World War II and in the decade that followed it. This interest found its expression in the increasing number of epidemiological studies of mental disorders, in the strengthening of the involvement of schools of public health in mental health, in the creation of non-governmental organizations focusing on mental health (rather than mental disorders), and in studies of functioning of mental health services. Gradually, the emphasis has moved to the study of specific diseases using biological methods and to issues related to the treatment of mental illness—both probably related to the introduction of new psychopharmacological agents in the treatment of mental disorders. Chlorpromazine and similar medications and, somewhat later, antidepressants, seemed to open the door to a psychiatry practised in a manner similar to other branches of medicine. Initially this new psychopharmacotherapy targeted symptoms; somewhat later, the indications for treatment were defined in terms of disorders. Many educational guidelines for practice described what needs to be done to recognize and manage specific disorders At the same time the general advances of medicine and the reduction of morbidity from communicable diseases gradually led to the disappearance of physical disease wards (for tuberculosis, cerebral malaria, encephalitis, etc.) that had been obligatory parts of mental hospitals until then. This trend contributed to the tendency to neglect comorbid physical illness in psychiatric practice. The neglect of comorbidity of mental and physical illness also reflected, in part, the traditional and enduring separation of psychiatry from other medical disciplines.

The descriptions of mental disorders in textbooks of psychiatry give an impression that diseases appear one by one: the notion that the form, treatment, and outcome of a disorder depend on what other conditions might be present received very little attention. The biopsychosocial approach introduced by Engel in the mid-1970s argued that psychological, biological, and social factors play a role in health and disease: but despite the apparent comprehensiveness of this approach the focus of much research and service development remained based on the paradigm of single-disease morbidity. Problem-based education introduced in some of the medical schools in the late 20th century did expect students to look at patients in their entirety; yet in most instances psychiatric problems were conspicuous by their absence in the descriptions of problems that were used in such training.

The neglect of comorbidity of mental and physical illness is harmful for patients, whether their 'primary' illness is physical or mental, and for the discipline of psychiatry.

The prevalence of comorbidity grows with age but it is present at all ages. It is now becoming closer to a rule rather than an exception. Yet psychiatrists seem to focus their attention on the comorbidity of mental disorders (to a large extent an artefact of the currently existing classification rules) and are reluctant to look for illnesses that are not their specialty. Specialists in other disciplines do the same, with consequent poorer outcome of treatment and a greater frequency of complications in the course of treatment (22–28) The single-disease paradigm needs to be discarded and replaced by a comorbidity paradigm. Findings of research in recent years indicate the high (and growing) prevalence of comorbidity, and experience from practice shows that a comprehensive approach covering all the diseases that a person might have at the same time is necessary. It is clear that the appropriate management of comorbidity will require major changes in the organization of services for people with mental illness and in the education of all types of health personnel. This is a challenge for governments but also for specialists of all types—a challenge that has to be met at a time when comorbidity is becoming more frequent, and while medicine is increasingly fragmented. For psychiatry this reorientation will be beneficial—not only because it will make it possible to provide better care to people with mental illness but also because a change of its practice will bring it back to other branches of medicine from which it has been separated for a long time—to the loss of both medicine and psychiatry.

The paradigm of parity of care for people with mental and those with physical illness

People with mental illness are disadvantaged in many ways. Stigmatization prevents their access to housing, employment, and social activities. The stigma of mental illness implies that people suffering from mental illness are of no value to society and that they will not recover from their illness. Medications which are used in the treatment for mental illness are wrongly considered to be very expensive (and governments are reluctant to provide them) although there are many other types of medications (e.g. medications used in the treatment of cancer) that are much more costly yet do not have the reputation of expensiveness. In many countries—including the United States until very recently—the treatment of mental illness is reimbursed less well than treatment for other diseases. Schooling for children with intellectual impairments is less well supported than schooling for children who suffer from other types of disability. The reimbursement for a day of treatment in a psychiatric institution is lower than that for other diseases. It is therefore not surprising that one of the paradigms of health care for the mentally ill today is that governments and insurance companies should introduce parity of care for people suffering from mental and other diseases. Parity in terms of reimbursement for treatment has been considered an important principle and achieving parity continues to be a goal of a number of non-governmental organizations.

Yet, that paradigm has also been gradually eroded. People with mental illness are often poor and less well educated than their peers. They frequently have few social skills and their families are more likely to be dysfunctional. Their knowledge of the law and of the regulations that govern health care are usually non-existent. Thus, even when equal access to health care is guaranteed by law and when services are available, people with mental illness will use them less well than people who have other illnesses. In addition the very symptoms of mental illness—and previous experience, sometimes of coercion and abusive treatment, in contact with health services—make many of those suffering from mental disorders reluctant to come forward and ask for help.

It follows that aiming at equal access to care is not enough: mental health services must have additional means to provide care and the goal should no longer be equal access to care (29)—but care sufficient in quality and quantity to arrive at the best possible outcome. This replacement of the paradigm of parity by a paradigm of sufficient care (or a paradigm of equal outcome) will require legislative and other action—but the first step should undoubtedly be the acceptance of the fact that the goal that was pursued with so much vigour in many places is not sufficient to offer an equitable model of health care.

The paradigm of psychiatry's responsibility for the promotion of mental health and the prevention of mental disorders

Public health is inseparable from politics, and nowhere is this truer than in mental health. For example, the cold war between the United States and the Soviet Union (and their respective allies) found its reflection in the definition of the legitimate area of psychiatry and of its methods of work. The emphasis on the biological origin of mental disorders and treatment using 'biological methods' was the accepted doctrine of treatment in the Soviet Union and its satellites, while psychoanalysis and other psychodynamic approaches predominated in the United States and Western Europe. In parallel with this difference of opinion was also the difference in the definition of the legitimate tasks of psychiatry. The prevention of mental disorders and the promotion of mental health were seen as essential components of psychiatry and mental health sciences in the West; in eastern Europe the promotion of mental health was seen as a task of the government whose duty was to create a health-promoting environment and to provide regulations that will optimize the physical, mental, and social development of the citizens and make them live a life of good quality. The difference between the Eastern and Western blocks also found its expression in the definitions of quality of life. In the Soviet zone of influence quality of life was defined as the satisfaction of (mainly material) human needs—such as shelter, food, health care—while on the other side of the Iron Curtain the definition emphasized the feelings of the individual whose quality of life was assessed, rather than the degree to which the human needs were met. Thus, for the Western scientists it was important to assess whether an individual is happy to have (or not have) a job, not only whether he has one. Some of the human rights were also interpreted differently, Thus, for example the right to work was interpreted in the Eastern block as the obligation of the state to provide jobs for everyone; in the Western block the right to work was interpreted as the right to be considered for a job and get it if qualified and if there is a job available.

The difference in the definition of psychiatry as a discipline was further confounded by the differences in the definition of the promotion of mental health. While the Western countries considered that promotion of mental health is best seen as an increase of the value that people give to their mental health, in the Eastern block the promotion of health meant a decrease of the prevalence and incidence of mental diseases.

Worldwide the prevention of mental and neurological disorders was given relatively little attention and the prevailing opinion was that little can be done to prevent these disorders. A notable exception to this position was the sterilization of the mentally ill in a number of countries, but this practice was gradually abandoned, particularly after the horrors perpetrated in this respect in Nazi Germany. Various other practices were supposed to prevent dysfunctionality of families and consequent higher risks for mental disorders in children, but there was little consensus about the best measures to take and little evidence that such interventions were useful.

In time it became accepted that most of the prevention of mental disorders cannot be the sole responsibility of mental health services, but rests mainly with other parts of the health and social system. In the 1980s a report to the World Health Assembly of WHO summarized possibilities for prevention of mental disorders (30–32). The report and its recommendations were well accepted by governments and a follow-up 2 years later indicated that some action was taken. The report drew attention to a variety of measures which could significantly reduce the incidence of mental and neurological disorders, including the provision of adequate perinatal care, prevention of brain injury by the obligatory use of helmets by cyclists and motorcyclists, provision of iodine to women before and during pregnancy, education of parents, arrangements for the education of children with intellectual impairments, correction of sensory deficits (e.g. of vision) and others—all with fairly good evidence of effectiveness. More recently a variety of other measures have been tested and recommended. The paradigm of responsibility of psychiatry for the promotion of mental health and the prevention of mental disorders will thus also need to be reformulated. Psychiatry can recommend measures and interventions to prevent brain injury and other risks to mental health, but the responsibility for the application of these measures has to be with the general health care and social service system. The promotion of mental health, in the sense of raising the value that people give to mental health, must also be the responsibility of other social agents such as schools, producers of educational media, parent organizations, and social services The formulation of legal instruments that will support the promotion of mental health and the prevention of mental illness will remain the area of responsibility of governments. Psychiatry can at best identify risk factors that may lead to mental disorder and draw attention to them so that appropriate action can be taken.

Coda

The past 50 years have been rich in events and developments that have affected psychiatry in developing and developed countries. Science has produced new knowledge about the functioning of the brain and put in place new methods of investigating its function. Psychopharmacology has created effective medications that can be used in the provision of mental health care. New and effective methods of psychotherapy (such as cognitive behavioural and interpersonal psychotherapy) have been introduced and it has been demonstrated that they can be used with significant effect in different social and cultural settings. The doors have thus been opened to further scientific investigations and to a major change in the practice of psychiatry.

These and other scientific and medical developments have been happening in the context of major changes affecting the world's societies. Among them, globalization, emphasis on economic productivity at the cost of social and cultural progress, rural–urban and intercountry migration, and changes of demographic structure of societies have been particularly important for psychiatry and its applications. They have led to an erosion of some of the paradigms on which psychiatry and mental health services have been based. Emphasis on community care, on parity of access to mental health services, and on shifting of tasks from specialized to general health services are among paradigms that need to be reviewed and revised—as well as those that emphasize single-disease morbidity in psychiatric practice and teaching and the primacy of primary health care.

It is clear that optimal approaches to mental health service development will not be immediately possible in all settings and that they may have to be somewhat adapted to fit local conditions. Yet, in contrast to what happens today, the inability (or reluctance) to immediately introduce the optimal solution would not lead to the acceptance of second-rate, suboptimal solutions but to efforts to make the application of the best possible. In a vast majority of countries the introduction of the correct answer to mental health problems is a matter of moving resources from one budgetary line to another; in some countries—and their number is very small—external help is necessary and could be requested on humanitarian and scientific grounds. An essential step in this strategy is to do whatever is possible to arrive at a consensus about the optimal solutions to mental health problems and disorders based on evidence and experience, and involving all concerned—the psychiatrists, other mental health workers, the mentally ill and their families, and general health care workers. It is to be hoped that reaching that consensus (which psychiatry has not even attempted to do so far) will be recognized as a priority for the further development of mental health care and psychiatry worldwide.

References

1 Sartorius N. (2009). Medicine in the era of decivilization. *Works of the Croatian Academy of Sciences and Arts* 504, Vol. XXXIII, Medical Science. Zagreb: Hrvatska Akademija Znanosti I Umjetnosti, pp. 9–28.

2 World Health Organization (1978). *Declaration of Alma Ata*. Report of International Conference on Primary Health Care, Alma-Ata, USSR, 6–12 September 1978, Geneva: World Health Organization.

3 World Health Organization (1981). *Global Strategy for Health for All by the Year 2000*. Geneva:World Health Organization.

4 Shorter, E. (1997). *A history of psychiatry*. New York: John Wiley and Sons.

5 Berios, G. and Porter, R. (eds) (1995). *A history of clinical psychiatry*. London:Athlone Press.

6 Scull, A. (2005). *Madhouse*. New Haven, CT: Yale University Press.

7 Leff, H. (1997). *Care in the community: Illusion or reality?* Chichester: John Wiley and Sons.

8 Kleinman, A. (2009). Global mental health: a failure of humanity. *Lancet* 374, 603–4.

9 Talbott, J. and Hales, R. E. (eds). (2001). *Textbook of administrative psychiatry: new concepts for a changing behavioural health system* (2nd edition). Washington: APPI Washington.

10 Thornicroft, G. and Tansella, M. (2013). The balanced care model for global mental health. *Psychological Medicine* **43**, 849–63.

11 World Health Organization (1984). *Mental health care in developing countries: a critical appraisal of research findings. Report of a WHO Study Group.* Technical Report Series 698. Geneva: World Health Organization.

12 Weiss, K. J. (2012). Psychiatry for the general practitioner. *Journal of Nervous and Mental Diseases* **200**, 1047–53.

13 Sartorius, N. and Harding, T W. (1983). The WHO Collaborative Study on strategies for extending mental health care, i: the genesis of the study. *American Journal of Psychiatry* **140**, 1470–3.

14 Eaton, J., McCay, L., Semrau, M. et al. (2011). Scale up of services for mental health in low-income and middle-income countries. *Lancet* **378** (9802), 1592–603.

15 Saraceno, B. and Dua, T. (2009). Global mental health: the role of psychiatry. *European Archives of Psychiatry and Clinical Neuroscience* **259**(Suppl 2), 109–17.

16 Levav, I., Kohn, R., Montoya, I. et al. (2005). Training Latin American primary care physicians in the WPA module on depression: results of a multicenter trial. *Psychological Medicine* **35**, 35–45.

17 Newell, K. (ed.) (1975). *Health by the people.* Geneva: World Health Organization.

18 Sartorius, N. (1997). Psychiatry in the framework of primary health care: a threat or boost to psychiatry? *American Journal of Psychiatry* **154**(6 suppl. Festschrift in Honor of Melvin Sabshin, MD), 67–72.

19 Leucht, S., Tardy, M., Komossa, K., et al. (2012). Antipsychotic drugs versus placebo for relapse prevention in schizophrenia: a systematic review and meta-analysis. *Lancet* **379**(9831), 2063–71.

20 Beldie, A., den Boer, J. A., Brain, C., et al.; Sartorius, N. (ed.) (2012). Fighting stigma of mental illness in midsize European countries. *Social Psychiatry and Psychiatric Epidemiology* **47**(Suppl 1), 1–38.

21 Thornicroft, G., Brohan, E., Rose, D., Sartorius, N., and Leese, M. (2009). Global pattern of experienced and anticipated discrimination against people with schizophrenia: a cross-sectional survey. *Lancet* **373**, 408–15.

22 Leucht, S., Burkard, T., Henderson, J. H., Maj, M., and Sartorius, N. (2007). *Physical illness and schizophrenia. a review of the evidence.* Cambridge: Cambridge University Press.

23 Katon, W., Maj, M., and Sartorius, N. (2010). *Depression and Diabetes.* Oxford: Wiley-Blackwell.

24 Glassman, A., Maj, M., and Sartorius, N. (2010). *Depression and heart disease.* Oxford: Wiley-Blackwell.

25 O'Hara, J., McCarthy, J., and Bouras, N. (2010). *Intellectual disability and ill health: a review of the evidence.* Cambridge: Cambridge University Press.

26 Gordon, A. J. (2010). *Physical illness and drugs of abuse: a review of the evidence.* Cambridge: Cambridge University Press.

27 Kissane, D. W., Maj, M., and Sartorius, N. (2011). *Depression and cancer.* Oxford: Wiley-Blackwell.

28 Kurrle, S., Brodaty, H. and Hogarth, R. (2012). *Physical comorbidities of dementia.* Cambridge: Cambridge University Press.

29 Johansen, C., Dalton, S.O. and Bidstrup, P.E. (2011). Depression and cancer—the role of culture and social disparities. In. Kissane, D.W., Maj, M. and Sartorius, N. (eds.) *Depression and cancer.* Oxford: Wiley-Blackwell, pp. 207–20.

30 **World Health Organization** (1988). *Prevention of mental, neurological and psychosocial disorders*. Report by the Director-General to the 39th World Health Assembly, and WHA resolution 39.25. Geneva: World Health Organization.

31 **Jenkins, R. and Ustun, B.** (1998). *Preventing mental illness*. John Wiley and Sons, Chichester.

32 **World Health Organization** (2004). *Prevention of mental disorders—effective interventions and policy options. Summary Report*. Geneva: World Health Organization.

Fifty years of mental health legislation: paternalism, bound and unbound

George Szmukler

As far as society is concerned, the insane are 'in it' but not 'of it' (1).

Introduction

This is the conundrum. A person seems badly in need of treatment, but fails to recognize it and rejects it. How can one reconcile involuntary detention and treatment with that person's right to liberty? From one perspective, treatment for which there are strong or even compelling reasons is obstructed by an anti-therapeutic legal straight-jacket. From the other perspective, legal protections are crucial as fundamental civil liberties are being violated in what looks like a form of social control. A distinctive mental health law has developed in most countries aiming to achieve an acceptable balance between these competing frameworks. This law attempts to construct and regulate relationships between those involved (2). Some argue that this legally formed 'mental health system' may no longer serve the interests of the mentally ill.

The focus of this essay is the law governing involuntary treatment. I restrict myself to the civil sphere and will not consider the law relating to mentally disordered offenders. Nor will I be dealing with medical law relating to such matters as confidentiality or negligence. As mental health law has been most elaborated in Europe, the United States, and Australasia, most attention will necessarily be devoted to these countries. However, I intend not to ignore their influence on, or relevance for, low-income countries.

To make sense of the changes in the law over the last 50 years or so, and the challenges it presents today, it is necessary to go back a century or so. Past solutions to the problems noted above shape the mental health laws of today. The same dilemmas trouble us. However, the old solutions now face major challenges—partly due to the changing spaces in which mental health care occurs, and partly due to changes in thinking about 'human rights'.

Another point seems worth making by way of introduction. This concerns variation. Much variation occurs in the specific content of mental health law between countries and states; this obviously reflects different social, cultural, and legal histories. But even more striking are differences in the rates of involuntary treatment. A 30-fold difference in rates has been found between states in the European Union (3). Even allowing for different national methods of data recording, the variation must remain large. There is also variation in rates of involuntary hospitalization between provinces within the same state having the same mental health law, and even the same service template—for example, a five-fold difference has been reported in Sweden. Clearly there is large variation in how a law is implemented, with large scope for discretion on the part of the actors involved.

A final question might be asked by the reader as we examine changes over time and in different places: what can we expect from such law?

The distinctive nature or 'exceptionalism' of mental health law

The general contour of today's law governing involuntary treatment emerged in the 19th century. Unsworth (1), following the French historian Castel, dates this from the early 19th century. The *'relation de tutelle'* was Castel's term characterizing a special legal structure for mental disorder (4). Set down in the law of 1838 in France, and reflecting an ascendant liberal-democratic order, it was a solution created to deal with a social problem—how to manage individuals who were unable to participate in rational exchange in a social contract, who at the same time cannot be held responsible for their actions. The tutelary relationship represented a 'special subordinate legal status', filling a space that law did not enter, in which the person became subject to a regime of (principally) medical paternalism. Unsworth offers a 'telling characterization of this relegated status' by quoting the Chairman of the 1924–26 Royal Commission on Lunacy and Mental Disorder, H.P. Macmillan, who stated 'that when the fate of the mentally disordered was in question, what was at stake was something more subtle than rights'.

The tutelary relationship defines the system of legal relations between family, doctors, administrators, and the judicial system. Over time, the balance of power within this set of relationships has see-sawed. The most prominent shifts have been in the range of discretion given to doctors against legal regulation (or 'legalism'). Instability in the system also arises around the boundary between those who should be accorded full legal status but are wrongly detained as 'insane'; or how far those designated as 'insane' nevertheless should be accorded full legal status.

This form of law has in essence endured; it is noteworthy in this regard that the French law of 1838 was not revised until 1990, and even then its form did not change very substantially. It was revised only in 2011 after being ruled by the Conseil Constitutionnel to be inconsistent with the constitution.

A brief look at the 19th and early 20th centuries

Lunacy treatment in the 18th century was diverse and essentially unregulated. Laws embodying the 'tutelary relationship' were developed in Europe and the United States in the setting of the expanding 19th-century asylum system. During this period insanity and detention were practically synonymous. The early enthusiasm for 'moral treatment' in the late 18th and early 19th centuries failed to live up to its promise, while, due to major social changes largely related to industrialization, the numbers of those detained in the asylums grew far beyond what was originally envisaged. While psychiatry established itself as a professional discipline in the context of the asylum, management became more and more custodial and scandals increasingly publicized. The view that insanity represented the late stages of an incurable degenerative process became common.

Admissions, generally effected under case law and involving the family and a doctor for those who could pay, or a magistrate and a doctor for paupers, were increasingly challenged. (In the case of the latter, the role of the magistrate was more about the allocation of public funds than the interests of the pauper.) The need to preserve the privacy of the family and to avoid shame was prominent. Earlier concerns about the protection of the sane from wrongful detention were, over time, joined by concerns about the protection of the insane while detained. Piecemeal accretions to the case law—such as regulations requiring signed medical certificates, medical entries in the records, or the establishment of inspecting bodies (such as the Lunacy Commission in 1845 in England[1])–were seen as inadequate, and eventually culminated in new statutes. The French law of 1838 was the first comprehensive statute of this kind. Most statutes were enacted in the late 19th century or early 20th century. Such statutes, in different states, established varying legal relationships between medical discretion, the administrative machinery (covering admissions, discharges, and inspections) and the judiciary (certification, notification of admissions, appeals).

While this turn to enhanced 'legalism' occurred in a number of jurisdictions, there were large differences between states. In the first half of the 20th century, in some countries medical judgement coupled with a family member's application for treatment continued to form the basis for admission, with discharge occurring when the family was ready to receive the patient. Medical paternalism was generally the dominant mode in European countries. Even in countries where a magistrate or court was involved, (e.g. Italy, Spain) what happened subsequent to admission was a medical responsibility. In the United States, the turn to legalism (or greater constraint on medical discretion) was more marked. A court hearing was usually required, while some states required a trial by jury before a mentally ill person could be involuntarily committed. Detention in jail prior to a hearing was common, especially in states without laws covering emergency admission. Procedures were often cursory, however; for example, the patient not being present at the hearing. Certification was generally tantamount to legal incompetence, depriving the person of control of all their significant affairs.

The history of *voluntary* inpatient treatment in a public mental hospital is relatively recent (for those who could pay, voluntary treatment was for a long time possible in the private sector). Jurisdictions began to introduce 'voluntary' status in the early 20th century, in part with the hope that early treatment would result in better outcomes. In the Netherlands this became possible in 1904; in Victoria, Australia in 1916; in England not until the passing of the Medical Treatment Act in 1930 (although there were ways of

---

[1] Scotland and Northern Ireland have had their own mental health laws since 1707 and 1921 respectively whereas Wales has shared the same laws with England; Wales is included in any reference to England in this essay.

achieving it earlier), and in Italy, not until a special decree in 1968. In the United States, most states provided for voluntary admission by the 1930s.

The situation in the 1950s

In 1950 legislation in Western countries comprised in varying combinations the following: the powers to detain and treat; for whom (though 'insanity' was generally undefined as it was presumably regarded as obvious); by whom (usually family, doctors, and an administrator—for example a préfet, mayor, or public prosecutor—and, perhaps later, a magistrate or judge); for how long (usually unspecified); checks on medical powers following admission (usually few); inspection regimes; reviews (usually reports to an administrative authority); appeals (usually none, although recourse could sometimes be taken to the law of habeas corpus, or its equivalent). Some statutes, like the Lunacy Act 1890 in England, included protections against legal action against doctors as long as they acted in good faith.

The 1950s saw a major change in outlook in some, mainly anglophone, countries on the proper balance of powers that should be in play. A new optimism emerged concerning the role of psychiatry, the effectiveness of treatment, and the likelihood that patients would be reintegrated into the community following a period in hospital. Outpatient clinics multiplied. Psychiatry received a boost to its legitimacy as a medical speciality founded on scientific principles following the introduction in the early 1950s of chlorpromazine, a drug that could reduce psychotic symptoms. The numbers of patients in asylums started to decline (arguably unrelated to medication) and admissions became shorter and much more likely to be voluntary. The antidepressants imipramine and iproniazid were introduced in later in the decade. New psychosocial interventions, such as the 'therapeutic community' and 'milieu therapy' also appeared promising. There was talk of a 'therapeutic revolution'.

Unsworth (1) argued that equally important, with England as an example, was the emergence of the 'welfare state'–a newly forged system of social and health reform aimed at ensuring a minimum of protection for all while putting an end to 'poor law' residues and their associations with stigma and disqualification. This shift in policy in favour of benevolent social interventionism involved substantial reliance on informal methods of control and a diminished emphasis on legal procedures. A 'therapeutic' optimism at the political level chimed well with that at the psychiatric level.

In England, a Royal Commission on the Law Relating to Mental Illness and Mental Deficiency, chaired by Lord Percy, sat from 1954 to 1957. It concluded that mental disorder should be regarded in the same way as physical illness, and that hospitals for mental illness should be run in much the same way as those for physical illness. The 1959 Mental Health Act, passed with substantial parliamentary consensus, reflected these principles. Judicial certification was seen as stigmatizing and was removed. Admissions to psychiatric hospitals were to be 'informal' wherever possible, without a patient signature confirming willingness. The emphasis on informal treatment supported an ideal of a contractual therapeutic relationship with the patient taking greater personal responsibility. A better outcome, sustainable on discharge to the community, would follow. Links between mental health services and social agencies were also addressed. Involuntary admissions were to be primarily a medical matter following an application from the nearest relative or a social worker, but the patient, if placed on a long-term treatment order, could appeal to a Mental Health Review Tribunal, chaired by a lawyer and having an independent psychiatrist member. 'Mental disorder' was defined as 'mental illness, arrested or incomplete development of mind, psychopathic disorder, and any other disorder or disability of mind'. Much discussion concerned 'psychopathic disorder'. It was eventually included if falling within the following definition: 'a persistent disorder or disability of mind . . . which results in abnormally aggressive or seriously irresponsible conduct . . . and requires or is susceptible to medical treatment'. The criteria for admission or treatment were that it was necessary in the interests of the patient's 'health or safety, or for the protection of others'.

A similar optimistic turn occurred in the United States. A Draft Act Governing Hospitalization of the Mentally Ill was published in 1949 (revised in 1952) by the National Institute of Mental Health as a model for state legislation. Voluntary treatment, it proposed, should be the norm. The process of admission should facilitate successful treatment, not impede it. Eliminating stigmatizing procedures characteristic of the criminal justice system was thus important. Recommended criteria for admission were either 'because of his illness the patient is likely to injure himself or others' or because the patient 'is in need of care or treatment . . . and because of his illness, lacks sufficient insight or capacity to make responsible application'. Hospitalization, the Draft proposed, should be placed in medical hands, two physicians certifying its need. Such hospitalization could be indefinite, but the patient could request a prompt court hearing, with legal representation, to consider the case for discharge. Emergency admissions could be effected by an application from any person and confirmed by a single physician. The Draft further proposed that patients could be sent home on convalescent status, from which they could be readmitted without judicial review. A number of states adopted the model almost entirely or in significant part (5).

A similar confidence in medical beneficence was evident in Australia. For example, the 1959 Mental Health Act in the state of Victoria empowered the superintendent of any hospital and the authorized medical officer to consent to any surgical or medical treatment on behalf of any patient, whether involuntary or voluntary, and without any need to determine whether the patient was competent to decide. The only external review of any decision to detain and treat was by way of habeas corpus proceedings in the Supreme Court.

In continental Europe at this time there appears to have been little legislative activity. For example, legislation in France, Belgium, Greece, and the Netherlands dated from the 19th century. If the optimism surrounding new psychiatric interventions did not lead to new legislation, then at least there seemed no reason to interfere with a general mode usually favouring medical paternalism.

Disillusionment, 'anti-psychiatry', and the civil rights movement: law reform in the United States

However, within a decade or so, strong winds began to blow in an opposing direction. The optimism of the postwar period began to appear misplaced. The United States was first to react (6).

Highly publicized scandals involving mental hospitals continued to occur. At the same time, evidence appeared in both the academic and popular spheres that 'total institutions' like mental hospitals, in which almost every aspect of the inmate's life is ordained according to the institution's aims, far from being therapeutic places, actually contribute to a dehumanizing erosion of identity encouraging dependence and disability. Goffman's 1961 *Asylums*, Barton's 1962 *Institutional Neurosis*, and Wing and Brown's 1970 *Institutionalism and Schizophrenia* were influential texts in this regard.

Joined to these criticisms was another set of voices doubting or denying the legitimacy of the psychiatric enterprise itself. Key figures in this 'anti-psychiatry' movement included three psychiatrists—Thomas Szasz, R.D. Laing, and David Cooper. Szasz held that 'mental illness' was a 'myth' and had no kinship with 'real' illness; what were called mental illnesses were 'problems of living', not brain diseases. They represented a designation by which society attempted to control through medicalization—including detention in hospital—people who were deviant through breaking social, moral, or legal norms. From a rather different perspective, Laing and Cooper also rejected the medical model of mental illness. They argued that insanity was in fact an understandable reaction of some people with heightened sensibilities to impossible family pressures or even to a world gone insane. The 'schizophrenic' experience, they claimed, handled correctly, could be transformative. Conventional treatment was certainly not the right way. These ideas fitted well with the anti-establishment 'counterculture' of the 1960s and 1970s from which they drew further support.

Another figure linked with the 'anti-psychiatry' movement was Michel Foucault. His *Histoire de la Folie*, first published in 1961, and translated in a much abridged form into English in 1965 as *Madness and Civilization*, carried in this translation a polemical introduction by David Cooper. Cooper was also invited by Foucault to give lectures at the Collège de France in the 1970s, and in his 1973 lecture series Foucault allied himself with 'anti-psychiatry'. He emphasized the power of the psychiatrist over madness—calling it 'illness' disqualified the patient's voice, and qualified the psychiatrist to intervene, diagnose, restrain, direct, and govern (7). However, *Madness and Civilization* was not conceived as an anti-psychiatry text, but as an exercise in historical epistemology—examining how the idea of 'mental illness' assumed the status of 'positive knowledge' in the context of changes in society and its expectations of productive citizenship. Although doctors had been closely involved with private madhouses in the 18th century, the asylum provided the condition for the development of psychiatry as a discipline. (This can be seen in the United Kingdom, for example, in the changing title of the journal for asylum doctors: *Asylum Journal* in 1853; changed to *Asylum Journal of Mental Science* in 1854; *Journal of Mental Science* in 1859; *British Journal of Psychiatry* in 1962.) Though it was presented as a medical discipline, Foucault argued its expertise was largely exercised through practices developed for the normalization of certain sorts of 'unordered' behaviours that transgressed social or moral codes. The book was a forerunner of Foucault's later work on forms of 'discipline' ('moral treatment' being an example), part of the machinery of social control in the modern bureaucratic state. At the very least, Foucault overturned a complacent narrative of the care of the insane as being unambiguously marked by progressive improvement.

Although these writers differed significantly in their approaches and theories, they had in common a critique of psychiatry's basic assumptions, its purposes, and of the institutions in which it was practised.

A further significant influence was the civil rights movement in the United States, increasingly effective in the 1960s and 1970s (6). Starting with the assertion of civil rights for African Americans, it spread to other groups subject to discrimination or social exclusion—prisoners, women, people with mental illness, and those with disabilities. An essential instrument in making progress was the law, with a number of key legal decisions ushering in changes in institutional practices. The US Supreme Court was roused into activity. In the case of mental illness, a new literature proliferated, while professorships in 'psychiatry and the law', later highly influential, were created. Increasingly publicized abuses of psychiatry in the Soviet Union during the 1970s and early 1980s seemed to point to the fact that unless involuntary hospitalization was the subject of special scrutiny, serious injustice could follow.

Finally, departments of health faced fiscal pressures arising from the need to refurbish decaying public hospitals neglected since the Great Depression and World War II. Added to the fact that the largest item on the state health budget was usually mental health, and the largest proportion of mental health expenditure was consumed by institutional care, a reduction of inpatient care was attractive. The landmark case of *Wyatt v Stickney* in the United States in 1972 that forced the state of Alabama to upgrade its substandard mental hospitals was further cause for fiscal alarm. The proposal from a number of eminent psychiatrists that outcomes would be better if treatment were focused in the community rather than in hospitals was also welcome. (Some have argued that professional support was driven significantly by the wish to resolve the contradiction between the therapeutic, 'truly medical' function of psychiatry and the distasteful custodial one.) One means of reducing hospitalizations was by tightening the regulation of involuntary admissions. The forces leading to the policy of deinstitutionalization here overlapped with those acting to reduce recourse to involuntary hospitalization. Some noted an 'unnatural alliance' between the civil libertarians, who distrusted the state and psychiatric expertise, and conservatives, who were concerned with the high institutional costs of mental health care.

The result of these forces was a radical overhaul of the laws governing civil commitment in the United States (6). Such action became limited, for example, only to individuals who were imminently likely to be dangerous to themselves or others, as evidenced by recent overt acts. Dangerousness to self could include an inability to meet basic needs (e.g. for food, clothing, shelter or personal safety) so severe that the physical health of the person was endangered. The historic 'need for treatment' standard was abandoned. In the mid-1960s new legislation was introduced in Washington DC and California. Soon state and federal courts in landmark decisions, such as *Lessard v Schmidt* in 1972, ruled that the 'need for treatment' standard was too vague. As well as the narrowing of criteria governing commitment, procedural safeguards were revised, adopting many of those characteristic of the criminal justice system. In both legal systems, it was argued, deprivation of liberty was at stake, and thus comparable rigour was necessary. Thus various combinations of features characterizing 'due process' such as rights to precommitment investigation for probable cause, subpoena of witnesses, representation by an attorney, right to silence, exclusion of hearsay evidence, and standards of proof from 'clear and convincing evidence' to 'beyond a reasonable doubt', were adopted. The concept of the 'least restrictive alternative' was widely accepted. By the end of the 1970s every state had greatly narrowed the legal criteria permitting involuntary commitment.

Soon, however, some US jurisdictions began to consider that narrow dangerousness-based criteria were excluding too many patients from hospitalization who seemed on commonsense grounds to require involuntary treatment. There was talk of patients 'dying with their rights on' and of psychiatry being 'belegalled'. In 1979 Washington was among the first states to relax its criteria to include persons whose deterioration to a dangerous level was predictable. The meaning of 'dangerousness' became subject to broader interpretation. Massachusetts legislation included within its scope a person who, based on treatment history, was in need of treatment to prevent further disability or deterioration predictably resulting in danger to self/others and was unable to make informed decisions concerning treatment. By 2005, while dangerousness remained the major grounds for detention, about one-half of the states had included eligibility criteria based on the need for treatment given the likelihood of relapse and danger of some kind (in Colorado extending to those in need of care because of pending loss of support from a relative who is a caregiver).

A further development in the United States was the realization that 'refusal of treatment' could be regarded as a separate action following the execution of involuntary hospitalization, one that required separate adjudication. Detention was seen as serving the state's interest in protection, which did not necessarily extend to treatment. Legislation thus provided for a separate decision about treatment competence that could be made by a court or an administrative process involving independent decision-makers. Thus a person could be detained, yet his or her treatment refusal, if made with decision-making competence (or capacity), might be respected. (The question of treatment refusal and consent is considered later.)

Reform beyond the United States

Europe

During the late 20th century, most western European countries also implemented reforms governing involuntary hospitalization and treatment, though generally adopting less narrow criteria than in the United States and less permeated by procedures imported from the criminal system.

Although the drivers of change were similar to those in the United States, a further influence on member states of the Council of Europe was, and continues to be, the European Convention on Human Rights (ECHR) drafted in the aftermath of World War II by the newly formed Council of Europe in 1950 (8). The ECHR is overseen by the European Court of Human Rights and the Council of Europe. Ratification is compulsory for all member states. Most pertinent have been articles concerning the right to liberty—subject only to arrest or lawful detention (including persons of 'unsound mind'); the right to a trial or hearing by an independent and impartial tribunal, within a 'reasonable' time for those detained; and the prohibition of torture or 'inhuman or degrading treatment'. A wide latitude has been granted thus far by the Court for the last, resting on the notion of 'medical necessity'.

Further international legal rights instruments exist, of course, most notably the two treaty-based binding United Nations covenants within the United Nations system of the International Bill of Human Rights. These are the Covenant on Civil and Political Rights and the International Covenant on Economic, Social and Cultural Rights, adopted in 1966 (though entering into force a decade later). They, however, do not focus explicitly on the rights of persons with mental disabilities. In 1991 the United Nations produced the non-binding Principles for the Protection of Persons with Mental Illness and for the Improvement of Mental Health Care ('MI principles'). (The 2006 *UN Convention on the Rights of Persons with Disabilities* is discussed later)

In some countries, another factor leading to reform was a dissolving consensus in the 1970s for the welfare state. A liberal, individualist, market-based philosophy began to emerge. A new legalism, aimed at limiting state intrusion in individuals' affairs, followed. England was the first to reform legislation. The 1970s saw an effective campaign led by Larry Gostin, an American civil liberties lawyer, who became the legal officer for Mind (a charitable organization providing a range of psychiatric services and representing the interests of patients). Patients came to be legally represented in some key test cases; both in domestic courts and the European Court of Human Rights, lawyers started to represent patients before Mental Health Review Tribunals, and a widely publicized Mind report, *A Human Condition*, set out the case for civil rights-based reform of the 1959 Mental Health Act. Indeed, mental health was at the forefront of test case advocacy both in the United Kingdom and in Europe. The result was the Mental Health Act 1983 for England and Wales. However, compared to changes in the United States, criteria were less dangerousness-based and procedures less legalistic. Involuntary hospitalization for treatment was justified if the person suffered from a mental disorder of a nature or degree making medical treatment in hospital appropriate, and admission was necessary for the 'health or safety' of the patient, or for the 'protection of other persons'. The review process was tightened—patients could appeal while on either short-term 'assessment' or longer-term 'treatment' orders, but if they did not do so, a hearing occurred automatically after 6 months. The review body was the three-person Mental Health Review Tribunal chaired by a lawyer. The 1983 Act also accorded roles to other professions—particularly, social workers and nurses, in effect acting as further checks on medical discretion.

Most European states passed new mental health legislation in the late 1980s and 1990s. That in Austria, Belgium, the Netherlands, Germany, and Northern Ireland most resembled US statutes with a relative emphasis on dangerousness, and court-ordered detention (9). In Germany and the Netherlands, as in in the United States, there was a separation of criteria for detention and treatment, with treatment refusal being possible for detained patients with mental capacity. On the other hand, countries including Denmark, Sweden, Finland, Norway, and Ireland passed laws during this period that allowed admission to be primarily founded on the 'need for treatment'. A routine judicial review, unless the patient appealed, might not occur at all in some countries, or if mandated, might not occur for between 1 and 3 months.

What constitutes 'mental disorder' or 'mental illness' in legislation has usually been more or less undefined and left to medical expert opinion. Sometimes the terms 'serious', or 'psychosis' appear, or some of the more disruptive clinical features generally associated with psychosis. Generally, a severity threshold has been denoted by a statement along the lines that the person's illness warrants treatment in hospital.

In general, forcible measures after involuntary hospitalization, such as restraint, seclusion, or medication, are not regulated by legislation; documentation (sometimes with requirements set out in supplementary regulations or forms of guidance), noting the reasons for the intervention and who made the decision, is the usual form of oversight.

A few countries deserve special mention for their unusual aspects. In France, the law of 1990 continued two separate pathways to involuntary detention (and treatment) first laid down in the law of 1838. The first, Hospitalisation à la Demand d'un Tiers (HDT), is at the request of a family member or a person acting in the interests of a person who requires immediate treatment in hospital but is unable to consent. The request must be supported by medical certificates attesting to the need. The second, Hospitalisation d'Office (HO), is carried out via a police order issued by a préfet (the State's representative in local government and responsible for security, safety, and ensuring respect for legality), and covers a person whose mental disorder jeopardizes law and order or public safety. Discharge from a HO is by the préfet. These two pathways distinguish the two elements that are usually combined in most mental health laws—the risk to self and the risk to others. A revision of the law in 2011 preserves the two modalities of admission but now includes a review by a judge if the patient is still detained continuously in hospital for 15 days.

In Spain, under a law of 1931, involuntary psychiatric admission required the authorization of a judge. However, since the introduction of a new health law in 1986, Spain has had no separate specific mental health law. The General Law of Health covers all illnesses. A patient's consent to treatment is not required when they are not capable of making such a decision. No special legal procedure is laid down. However, under the Civil Code, deprivation of liberty, as in involuntary admission to hospital, cannot occur without judicial authorization. A judge visits and examines the patient in hospital.

Italy stands out for its radical mental health reform in the late 1970s (10). Law 180, passed in 1978 (replacing legislation of 1904), stated that involuntary treatment must be used only as a last resort, and is only applicable for those in imminent need of treatment who refuse it and where no less restrictive alternative exists. Dangerousness to others was explicitly eliminated as a criterion. The law also ordered a process of deinstitutionalization; construction of new mental hospitals was prohibited, and a deadline was to be set beyond which new admissions could not occur to such hospitals. This law was inspired by the charismatic Dr Franco Basaglia. Like Goffman, he concluded it was impossible to separate the damage due to mental illness from the segregation, exclusion, and dehumanization of the hospital. Simply unlocking the doors of the asylum was insufficient; new ties had to be established with the community. Through alliances with trade unions, progressive political parties, and neighbourhood organizations, relations between patients, staff, and the community were transformed. Eventually his hospital at Gorizia closed and became a new social space for general community activities.

Other countries

Statutes in Australasia in the 1980s and 1990s, in general, followed similar lines to those in England (though New South Wales was more like the United States in being more oriented towards the risk of serious harm and formal due process). Criteria for involuntary admission and treatment in 12 mental health acts in Canada covered a similar range as in Europe, though probably being more dangerousness oriented and 'due process' based (as in the province of Ontario) than European states. An analysis of mental health legislation from diverse Commonwealth jurisdictions showed a clear trend over time in favouring protections for patient 'autonomy' (11).

However, beyond westernized, high-income countries (and some of their former colonies), legislation did not develop in similar ways—or at all. The World Health Organization (WHO) in 2005 reported that 22% of 173 countries (accounting for 30% of the total world population) did not have mental health legislation. Only one-half had laws passed after 1990, and nearly one-sixth had legislation dating back to the pre-1960s. This was despite binding international 'rights' instruments mentioned earlier, and including regional charters such as the African Charter on Human and People's Rights (1981), and the evidence that mental disorder carries a huge burden of disease. In introducing a *Resource Book on Mental Health, Human Rights and Legislation* in 2005, WHO painted the worldwide picture in stark terms:

> There are more than 450 million people with mental, neurological or behavioural problems throughout the world. In many countries, they are among the most vulnerable and the least legally protected. . . . In some communities, people with mental disorders are tied or chained to trees or logs. Others are incarcerated in prisons without having been accused of a crime. In many psychiatric institutions and hospitals, patients face gross violations of their rights. People are restrained with metal shackles, confined in caged beds, deprived of clothing, decent bedding, clean water or proper toilet facilities and are subject to abuse . . . people with mental disorders often face social isolation and severe stigmatization . . . including discrimination in education, employment and housing. Some countries even prohibit people from voting, marrying or having children.

A shadow over the practice of psychiatry

A shadow was cast over the practice of psychiatry by its systematic abuse for political purposes in the former Soviet Union. Mounting evidence emerged in the 1970s of the involuntary incarceration of political dissidents labelled as suffering from mental illness (12). Following discharge 'patients' could be placed on a psychiatric register and were then subject to compulsory recall for examination. According to the journal *Ogonek*, in 1988 there were 10 million names on this register.

There was no formal mental health law; civil commitment was based on various administrative orders and decrees issued by the Ministry of Health in coordination with the Procurator's Office and the Ministry of Internal Affairs, most of which failed to conform to the USSR constitution. Vaguely described conditions or 'illnesses' associated with 'social danger' were listed. A single doctor, above any objection by the family, could order admission, but this had to be later approved by a panel of three psychiatrists. No judicial review was available. Criminal commitment procedures were subject to cursoriness where 'mental illness' was concerned. Podrabinek (13) stated there was an official view that in criminal cases the defence has no need for psychiatric witnesses of its own, because 'there is no reason to doubt the impartiality of the psychiatrists assigned by the Ministry of Health'.

Bonnie (14) identified two factors as especially significant in understanding the coercive behaviour of psychiatrists in the Soviet Union; psychiatrists were state employees who were regarded as having a special responsibility to the state (e.g. expressed in an oath swearing guidance by the 'principles of communist morality'), and the absence of a professional identity with an explicit or implicit code of practice.

With perestroika came an admission of abuses. An interim mental health law in 1988 was followed by a comprehensive Law on Psychiatric Care in 1992 containing a full range of procedural safeguards, advocacy, reviews, and so on. A report in 2004, *Human Rights and Psychiatry in the Russian Federation*, compiled by the independent Moscow Helsinki Group, concluded that in the majority of centres judicial control was not working. Given resource-starved services it is not surprising that the survey concluded there was a 'violation of not only the right to decent living conditions and adequate therapy, but also the violation of even the most fundamental rights to safety, voluntarism, and human dignity'.

Most eastern European countries now have mental health laws, often modelled on those of the West and variably compliant with the ECHR. But procedures tend to be cursory. Lack of resources allocated to mental health services lead to continued unacceptable practices, some of them gross. Particularly troubling are the conditions in long-stay 'social care homes' where many residents are subject to arbitrary detention and degrading treatment (15).

Addictions

There is not the space to deal in detail with legislation specifically directed at the involuntary treatment of people with addictions. While a substantial minority of countries have legislation of this type, there is enormous variability in intent (for treatment of acute problems or for long-term rehabilitation) and even if the legislation exists, its implementation. An influential historical example was legislation in California and New York in the 1960s associated with the establishment of so-called 'narcotic farms' for long-term treatment of addicted persons. These were abandoned after becoming essentially custodial, expensive, and of uncertain value in terms of achieving improvement. In some countries, mental health law excludes people from involuntary treatment on the basis solely of an addiction (in the absence of a supervening complication such as delirium, psychosis, or depression). In most countries, mandatory treatment for addictions is mainly exercised through the criminal justice system, usually via the courts following conviction for an offence. 'Drug courts', where the person is given the option of treatment instead of the usual penalty, are becoming increasingly common. An important tension has existed, especially since the early 20th century, between the view that the addicted person is sick and needs treatment (advocated for the past half-century by WHO), or is a free agent who has made a morally culpable and punishable choice. A coherent approach to involuntary treatment has consequently been difficult to establish.

A new development: involuntary outpatient treatment

Since the 1980s it has been increasingly agreed that the law needs to change if it is to keep pace with developments in psychiatric practice. In keeping with a growing focus on care in the community, provisions for involuntary treatment outside hospital have been introduced in a number of jurisdictions. By 2011, 42 States in the United States, 5 countries in Europe, and most states in Australasia and provinces in Canada had specific involuntary outpatient treatment (IOT) statutes. In some other countries, older legislation has been used, sometimes controversially, to achieve similar ends.

Some forms of IOT constitute a 'less restrictive alternative', allowing commitment to outpatient treatment instead of inpatient treatment, or by permitting earlier conditional release from inpatient commitment. Other forms of IOT may allow 'preventive commitment'. This is the most controversial since it may allow the compulsory treatment of a patient who is not currently at risk. Based on recurrent relapses following treatment discontinuation, and of dangers previously evident when ill, compulsion is used to avert future anticipated risk.

The scope of IOT powers varies widely. They nearly always include a requirement on the patient to accept treatment (even if this is not matched by a power to forcibly medicate the patient in the community). They may include a direction that the patient accept visits from clinicians and attend appointments; a direction as to where the patient should reside (e.g. in a hostel); an authority for a clinician to enter the patient's residence at reasonable times and for purposes directly related to treatment; the power to recall the patient to hospital (e.g. if compliance with conditions placed on the patient by the IOT order are breached, or if early signs of relapse are detected); and, to provide involuntary treatment in a hospital or clinic where such treatment may be safely and appropriately be given.

The transition from an asylum to a post-asylum phase of psychiatric treatment taxes conventional thinking about the limits of involuntary treatment. Ethical criticisms have included potential violations of human rights, such as privacy; the potential to distract attention from the quality of community services and to undermine the development of non-coercive approaches for engaging reluctant patients; the possibility that fears of involuntary treatment may deter patients from seeking treatment; and the limited range of treatments that can be enforced, some being perhaps suboptimal (e.g. relying on drugs that can be given by intramuscular injection). There are also concerns (supported by some evidence) that outpatient orders may lead to an increase in the overall use of compulsion, since unlike inpatient commitment, there is no 'ceiling' imposed by a finite number of available beds on the numbers on compulsory orders. The elasticity of the concept of 'risk', and its potential to encompass a broadening range of behaviours seen by the community as troubling and needing to be controlled, is a further concern.

It is noteworthy that in relation to IOT a new kind of discourse on legal interventions has arisen in public debate—the 'evidence base' for its effectiveness. The 'therapeutic jurisprudence' movement has argued for some years for looking at evidence of the impact of the law on the health of those subject to it, aiming to minimize the harms and maximize the benefits. However, this kind of discussion has not been widely adopted. Despite attempts to evaluate the evidence in relation to IOT there has been a lack of agreement about what it says concerning its effectiveness in, for example, reducing admissions, reducing patient violence, or improving psychosocial outcomes. The same studies, including randomized controlled trials, are interpreted quite differently by different investigators (16). One begins to wonder whether, when feelings run high on opposing sides, any consensus on evidence is possible.

How significant the evidence base should be as an argument for the use of a species of legal instrument in which moral issues (such as liberty) are central is another question. It could be argued that if no benefit is gained, the case against is much strengthened; however, if some benefit is shown—to society as a whole, perhaps by reducing violence—does such a finding have justificatory value?

The start of the 21st century: autonomy, rights, and non-discrimination

Informed consent (or its converse, refusal), as understood in general medical practice, has played a subsidiary, or commonly, no role in relation to involuntary treatment in psychiatry. The 'exceptionalism' of mental health legislation to which attention was drawn at the beginning of this essay resides in large part in this absence—an absence that is understandable if we recall the social context of the 19th-century origins of this kind of law.

We have seen there are some jurisdictions where there is a separation of detention and involuntary treatment, and where the patient does have the right to refuse treatment even though involuntarily hospitalized. The patient's capacity to refuse is separately determined and if the patient is found incompetent, non-consensual treatment can be given. There are two difficulties here: first, what is the justification for detention in a hospital, presumably thus serving a health interest, if treatment cannot be given; and, second, in what sense can a patient who is detained in hospital, 'voluntarily' consent to treatment? In the view of many, myself included, this practice is difficult to justify.

In some jurisdictions, where detention and treatment are not separated, the inability of the patient to consent (usually vaguely specified) may sometimes be a criterion for involuntary treatment, but it is nearly always the risk of harms that is determinative (17). The major international instruments—the UN Principles for the Protection of Persons with Mental Illness, the ECHR, and the 2004 Council of Europe Recommendations concerning the human rights and dignity of persons with mental disorder—affirm the primacy of risk in relation to involuntary hospitalization.

But when considered in the context of general medicine, current practices of involuntary treatment, with or without a separation of detention and treatment, are frankly discriminatory. Such recognition has led to proposals that decision-making capacity, and the respect for the 'autonomy' or self-determination of the person that this serves, should be at the heart of a determination that involuntary treatment is justified (18,19).

Before examining this issue further, I need to briefly touch on a complex area. The *relation de tutelle*, originating in the 19th century and mentioned in the introduction, placed the person in the asylum more or less fully under the supervision of the doctor who could then effectively make decisions for the patients concerning virtually all of their affairs—medical, financial, social, and so on. In many jurisdictions in Western countries, usually in the later decades of the 20th century or early 21st century, the control of matters unrelated to treatment has been separated off, and is usually dealt with under a form of 'guardianship'. For example, this occurred in France in 1968 in relation to the law of 1838. The Mental Health Act 1983 in England and Wales narrowed the sphere of guardianship permitted under the 1959 Act, and in 2005 a Mental Capacity Act was passed dealing comprehensively with the interests of such persons. The point here is that impaired decision-making capacity, nowadays assessed separately for each specific decision required of the person, is the key justification for guardianship. Such law, whether through statute or through case law, usually covers the non-consensual treatment of persons with an impairment or disturbance of mental functioning when the condition is 'physical' (non-psychiatric) and is considered by doctors to be in the person's best interests: an example would be the amputation of a leg due to gangrene in someone who is confused and resisting following a head injury sustained in an accident. (It must be added though, that the articulation between civil commitment and 'guardianship' legislation, where the two coexist, can be ambiguous.)

When comparing the legal criteria for the involuntary treatment of persons with 'physical' disorders and 'mental' disorders, we note a divergence. The former patients can only be treated against their will if they lack the capacity to make a treatment decision, and then, only if the treatment is in their 'best interests'. Notions of 'best interests' vary, but behind them in most conceptualizations is the idea that it is the patient's perspective that counts. For example, were the patient able to consider their current predicament while, hypothetically, briefly recovering capacity, would they accept the treatment? Or, through consulting with those who know the patient well, could one deduce what the patient would have chosen in the light of their previously expressed values and preferences? An advance directive obviously provides strong support. (It is interesting to note here that the majority of states in the United States have introduced 'psychiatric advance directives'. However, the patients' instructions can be 'trumped' by civil commitment laws. Furthermore, in many cases they can be overridden by the clinician if following those instructions were to lead to a failure to match 'acceptable' standards of treatment. Obviously, the force of the advance directive is thus considerably weakened, while raising the question of why such a limitation should be placed on psychiatric advance directives, and not on those made by other patients receiving medical care. The subject is highly controversial.)

It is increasingly being asked why there should be a difference in the approach to patients with mental disorder compared to those with a physical disorder? Why are the criteria based on 'risk' for the former, and not decision-making capacity? Why is autonomy not respected in the same way? Seen from this perspective, conventional mental health legislation discriminates unfairly against people with mental illness. What justification can there be for a health interest intervention in a person's life, against their wishes, other than an impairment of their autonomous decision-making capacity? The person with capacity is best placed to decide what is in their best interests, all things considered.

The argument then is for capacity-based legislation. But it can go further. If lack of capacity similarly justifies involuntary treatment for both physical and mental disorders, it may not be necessary to have separate mental health legislation at all; all that is required is a single statute that covers involuntary treatment (in the best interests) of any person who lacks decision-making capacity, from whatever cause (dementia, head injury, schizophrenia, delirium, confusion following haemorrhage) and in whatever health care setting, indeed including the community (as in IOT). Such legislation would be non-discriminatory and spell the end of the 'exceptionalism' of mental health law and vestiges of the old tutelary relationship.

The theme of discrimination is further evident in developments in thinking about human rights. The UN Convention of the Rights of Persons with Disabilities 2006 (CRPD) gives clear expression to these in relation to people with mental disabilities, including mental illness. It contains the classic array of liberal rights, such as the right to liberty, integrity of the person, freedom from torture and inhuman treatment, as well newer socio-economic rights that have come to prominence since World War II, including the right to home and family life, to education, and to health. There is also a specific collection of rights particularly relevant to people with disabilities, including the right to independent living and community inclusion, to work and employment, and to be free from exploitation and abuse. Two articles are especially relevant to involuntary treatment—all persons shall 'enjoy legal capacity on an equal basis with others in all aspects of life'; and, 'the existence of a disability shall in no case justify a deprivation of liberty'. Considering the application to psychiatric detention, the Office of the UN High Commissioner for Human Rights stated in 2009:

> . . . this must include the repeal of provisions . . . authorizing the preventive detention of persons with disabilities on grounds such as the likelihood of them posing a danger to themselves or others, in all cases in which such grounds of care, treatment and public security are linked in legislation to an apparent or diagnosed mental illness . . . the legal grounds upon which restriction of liberty is determined must be de-linked from the disability and neutrally defined so as to apply to all persons on an equal basis.

Most current mental health legislation would thus be ruled out. A comprehensive capacity-based statute would, it could be argued, constitute a 'neutrally defined', non-discriminatory basis for involuntary treatment. All persons, whether they have a pre-existing disability or not, may develop a lack of capacity as a result of an illness causing a disturbance of mental functioning. However, some mental health advocacy groups have gone as far as to argue that the CRPD effectively abolishes involuntary treatment altogether.

Reference to advocacy groups draws attention to another significant development, especially since the 1990s: the emergence of the 'voice' of the patient (also referred to as the 'consumer' or 'service user'). I can do no more here than briefly mention what may become a growing influence on mental health policy and service development. This voice can be seen as linking back to a key criticism of psychiatry by the 'anti-psychiatry' movement. Foucault, for example, can be seen as being concerned with the silencing of the patient's voice. How powerful this voice will be in affecting changes in mental health legislation remains to be seen. To date the influence in this particular respect (in contrast to its significant effects on the shape of mental health services) has been quite minor.

There is a sociopolitical development essentially acting in an opposing direction to legislation supporting autonomy, rights, and non-discrimination. This is the emergence of what has been termed by sociologists, such as Beck (20) and Giddens (21), the 'risk society'. A feature of 'modernity' is that societies are changing at an unprecedented rate, generating insecurities about 'manufactured' hazards, that is, those resulting from human agency. Consequently there is a growing orientation to the future and safety. A good deal of political decision-making is concerned with managing risks, even risks that do not originate in the political sphere. Risk thinking is clearly evident in mental health policy, especially in England, the United States, Australia, and more recently, France. Risk in psychiatry is perceived as deriving from the shift from institutional to community care. A preoccupation with preventing bad things happening leads to legislation characterized by provisions for detention, registers, surveillance, monitoring, and supervision for people judged as 'risky' (22). Professional practice changes in ways that are beyond the control of its practitioners, as mechanisms of accountability are imposed to reassure the public that protective measures are fully engaged. The increasing prominence given to training in 'risk assessment' is an example.

Persons with mental illness often enter the frame for such an attribution of 'risky', reflecting the commonly held stereotype that they are dangerous. Amendments to the Mental Health Act in England and Wales in 2007 reflect an increasing concern with public protection: criteria for compulsion have been broadened (e.g. now including personality disorder, without qualification as in the previous Act) while considerable discretion is given to doctors in authorizing involuntary treatment in the community and its associated conditions (e.g. requirements to take medication, not to use drugs or alcohol, place of residence). The risk-based criteria in mental health law that govern inpatient involuntary treatment do not translocate readily into community settings. Such criteria, for instance, as 'the health or safety of the patient' or 'the protection of others' formerly had to reach a level that warranted detention in hospital, but when they can be applied to what is acceptable in the community, may assume a very broad meaning.

Conventional mental health legislation, when using 'risk to other persons' as a criterion for involuntary admission or treatment, again discriminates against people with a mental disorder. In liberal-democratic states the law generally only allows detention of people after they have committed an offence (or are seriously suspected of having done so). But people with a mental disorder constitute an exception—they can be detained (in hospital) solely on the basis of the risk they are deemed to pose. However, if detention is to be regarded as acceptable on the basis of putative 'risk' alone, then the level of that risk should determine liability to detention, not whether the person has a 'mental disorder' or not. Fairness demands that all people presenting an equal risk should be equally liable to detention. Then, what should be done to reduce that unacceptable risk should depend on the characteristics of the person: if the person has a treatable illness and lacks capacity—or retaining capacity, consents to the treatment—this would be the course to take. If the person did not have a mental illness, another course of action would be required—for example, anger management training for a spouse abuser, an alcohol programme for a habitual drunken driver, or a custodial sentence for a suspected terrorist. Fairness then entails some form of generic preventive detention legislation—or no preventive detention for anyone, including those with a mental disorder.

Concluding remarks

The last half-century has witnessed significant shifts in the balance of power between actors involved in involuntary admission and treatment. In the 1950s medical discretion was often favoured, but by the 1970s a new 'legalism' became more prominent. The extent to which legalism outweighed medical paternalism varied in different jurisdictions, reflecting a range of historical, social, cultural, and political factors—for example, libertarian traditions, the perceived legitimacy of psychiatry, hospital scandals, confidence in the welfare state, traditions of resistance to state intrusions, the pace of deinstitutionalization, the place given to mental health in social policy agendas, fiscal pressures, and so on. However, few jurisdictions remained untouched. In the latter years of the 20th century and early 21st century, criteria were sometimes relaxed, while psychiatry gained more respect as new research technologies (e.g. in genetics and brain imaging) made their mark. The introduction of involuntary treatment in the community marked a major transition in the psychiatric legal landscape, highlighting important questions concerning the translation of regulations appropriate to a hospital era to the community. At the same time, a significant number of countries remain without civil commitment legislation.

To what extent, though, do changes in legislation affect practice? Studies in the 1970s and 1980s examining the impact of new dangerousness-based civil commitment in the United States and Canada found a reduction in the number of involuntary admissions in the short-term, but after 2 years or so, numbers were back to previous levels (6,23). It appeared that decisions were being made according to intuitions about what was appropriate, with wide latitude in how the legislation was interpreted. This applied as much to judges and legal representatives as to psychiatrists. Some have argued that an increase in the mentally ill homeless and imprisoned resulted from restrictions on civil commitment. However, this does not sit well with the research evidence above, and is more likely to reflect concurrent changes in mental health services, especially reductions in the number of hospital beds, tighter admission policies, and briefer stays. But causal relationships are not straightforward. Despite unchanged legislation, England saw a 60% increase between 1987 and 1997 in the number of involuntary admissions. A 'moral panic' about the risk posed to the public by mental patients 'released' as a result of community care was probably significant here. At the same time there was a 40% reduction in compulsory admissions in Sweden. Some provinces in Italy, mainly in the north, saw a reduction in involuntary admissions following the Law of 1978, but there were concomitant service changes demanded (but not always met) by that law. In all places, the social construction of what counts as 'mental disorder' that needs containment will influence which (troublesome) groups of people may be so designated. The impact of legislation on involuntary detention is thus complex, is probably not major, and depends on the nature of services as well as the social context.

Looking at mental health legislation across time and place, it becomes clear that its impact depends fundamentally on the quality of available mental health care. Where services are rudimentary and resources lacking, legislative intentions may be short-circuited or even ignored. In such places the 'voluntary' admission rate may approach a difficult-to-believe 100%. Well-constructed legislation in the absence of decent mental health services is like 'mustard without the meat'. Across the European Union, spend on mental health varies from 2% to 14% of the health budget. We have seen that in states where human rights are not high on the agenda, legislation has provided few safeguards.

What about prospects for the future? As described in the previous section, there are now two major currents in mental health legislation. The first flows in the direction of patient 'autonomy' and, as in the UN Convention on the Rights of Persons with Disabilities, emphasizes legal capacity, non-discrimination, and 'positive' socio-economic rights. Stronger voice is given to the patient. The 2005 WHO *Resource Book on Mental Health, Human Rights and Legislation* argues for the routine incorporation of rights clauses in mental health legislation. Whether this might be effective in improving the position of people with mental disorders is uncertain. It may instead amount to not much more than an expression of a reformist ideology of mental health care or a rallying call for ethical practice. Participation in the community requires access to goods, services and supports—'socio-economic' rights—that were not much addressed when care was hospital based. However, rights legislation to date, such as the ECHR, has been better at protecting people from state intrusion (supporting so-called 'negative' rights), for example, by strengthening safeguards against inappropriate detention, than in ensuring the provision of 'positive' rights. It is also unclear how far the law should venture into standard setting; resources thus diverted by the law into one service area may mean less being available for others, including some that may be just as important, or even more so.

The second current pushes in an opposite direction, emphasizing the reduction of 'risk'. To date 'risk' has exercised some societies more than others, but if the sociologists are right, is likely to spread in 'late modern' societies. Legislation influenced by risk emphasizes formal risk assessment, risk management, prevention, incapacitation through detention, monitoring, and surveillance—thus restricting rights supporting autonomy and self-determination. A proposal in England in 1999 for the indeterminate detention, even in the absence of effective treatments, of persons with 'dangerous severe personality disorder' is an example. The emphasis on risk changes professional practice, imposing new obligations and accountabilities. A risk 'lens' also affects patients and their carers in subtle ways—for example, through a 'looping effect' (24), where classifications of people affect the way those classified come to understand themselves and to behave accordingly, and the way others come to understand them and behave towards them. Little appreciated is the huge overestimation of risk, where even the best instruments are wrong more than 9 times out of 10 for cases of serious violence (25). The debate in England, starting in 1999 and lasting almost a decade, about the form new mental health legislation should take, and which ended with a set of amendments rather than a new Act, illustrates the tension between the two currents (26).

Predicting the direction the law will take is foolhardy, particularly as it will be subject to unforeseeable social changes in highly uncertain times. If forced to bet, I think reducing risk will outweigh other considerations. Unsworth (1) concludes his political-historical investigation thus:

> It would seem that legalism is resorted to at times of pessimism or uncertainty about how society should respond to the problems posed by mental disorder. Faith in procedure provides a substitute for conviction as to the 'solution' to these problems.

I am unsure whether a future risk policy will lean on legalism in this manner, or whether it will be judged as better served by allowing greater professional discretion but effectively reined in and controlled through tight accountability mechanisms, such as standardized assessments, forms, certificates, documentation, audit, and so on. This is the genre adopted in the amended English Mental Health Act in 2007. Whichever approach is adopted, the rights of persons with mental illness are likely to suffer. As discussed above, an emphasis on reducing risk is usually associated with the discounting of the rights of persons with mental illness.

What can be predicted with confidence is that the subject of involuntary treatment will continue to generate much controversy.

References

1 Unsworth, C. (1987). *The politics of mental health legislation.* Oxford: Oxford University Press.

2 Fennell, P. (1986). Law and psychiatry: the legal constitution of the psychiatric system. *Journal of Law and Society* **13**, 35–65.

3 Salize, H. J. and Dressing, H. (2004). Epidemiology of involuntary placement of mentally ill people across the European Union. *British Journal of Psychiatry* **184**, 163–8.

4 Castel, R. (1976). *L'ordre psychiatrique: l'âge d'or de l'aliénisme.* Paris: Éditions de Minuit.

5 Appelbaum, P. S. (2000). Commentary & analysis: the Draft Act Governing Hospitalization of the Mentally Ill: its genesis and its legacy. *Psychiatric Services* **51**, 190–4.

6 Appelbaum, P. S. (1994). *Almost a revolution: mental health law and the limits of change.* New York: Oxford University Press.

7 Rose, N. (1986). Psychiatry: the discipline of mental health. In: Miller, P. and Rose, N. (eds.) *The power of psychiatry.* Cambridge: Polity Press.

8 Bartlett, P., Lewis, O., and Thorold, O. (2007). *Mental disability and the European Convention on Human Rights.* Leiden: Martinus Nijhoff.

9 Salize, H. J., Dreßing, H., and Peitz, M. (2002). *Compulsory admission and involuntary treatment of mentally ill patients—legislation and practice in EU-member states.* Final Report. Mannheim: Central Institute of Mental Health.

10 Scheper-Hughes, N. and Lovell, A. M. (1986). Breaking the circuit of social control: lessons in public psychiatry from Italy and Franco Basaglia. *Social Science and Medicine* **23**, 159–78.

11 Fistein, E. C., Holland, A. J., Clare, I. C., and Gunn, M. J. (2009). A comparison of mental health legislation from diverse Commonwealth jurisdictions. *International Journal of Law and Psychiatry* **32**, 147–55.

12 Bloch, S. and Reddaway, P. (1977). *Russia's political hospitals: the abuse of psychiatry in the Soviet Union.* London: Victor Gollancz.

13 Podrabinek, A (1980). *Punitive medicine.* Ann Arbor: Karoma.

14 Bonnie, R. J. (1990). Soviet psychiatry and human rights: reflections on the report of the U.S. Delegation. *Law and Medical Health Care* **18**, 123–31.

15 Lewis, O. (2002). Mental disability law in central and eastern Europe: paper, practice, promise. *Journal of Mental Health Law* **6**, 293–303.

16 Churchill, R., Owen, G., Singh, S., and Hotopf, M. (2007). *International experiences of using community treatment orders.* Department of Health: www.dh.gov.uk/en/ Publicationsandstatistics/Publications/PublicationsPolicyAndGuidance/DH_072730.

17 Dawson, J. and Kampf, A. (2006). Incapacity principles in mental health laws in Europe. *Psychology, Public Policy and Law* **12**, 310–31.

18 Campbell, T. and Heginbotham, C. (1991). *Mental illness: prejudice, discrimination and the law.* Waterbury, VT: Dartmouth.

19 Dawson, J. and Szmukler, G. (2006). Fusion of mental health and incapacity legislation. *British Journal of Psychiatry* **188**, 504–9.

20 Beck, U. (1992). *Risk society: towards a new modernity.* London: Sage.

21 Giddens, A. (1990). *The consequences of modernity.* Cambridge: Polity Press.

22 Rose, N. (1998). Governing risky individuals: the role of psychiatry in new regimes of control. *Psychiatry, Psychology and Law* **5**, 177–95.

23 Bagby, R. M. and Atkinson, L. (1988). The effects of legislative reform on civil commitment admission rates: A critical analysis. *Behavioral Sciences and the Law* **6**, 45–61.

24 Hacking, I. (2002). *Historical ontology.* Cambridge, MA: Harvard University Press.

25 Large, M. M., Ryan, C. J., Singh, S. P., Paton, M. B., and Nielssen, O. B. (2011). The predictive value of risk categorization in schizophrenia. *Harvard Review of Psychiatry* **19**, 25–33.

26 Richardson, G. (2007). Balancing autonomy and risk: a failure of nerve in England and Wales? *International Journal of Law and Psychiatry* **30**, 71–80.

The ethical dimension in psychiatry

Stephen A. Green and Sidney Bloch

Introduction

The origin of medical ethics dates back to the 4th century BC in the form of the Oath of Hippocrates; although the document covers a range of clinical situations, none of them refers to the treatment of the mentally ill (1). Over the next millennium professional and lay attitudes towards mental illness developed erratically, with paternalism as the dominant paradigm. An enlightened approach evolved during the golden era of Arab medicine, in contrast with the later Christian view of madness that focused on witchcraft and demonization. Little attention was paid to ethical considerations of psychiatric care until the evolution of the asylum era in the 18th century. Begun as a well-intentioned transfer of the insane from the street to places of refuge, it degenerated into cruel and dehumanizing treatment. Any benevolent paternalism evaporated as the pressure of growing numbers of patients vitiated what could be offered professionally (2). In stark contrast to what prevailed generally, there were isolated examples of humanism; for example, Philippe Pinel removed patients' chains at the Salpetrière and Bicêtre in Paris, and the Quakers established 'moral treatment' in their own newly-established institution, the York Retreat, in the north of England (3).

In 1791 Thomas Percival (4), a Manchester physician, drafted a code of medical practice that included specific mention of desirable attitudes towards the mentally ill; they were to be treated with 'tenderness and indulgence'. Many of his precepts were replicated in the American Medical Association's (AMA) inaugural code of 1847. More than a century on, this formed the basis of the American Psychiatric Association's (APA) foundation code of ethics in 1973 (5). A couple of years later, the World Psychiatric Association (WPA) launched their first ever initiative in the sphere of ethics, culminating in the Declaration of Madrid, a duty-based code comprising guidelines regarded as fundamental to the ethical practice of psychiatry. This occurred in the context of the systematic abuse of psychiatry in the former Soviet Union, a state-led policy to quell political and religious dissent and render powerless human rights activists.

The 1970s ushered in a small number of publications, including articles by Braceland, Redlich and Mollica, Moore, and Szasz in the United States and a thought-provoking book by Anthony Clare in the United Kingdom. Among the themes canvassed in this literature were informed consent; the right to be treated or to refuse treatment; conflict of interest; confidentiality; the influence of values and the boundaries of mental illness. The next decade witnessed the first textbook, edited by Bloch and Chodoff and devoted exclusively to these and other themes. This multiauthored volume of

18 chapters appeared in 1981 and had gone through four editions by 2009. Following this rather erratic initial phase, the number of publications on diverse aspects of psychiatric ethics has mushroomed to the extent that the first anthology appeared in 2006, reflecting its growing relevance to clinicians and researchers, and signifying a significant academic pursuit in its own right. Due to space constraints the ethical dimension of psychiatric research will not be discussed here; it is well-detailed in *An Anthology of Psychiatric Ethics*, among others (6–13).

Three critical factors which influence psychiatric ethics

Our first step is to introduce three critical factors underlying ethical dilemmas specific to the practice of psychiatry: ill-defined boundaries of the psychiatric profession, the subjective nature of diagnostic criteria, and the inherent power differential in the clinician–patient relationship.

First, the absence of a well-demarcated professional boundary leads to a nebulous role for psychiatrists in terms of what constitutes their legitimate function. The views expressed by two former presidents of the APA reflect this well: Ewald Busse argued for a limited role in which clinicians restrict their attention to the suffering patient, whereas a year later Raymond Waggoner called on his colleagues to pursue lofty 'social goals' and concern themselves with society at large (14, 15).

Secondly, despite the evolution of psychiatry as a scientific discipline since the early 19th century, the profession has continued to grapple with the question of how to define mental illness. In contrast to other branches of medicine, many diagnoses within psychiatry depend only on clinical observation. Inadequate objectivity, dubious reliability, and shifting diagnostic criteria have led to pervasive inconsistencies. For example, the APA resorted to a poll in 1973 to determine the fate of homosexuality as a clinical entity, and intense debate has continued for many years over whether hyperactivity coupled with inattention and lack of persistence in children is a valid diagnosis.

Thirdly, the psychiatrist has been permitted by law to mandate involuntary treatment of some people who suffer or are suspected of suffering from a mental illness. Although commitment statutes have been subject to greater scrutiny in recent decades, uncertainty persists regarding the criteria that should be satisfied for compulsory treatment and whether such compulsion should also be applied in the community setting (16). Moreover, psychiatrists have often had to judge people's clinical needs at the same time as safeguarding their human rights. Civil libertarians have argued that an inalienable right to liberty is paramount in these circumstances, whereas their opponents have asserted that psychiatrists should be able to take measures, including coercion, to protect the interests of both patient and society.

Several issues arising out of the three cardinal features noted above have been addressed by both practitioners and academics, including the professional relationship, the nature of diagnosis, the issue of confidentiality, and several facets of the therapeutic dimension. We will now explore these topics in the context of a long-standing notion of ethics resting comfortably in the paternal arms of Hippocrates but in recent years buffeted by rapidly changing technological, moral, and social forces.

The professional relationship

Ethical values inherent in the relationship

It was not until the 20th century that the moral complexities of the interaction in delivering mental health care were specifically considered. Freud was one of the first to shed light on this in his evolving description of the transference (i.e. redirecting unconscious feelings, thoughts, and fantasies originating in the patient's personal life to the figure of the therapist); his observations highlighted the covert forces and their ethical implications that underpin the association between psychiatrist and patient. Gutheil and Gabbard (17) elaborated on Freud's account and offered supporting guidelines, such as establishing therapeutic neutrality; providing a consistent, private, and professional setting; defining the time and duration of sessions; and minimizing physical contact. They also distinguished boundary 'violations' that fulfil therapists' needs but harm patients, from a benign variant of boundary 'crossings'. An example of the latter is the offer to a patient of a ride home in a blizzard if she has no other means of transport and does not feel coerced. Boundary violations include use of abusive language rationalized as therapeutic confrontation, eliciting compliments or gifts, and sexual exploitation. Given the ongoing asymmetrical quality of the power relationship between patient and therapist, any sexual liaison between a therapist and patient, current or former, has been deemed unethical by several psychiatric and psychotherapeutic organizations.

The role of guild interests

The relationship between patient and therapist is, in addition to ethical guidelines, influenced by the latter's membership of the medical profession. Robert Fullinwider (18), a social philosopher, has defined a profession in terms of three core features. First, its members undergo specialized training, revolving around the acquisition of relevant knowledge and explicit skills. Given this expertise, its bearers anticipate that their recommendations will be addressed. Secondly, professionals assist people who are vulnerable and dependent. Thirdly, 'a trustworthy and effective' group of knowledgeable and skilled experts tend to serve the common good, thus enhancing societal well-being.

For centuries the medical profession determined the degree to which paternalism should pervade their work, resulting in what Katz (19) dubbed 'a silent world' that fostered an enormous power differential between patients and physicians. He rejected the assertion that 'altruism protects patients from abuse of that authority', and argued for promoting patients' autonomous wishes through the process of informed consent.

The profession's selection of educational goals also conveys values that directly affect patients. For example, the re-medicalization of psychiatry in the 1970s, typified by a cleavage between 'psychological' and 'biological' positions, influenced training and the form of care provided by graduates. This was vividly captured in the Osheroff debate (20, 21), which centred on the extended, ineffective psychoanalytic treatment of a patient suffering from severe depression (discussed later in the essay).

Another vital professional responsibility concerns enforcing standards of practice by monitoring members. Since a profession's established values for acceptable and unethical behaviour may be at variance with those held by non-professionals, its guild-based goal to maintain public trust is grounded in procedures designed to preserve organizational integrity.

The tension between ethical values and guild interests within the doctor–patient relationship

Through much of the 20th century medicine remained a self-regulating profession, except for some duties of the modern state such as sanctioning physicians engaged in criminal or negligent practices. Responsibility for monitoring ethical standards has basically occurred within the profession in the context of the interaction between physicians and patients. However, medicine's growing complex association with third parties (e.g. government agencies, private insurance companies), has transformed the therapeutic relationship into one that also includes aspects of the interaction between consumers and providers of health care. The transition to a triadic configuration—psychiatrist/patient/third party—highlights the tension between the goals of maintaining professional values and promoting guild interests. Many clinicians who 'serve two masters' (22) are confronted with ethical challenges that are inherent in these conflicting obligations.

Chodoff (23) discussed the issue specifically in terms of its impact on individual psychotherapy. Acknowledging that most therapists concede a legitimate claim by insurance carriers for particular clinical details about the cases for which they are authorizing payment, he observed how the requirement could undermine patients' trust in therapists not to disclose privileged information. Chodoff's statement was prescient, foreshadowing a slippery slope that resulted in a fundamental change in the trust-based nature of the therapist–patient relationship. Growing incursions into its traditional nature have also curtailed the process of obtaining fully informed consent from the patient by imposing 'gag rules' on the psychiatrist, and limited delivery of necessary care when 'gatekeepers' have refused to authorize certain mental health treatments (24, 25). Moreover, confidentiality has been breached by insurance carriers who require patients to sign blanket disclosure forms, thereby making them (and their therapists) unaware who has access to their medical records (26).

An extreme manifestation of dual or multiple loyalties relates to the role of psychiatry in a totalitarian state. As illustrated by the Nazi experience, the compromise of basic ethical principles that guide the doctor–patient relationship can culminate in horror. Proctor's (27) study of 'racial hygiene' described the situation as it applied to medicine in general, and psychiatry specifically, promoting a philosophy that 'medicalized' anti-Semitism and also resulted in the so-called euthanasia of thousands of mentally ill adults. Cocks (28) provided a detailed account of the perversion of psychiatry by the Third Reich, revealing how patient care and health policies were corrupted by governmental pressure and influenced adversely by clinicians committed to Nazi ideology.

In summary, psychiatry maintains a guild-like insularity, formulating self-defined guidelines that involve ethics in all aspects of professional development—entry requirements, standards of training and practice and criteria for enforced expulsion. Dyer is correct in observing that ethical issues are implicitly but persuasively involved in 'socialization to the norms of the profession' (29).

Confidentiality

The Oath of Hippocrates states: 'What I may see or hear in the course of the treatment or even outside of the treatment in regard to the life of men which on no account one must spread abroad; I will keep to myself holding such things shameful to be spoken about' (1). Accordingly, psychiatrists assure patients that whatever transpires between them will remain confidential. In recent years, however, many forces have limited the capacity of psychiatrists to guarantee absolute confidentiality, and have even raised questions about the moral basis of such assurance.

Bok outlined four premises for justifying confidentiality, beginning with respect for autonomy (30). A person is entitled to have secrets, save when a potential danger threatens; for example, bearing a contagious disease calls for respecting the interests of others. The second premise relates to shared secrets as exemplified in an intimate marriage, although circumstances may arise which warrant disclosing such a secret to other parties. A third premise deals with keeping a promised confidence, but questions may arise concerning situations that could override the obligation. The last premise focuses on professional relationships such as those with priests, lawyers, and doctors who commit themselves to keeping secrets disclosed to them. In the last case, the value of confidentiality is made explicit in that a person is likely to seek help rather than be fearful to ask for it when they are assured of the confidence of their disclosures.

Confidentiality has special relevance in psychiatry. Patients' disclosures are frequently exquisitely personal (e.g. an account of sexual abuse or a shameful act) and psychiatrists are commonly the first and possibly the only recipients of these revelations. The US Supreme Court recognized the centrality of this concept in *Jaffe v. Redmond* in 1995 (116 S. Ct. 1923, 1996). Mary Redmond, a policewoman, had shot and killed a man while on duty, and subsequently began psychotherapy to deal with the trauma. The deceased's relatives sued Ms Redmond and asked to access the therapist's notes; this request was denied on the grounds of the privileged status of the material. The Court ruled that communication between therapist and patient is '... rooted in the imperative need for confidence and trust'.

Despite the *Jaffe* case profession-based confidentiality cannot be absolute, which has raised genuine ethical dilemmas. Topics that have challenged the psychiatrist particularly are a potential breach when a patient threatens to harm another, sharing information with the family carer of a psychotic patient, and tension between the patient's need for complete privacy and the professional's need to advance the field.

The risk of harm to others is arguably the most challenging of these scenarios. In this context, having obtained the patient's informed consent makes a psychiatrist's potential for breaching confidentiality considerably easier to handle since the action stems from a partnership. By contrast, when the patient prohibits the psychiatrist from divulging any personal information or lacks the capacity to arrive at a sound judgement, ethical complications arise. The *Tarasoff* case (131 Cal. Rptr 14, 17 Cal. 3d 425, 551P. 2d 334, 1976), a landmark judgement regarding this issue, was decided by the Californian Supreme Court in the mid-1970s. Tatiana Tarasoff was murdered by a fellow student, Prosenjit Poddar, who had revealed his intention to do so to a psychologist 2 months earlier. Concerned by the prospect of harm befalling Ms Tarasoff, the therapist consulted his colleagues and the police. The latter questioned Mr Poddar and concluded that he did not in fact constitute a threat. A court decision found that in the event of a patient intending to harm an identified person, 'protective privilege ends when the public peril begins'. In other words, the therapist is duty-bound to protect an intended victim if that person can be identified. Criticism of the opinion revolved around the threat *Tarasoff* posed to the integrity of the therapeutic relationship. As Stone (31) proclaimed, imposing a duty to protect would undermine a patient's expectation of confidentiality and so jeopardize treatment.

Although *Tarasoff* became a legislative feature of many jurisdictions in the United States, the precedent has continued to confuse and confound. For example, in the state of Iowa a patient held her own psychiatrist negligent in not preventing her from murdering her first husband; recommended appropriate responses to the duty to protect have brought reason to this complicated picture. Possibly anticipating the uniqueness of each *Tarasoff* situation, jurisdictions outside of the United States, among them the United Kingdom, Canada, and Australia, shied away from legislating or setting a precedent. In the United Kingdom, the Royal College of Psychiatrists produced a series of guidelines designed to assist the clinician to make the best possible judgement. The decision might be finely balanced but had to take into account a range of factors including the duty to maintain confidences, an interest in a health service preserving such confidences, the scope of an actual disclosure, the risk of not disclosing (e.g. death or serious harm), and the ability to identify an intended victim.

Psychiatrists face other quandaries concerning the limits of confidentiality when a threat to an identified person exists (e.g. potential transmission of HIV), or when actual harm has occurred (e.g. child abuse). HIV infection and AIDS have generated challenging ethical dilemmas for the clinician. Kelly (32) argued for respecting confidentiality except in a few limited circumstances: a past sexual partner of a carrier should be notified of exposure in order to prevent the spread of the virus; a potential sexual partner or spouse of a carrier should be advised about the risk of infection; and medical staff in contact with infected body fluids had a right to know this in order to take protective measures. In 1993 the APA issued a policy statement concerning AIDS and disclosure (33) that encompassed the following guidelines: there were specified limits of confidentiality concerning HIV/AIDS; the law might require reporting names of HIV-positive patients; patients placing others at risk of infection should be counselled to cease that behaviour or inform the person/s concerned; it was justifiable in the case of a uncooperative patient to notify identified people at risk or to request a statutory health authority to do so; it was legitimate to contact an authority when the risk was to unidentifiable persons; hospital commitment was permissible when hazardous behaviour was the result of a mental illness; psychiatrists should counsel HIV patients to inform past contacts or ask a relevant health authority to do so (if the patient refused or was unable to do this, the psychiatrist was justified to notify the authority). In the United Kingdom, an independent working party launched its consideration of the interface between confidentiality and HIV/AIDS, arriving at similar recommendations.

In the case of child abuse, many enlightened societies have legislated mandatory reporting of child abuse to relevant authorities, though ethical dilemmas still arise. In one instance, for example, a mother and daughter disclosed to their general practitioner (GP) the continuing sexual abuse by the stepfather (also a patient of the GP), while insisting upon absolute confidentiality (34). Discussion of the case yielded a consensus of an overriding obligation to the patient since the safety of the child was paramount in all circumstances.

Other factors that threaten the therapeutic sphere of privacy include: the interaction between confidentiality and the law; clinical record-keeping (especially problematic in an era of advanced information technology and computerized transfer of data); the requirements of, and pressures from, third parties (e.g. insurers, employers, and statutory authorities); psychiatric genetics; group, family and couples therapy; multiple clinicians; teaching; and medical writing.

The family and confidentiality

Concurrent with the community psychiatry movement of the 1970s, there evolved an examination of the role of the family as informal carer for patients with enduring or recurring mental illnesses. The question of how family members should be involved in the care of their relative-patient has been much influenced by ethical forces. Given the considerable research supporting help from relatives to treat patients with psychosis though psycho-education, counselling, and the opportunity to obtain pertinent information, it would appear counterproductive to be thwarted by a patient's insightless refusal to consent. Yet to act against the patient's wishes places the therapeutic relationship in jeopardy.

Szmukler and Bloch (35) have addressed this ethical dilemma with a premise that a morally neutral encounter with patient and family is fanciful. Values are central, particularly their influence on how to balance the interests and needs of all members. Informed consent is the cornerstone upon which ethically sound care of patients and their families may occur, a process involving a continuing dialogue between clinician, family, and the patient; ethical dilemmas multiply when it is inoperative. The authors concluded that justification for disclosing information to the family, contrary to the patient's wishes, is most robust when the harms to be avoided are serious and likely; acceptable alternatives are unavailable; the capacity of the patient to assess self-interest is impaired; the family's values embrace mutual concern; and non-involvement of the family will lead inevitably to even greater restrictions on liberty.

Individual case material and confidentiality

Psychoanalysis grew out of the individual case report, beginning with Freud's classic studies at the turn of the 20th century that ushered in a novel way to understand the underlying dynamics of neurotic symptoms. In the Dora case, Freud acknowledged concerns about confidentiality when he pronounced that it was a doctor's duty to publish material about his patients as long as he was in a position to avoid causing them any harm.

The case report remains a respected means to share ideas in many journals, especially those of a psychotherapy type; however, the issue of preserving confidences persists. Glen Gabbard (36), co-editor of the *International Journal of Psychoanalysis*, depicted it as a conflict of interest between safeguarding privacy and facilitating scientific progress. In the late 1990s a number of journal editors began to articulate an ethically based policy, such as the requirement by the *British Journal of Psychiatry* that informed consent should be obtained from the patient or, if that was impossible, from an 'authorized person'.

This matter came dramatically to the fore in the case of Anne Sexton, a celebrated American poet, whose psychoanalytic sessions were audiotaped so that she might make better use of the process. Years later, (following her death by suicide), her psychiatrist permitted a biographer, in conjunction with the patient's daughter, to use the material. Some psychiatrists agreed with this course on utilitarian grounds, namely that it might promote knowledge potentially useful to future patients and society generally. Others argued that people have a right to privacy and therapists a corresponding duty not to undermine it. The Sexton biography serves to sensitize therapists to the complex nature of the trust patients place in them.

The perils of diagnosis

A huge effort has gone into elaborating objective criteria of mental illness since the 1960s, but controversy still prevails about the legitimacy of many categories. Concerns about the intrusion of value judgements into classifications have led to charges that a number of diagnoses reflect pejorative labelling and, therefore, are ethically questionable. For example, Kaplan (37) asserted that masculine-based assumptions had led to an array of behaviours in women incorrectly codified as valid. Thomas Szasz dismissed an ethical dimension of diagnosis, claiming that mental illness does not exist and that mental symptoms should be viewed exclusively in terms of physical cause. He argued that diseases of the mind reflect social values and are created by society in association with the medical profession to explain away 'problems of living' (38).

The position that mental illnesses are social constructs and cause harm to those labelled with a diagnosis was enunciated by a group of 'antipsychiatrists' during the 1950s and 1960s. One of the proponents of this position, R.D. Laing, viewed features of schizophrenia as a reasonable reaction to 'insane' environments, particularly those characterizing dysfunctional families. Those called 'schizophrenic' were 'divided selves', defending themselves against noxious circumstances (39, 40). Mental health professionals have undoubtedly been guilty of purposefully inventing the disorders they attribute to patients. As mentioned earlier, Proctor (27) highlighted chilling examples of this phenomenon when describing Nazi social policy towards citizens leading 'lives not worth living' due to physical or mental handicaps. In the former Soviet Union, the vague construct of 'sluggish schizophrenia' was employed to quash political and other forms of social dissent (41).

In contrast to deploying such value-laden criteria for psychiatric diagnoses, some leading figures in nosology have argued for an objective procedure to ascertain whether a person is mentally ill or not. Robert Kendall (42) conceptualized illness as a condition producing 'significant biological disadvantage', and included mental disorders in this spectrum (e.g. schizophrenia, bipolar illness, and drug dependence). Boorse (43) also adhered to a biological conception, broadening Kendall's view with a proposal that certain mental processes (e.g. perception, intelligence, and memory) are needed to support adaptive behaviour, thereby conceptualizing mental diseases as similar to physical ones.

Wakefield (44) proposed a way to reconcile the value versus biological basis of mental illness with his concept of 'harmful dysfunction'. To him, dysfunction, a scientific term based in biology, refers to the failure of an evolutionary mechanism to perform a natural task for which it is designed. On the other hand, 'harmful' is value-oriented in quality and covers the consequences of the dysfunction that are deemed detrimental for the person in terms of sociocultural norms. Applying this to mental functions, Wakefield described the benefits of natural mental mechanisms like those mediating emotional regulation; their dysfunction becomes harmful when they yield sequelae which are not valued by society (e.g. self-destructive acts). Thus, the inability of a mechanism to perform its natural function to the degree of causing harm to the person warrants diagnosis. Wakefield also argued that the 'harmful dysfunction' paradigm is justified by theories that point to psychological and genetic causes of psychiatric disorders. In terms of the former, dysfunction of the ego's defences leads to harm that bolsters claims for a disorder. Repression, for example, is a necessary mental mechanism that helps ward off painful feelings that could disrupt customary functioning. Fulford (45) has addressed Wakefield's harmful dysfunction concept by applying what he calls a 'fact-plus-value' approach, arguing that all diagnoses, whether physical or mental, are value-laden.

The legitimacy of psychiatric diagnosis has varied ethical implications. For instance, is a person diagnosed with an impulse-control disorder expressing itself as kleptomania legally culpable for shoplifting if the behaviour is viewed as having a predominantly physical, as opposed to psychological, cause (46)? And, as Halasz has discussed (47), a 'mistaken diagnosis' of attention deficit hyperactivity disorder (ADHD) can result in excessive, possibly harmful, pharmacological treatment of children. A related issue concerns the determination of treatment versus enhancement—should medications be prescribed in the absence of a definitive psychiatric diagnosis? And, as Chodoff noted (23), there are financial implications of psychiatric diagnoses. He describes an inexorable intrusion of third parties into the therapeutic relationship, providing greater incentive for clinicians to assign diagnostic labels to patients in order 'to qualify [them] for insurance reimbursement'. Indeed medical practitioners have acknowledged the 'gamesmanship' of manipulating diagnoses in their reports to insurers (48, 49), judging patients' welfare of greater value than telling the truth to third-party payers.

A final issue concerning ethics and psychiatric diagnosis is the influence of cultural factors. Wallace explored the topic theoretically and historically, noting that psychopathology can be shaped by a group's prevailing ways of schematizing abnormal experiences and behaviours. Leff, on the other hand, examined empirical data arising out of observations of Afro-Caribbean patients in the United Kingdom that demonstrated clinicians' lack of understanding of culture-specific abnormal bodily activities that dominated psychotic presentations (50, 51). One consequence was their difficulty in differentiating, particularly in women, between schizophrenia and mood disorders.

Psychiatric treatment

In addition to the need for a trusting alliance, psychiatric treatment depends on the therapist obtaining informed consent whose pivotal components are the capacity to understand the information about relevant treatment(s); to appreciate the implications of each potential therapeutic option for herself; and to agree to receiving treatment without being coerced, explicitly or subtly, by the therapist. A large proportion of patients are able to make decisions about treatment when presented with all pertinent options (52). However, since the source of rational decision-making is the same one that is functionally impaired in most psychiatric conditions, profound ethical complications can arise.

Managing the care of patients becomes ethically challenging and complex when the patient lacks the critical faculty to participate in the consenting process and enforced treatment is required to promote their interests and also to safeguard those of society. The intertwined rights to receive treatment, to refuse treatment, and to receive the correct treatment must then be carefully appraised. We now address the circumstances of compulsory treatment within the setting of a hospital as well as in the community.

Involuntary treatment

A consensus has prevailed for generations that a proportion of patients lose the capacity to discern what is in their best interests as a result of their disturbed mind; they then become vulnerable to harming themselves and/or others, acting in ways they will come to regret (e.g. sexual indiscretions, squandering financial resources), and suffering from self-neglect (e.g. homelessness, malnutrition, physical ill-health). What has not been universally agreed upon is how best to deal with such vulnerable people. Many jurisdictions have formulated legal measures to protect this group; however, variations in mental health law have been legion, reflecting, in part, the ethical complexity of the process. Consequently, psychiatrists and society have required robust arguments as to the principles they should heed.

J. S. Mill (53) highlighted the libertarian position in his essay, *On Liberty*:

> The only purpose for which power can be rightfully exercised over any member of a civilised community, against his will, is to prevent harm to others. His own good, either physical or moral, is not a sufficient warrant. He cannot rightfully be compelled to do or forebear because it will be better for him to do so, because it will make him happier, because, in the opinion of others, to do so would be wise or even right (51, p. 15).

Mill added a critical caveat—an exception is mandatory in the case of children and mentally disturbed people. As he put it, a person who is 'delirious' or in a 'state of excitement or absorption incompatible with the full use of the reflecting faculty' can legitimately be assisted. Mill's rationale is clear—such a person is not aware of the risks to which he exposes himself, and is therefore not experiencing true freedom.

Chodoff (54) argued eloquently regarding the awesome issue of depriving a person of his liberty on the grounds of mental illness. He proposed a 'chastened and self- critical' form of paternalism, encompassing 'strong safeguards against abuse' and a humanistic stance epitomized in his observation that involuntary admission to a hospital was not a conflict of right versus wrong but rather a conflict over the right to remain at liberty against the right 'to be free from dehumanizing disease'. The emphasis on humanism is not merely an example of piety. Procedural justice came into its own in the 1990s with an explicit argument for the need to detain certain patients as an inescapable duty of the psychiatrist that should always be accompanied by respect for the patients' dignity. Loss of critical faculties, as cited by Mill, may be a unifying feature in imposing involuntary treatment, though ethical factors may vary according to the particulars of a patient's state. An obvious example is suicidal behaviour. Szasz (55) viewed suicide as the voluntary act of a moral agent consistent with an 'ethic of self-responsibility', and objected to the state empowering itself to prevent self-killing; that is, everyone has the right to end their life according to their own personally held beliefs. On the other hand, he did concede that professional intervention (albeit informal and brief) is permitted in a case where objective evidence points to brain dysfunction and when a person has prepared a 'psychiatric will' that states unambiguously his wish to submit to involuntary intervention under specific circumstances.

The distinction between brain malfunction and other clinical circumstances in which suicidality is prominent is, for critics of Szasz, spurious and unworkable. This is not to argue that all suicidal behaviour reflects a disordered mind. For example, in his suicide letter the philosopher and author Arthur Koestler makes it explicit that his decision was coherent and rational. Suffice to say the suicidal patient highlights the psychiatrist's situation in having no choice but to foist treatment in specific clinical circumstances and declare a person unable to make rational judgements, as Heyd and Bloch (56) have discussed in their account of ethical aspects of suicide.

The issue of involuntary treatment became more challenging in the 1990s when several jurisdictions introduced compulsory treatment carried out in the community, and potentiality for extended periods, albeit subject to regular review and the option to appeal. The criteria applied to justify detention in a hospital were extrapolated to the community setting, given that similar restrictions on liberty lie at the heart of the moral dilemma when the psychiatrist has to assess the patient's competence. Munetz and his colleagues (57) tackled enforced community treatment applying utilitarian, communitarian, and beneficence arguments and concluded that all support the practice. Utilitarianism looks to the outcome of such an intervention; compulsory community treatment is justified if it reduces the rate of readmission to hospital and promotes the cooperation of patients and their families. The communitarian position revolves around the benefits generated for society, such as upholding humanistic values and creating a safe environment. A corollary, however, is that the community must respond to the needs of the mentally ill by formulating appropriate treatment plans and committing the necessary resources. Beneficence relates most directly to incapacity in that the state is obliged 'to make decisions on behalf of individuals who are unable to make informed decisions for themselves'. Patients who are definitely in need of treatment are thus assured of obtaining it.

The right to treatment

The asylum era was marked for the most part by tragic neglect of the needs of patients. It took a plaintiff, Kenneth Donaldson, to assure that an involuntarily committed person had the 'right to receive such individual treatment as will give him a reasonable opportunity to be cured or to improve his mental condition' (*O'Connor v. Donaldson*, F.2d 5th Cir, 26 April 1974; 422US. 563, 1975). His case arose from the claim that he received minimal treatment for a decade and a half after being admitted to the Florida State Hospital in 1957. The US Supreme Court concluded unanimously that a patient who did

not pose a danger to himself or to others, and did not receive treatment, had a constitutional right to be released if able to live safely in the community. Donaldson's victory
occurred in the context of a decade of civil rights campaigning that included respect
for the rights of the mentally ill. Indeed, a few years earlier, in 1971, a class action in
Alabama (*Wyatt v Stickney*, 325F Supp 781, 1971; 344 F Supp 373, 376, 379–385,1972)
led Judge Johnson to declare that due process was violated in circumstances where a
citizen was confined to a mental hospital ostensibly for humane purposes, but then not
given adequate treatment.

The right to effective treatment

The right to treatment has been revisited in other judgements since *Donaldson*, decisions that did not address a requirement that patients receive *effective* treatment.
The right to such care was explicitly examined when Dr Rafael Osheroff, mentioned
earlier, sued a psychiatric hospital for failing to provide antidepressant medication
in the face of his deteriorating mental state. The staff's continuing application of
psychoanalytic psychotherapy to treat his mood disorder was judged to constitute
malpractice. The decision was hotly debated by prominent American leaders of psychiatry. Gerald Klerman (21) argued that providing the most effective treatment was
feasible in the wake of sound scientific evidence, therefore obligating the clinician to
use only evidence-based care. Alan Stone (20) contended that Klerman's position was
tantamount to '. . . promulgating more uniformed scientific standards of treatment
in psychiatry, based on . . . opinion about science and clinical practice'. He believed
psychiatrists should depend on what he referred to as 'the collective sense of the profession' but also respect innovative treatments which might prove beneficial.

The right to refuse treatment

As a voluntary patient, Osheroff could have refused treatment as part of the process of
informed consent, but could not have done so had he been an involuntary patient. The
right to refuse treatment when hospitalized against one's will loomed large as an ethical question for several years, and was ultimately settled in 1979 in the case of *Rogers
v. Okin* (478 F Supp. 1342, D Mass., 1979; *Rogers v. Commissioner of the Department of
Mental Health*, 458NE 2d 308, Mass. Sup. Jud. Ct., 1983). The State Supreme Court of
Massachusetts ruled that detained patients had a constitutional right to refuse treatment, a decision coinciding with changes in many commitment laws from criteria linking the need for treatment to the level of danger posed by the patient to self and/or
others. All psychiatric inpatients, whether competent or not, had a right to refuse antipsychotics, except in an emergency. In the case of refusal, a substituted legal judgement
was indicated, namely that a court had to take into account what the patient would have
preferred had he the capacity to make a decision.

The ethical repercussions of *Rogers v Okin* were profound. If psychiatrists were legally empowered to detain patients, was it not a contradiction in terms if they were
then unable to offer treatment in the face of refusal? The argument rested on the premise that a person sufficiently disturbed to warrant involuntary admission is automatically entitled to treatment and the consulting psychiatrist suitably placed to provide it.

Without this arrangement the psychiatrist's job would be restricted to that of custodian. A countervailing argument was grounded in constitutional rights. Merely because people were committed did not mean that they were incapable of consenting. In the event that they failed to appreciate the rationale for a course of action, the argument followed, a form of substituted judgement could be used, so ensuring that rights remained in the foreground.

An assortment of legal remedies evolved in an effort to resolve this ethical quandary, ranging from a full adversarial process to reliance on a guardian's decision. Appelbaum (58) shared his predilection for a treatment-driven model in which patients should be committed on the grounds that their capacity to decide about treatment was lacking as part of their disturbed mental state. On the other hand, a question remained as to whether a single psychiatrist should be given complete discretion in this matter. As an alternative, an independent review to safeguard patients' rights (e.g. various types of legal guardianship) was suggested. It was also proposed that the question of competence could be legally dealt with prior to compulsory admission since addressing commitment and competence to reach a decision about treatment simultaneously would obviate the problem of compulsory hospitalization without treatment. The difficulty here is the fluidity of the mental state; what patients think about treatment during the maelstrom of being detained could well change once they are hospitalized.

The role of advanced directives

An ingenious idea emerged in the 1980s to deal with many of the aforementioned ethical issues—variously named an advanced directive, a Ulysses contract, a self-binding contract, and advanced treatment authorization. In summary, patients prone to a recurrence during which they might be too disturbed to consent to treatment would reach prior agreement with their psychiatrist about what constituted the best course of action should they suffer a future episode and find it difficult to decide what treatment was in their best interest.

Two methods were proffered as to how the process might be expedited—instructional and proxy. In the former, patients would specify a set of instructions when competent concerning, *inter alia*, use of drugs, electroconvulsive therapy (ECT), seclusion, people to be contacted, location of treatment, and financial aspects. A limitation of this approach was the difficulty of anticipating all contingencies, a hurdle partially overcome by the proxy method. Here, patients assign consent to a designated person who then uses what has been referred to as substituted judgement. Thus, a decision about treatment would be made in accord with what the patient would probably have preferred were he able to express it. An alternative to substituted judgement is the best interest approach in which the proxy would declare what he believed was in the patient's best interest.

Henderson et al. (59) examined the efficacy of advanced directives with a single-blind randomized controlled trial, in which 160 people diagnosed with a psychotic disorder or non-psychotic bipolar illness who had been hospitalized in the previous 2 years were randomly allocated to either an intervention or a control condition. In the former, a joint plan was devised, specifying the patient's treatment preferences. Over 15 months of follow-up the rate of compulsory admission was substantially less in the intervention group. The study is clearly pertinent as it demonstrated that an advanced agreement could reduce the rate of legal compulsion in treating the severely mentally ill.

Ethical aspects in using medication

Many issues discussed above entail the use of psychotropic medications, but more specific ethical challenges exist concerning psychopharmacological treatment.

The concept of the 'therapeutic orphan' captures the dilemma of the unavailability of research data for use in determining effectiveness and safety of drugs in children. Whereas we have built up a reasonably accurate picture of the proper place of antipsychotic and antidepressant agents in adult patients (less so in elderly people), the situation is less clear in younger people given that pharmaceutical companies commonly test products only in adults; obtaining consent from children and young adolescents is ethically much more complex. As a result, clinicians struggle with what to do when facing a young person presenting with moderate to severe depression whose adult counterpart would be prescribed a selective serotonin reuptake inhibitor (SSRI). Conflicting data spurred debate about the potential for increased rate of suicidal thinking and self-harm in children and teenagers on antidepressants. In the United Kingdom, for example, the Committee on Safety of Medicines (CSM) examined published and unpublished material and, as a result, introduced a warning to the effect that SSRIs, with one exception, were contraindicated in children. Responses to this dilemma have included a ban on prescribing until solid data become available; the use of the psychotherapies in place of medications on the grounds of safety, even though medication could well be beneficial; combining medication and psychotherapy; the requirement that pharmaceutical companies be legally compelled to conduct therapeutic trials in all age groups; and prescribing in the absence of robust research findings on the assumption that potential benefits outweigh possible harms.

In a well-balanced and pragmatic overview of the role of psychotropics in young children, Peter Jensen (60), a prominent child and adolescent psychiatrist in the United States, called for '. . . caution and an in-depth evaluation of the possible alternatives for each child'. He concluded that '. . . appropriate and judicious use, even in the absence of safety and efficacy data, may be warranted'. This was particularly so in the case of continuing substantial impairment.

Stimulants and attention deficit hyperactivity disorder

Although ADHD has been recognized as a clinical entity for decades, it has remained a controversial diagnosis principally because of the stimulant drugs used to treat it. Eisenberg (61), in 1971, addressed four key dimensions of the issue which continue to be contentious: limited research knowledge; the risks of adverse effects with long-term use; the question of whether it was the child being treated or another party such as parents, teachers, or the courts; and the social costs inasmuch as medication use might lead to a relative neglect of counselling parents or instituting remedial educational programmes.

The debate became more heated in the 1990s in the wake of the massive escalation in the number of children prescribed medication. Larry Diller (62, 63) estimated that stimulant use soared by several hundred per cent, with over 4 million children in the United States, mostly boys aged between 6 and 13, taking methylphenidate or amphetamines. This vast increase in prescriptions also occurred in Canada and specific regions of Australia. Whether medication has been overused depends on the rate of ADHD in these countries, but objective biological or psychological tests to confirm its presence have been unavailable, and variation in diagnostic practice has led to both over- and underdiagnosis. The argument has been made that sound judgements about the need for medication require comprehensive assessment of the child, family members, and relevant others, such as teachers. The Great Smoky Mountain Study in the United States (64) identified therapeutic implications of an inadequate assessment. The researchers found that 5% of more than 4000 children were diagnosed with ADHD, 7% of the sample was receiving stimulants, but over one-half of the children on medication did not satisfy accepted ADHD criteria. They evidently exhibited a range of behavioural and learning difficulties, highlighting Eisenberg's point of 'who is being treated'?

'Cosmetic' psychopharmacology

Should psychotropics be used in people who experience psychological states, such as tension, melancholy, and insomnia, that are customarily construed as reasonable responses to the vicissitudes of daily life? Klerman (65), in the early 1970s, raised the question in his article, 'Psychotropic hedonism vs. pharmacological Calvinism'. The Calvinist extreme of the prescribing continuum holds that drugs should only be used to treat states of mind scientifically determined to constitute psychiatric maladies (e.g. schizophrenia, bipolar disorder). Protagonists at the other end of the spectrum argue that psychotropics have the potential to play a role in promoting a sense of calm, boosting self-confidence, or facilitating social relationships. Psychiatrists often struggle as to where to draw the line between prescribing for legitimate clinical needs or as a form of palliation, particularly when pharmaceutical companies broaden indications for their products such as extending psychotropic use from generalized anxiety to social anxiety and even shyness.

Carstairs's (66) position in this debate was to warn clinicians of the 'tranquillizing anodyne' and the 'aberration' of public thinking that '. . . everyone nowadays expects to be happy' despite the fact that 'suffering, like pain, is part of the human experience'. The argument for and against this position has continued for decades without resolution. *Listening to Prozac*, by Peter Kramer (67), provoked much debate, beginning in the 1990s. He raised the ethical question of using a medication to shift one normal psychological state into another in the case where the latter has more beneficial qualities and there is no evidence of mental illness (e.g. altering facets of a person's temperament). The ethicist Carl Elliot (68) categorically rejected such usage. Echoing Carstairs's repudiation of a tranquillizing solution, he described how people generally grapple with a sense of personal, cultural, and existential alienation that medication cannot possibly alter.

Ethical aspects of electroconvulsive treatment

Max Fink, a leading figure in research on ECT, has described how the treatment seems unable to shed its controversial status, notwithstanding its long-standing demonstrable utility in treating melancholia and psychotic depression. Multiple myths about ECT and the stigmatization it provokes persist, even in the face of well-conducted trials since the 1980s (69, 70). One criticism is grounded in it being a form of physical manipulation of the brain whose rationale has never been determined, another because it is applied to normal brain tissue and not an identified pathological lesion (e.g. a brain tumour), and a third that it acts by causing an epileptic seizure.

Since it has provoked continuing and intense controversy, ECT warrants sophisticated ethical deliberation. The principal issue has revolved around informed consent (71–74); some patients with profound melancholia lack insight to comprehend information about the nature of the treatment and/or appreciate the implications of agreeing or refusing to have it. In these instances Culver et al. (75) have recommended proxy consent by relatives or guardians. Legally mandated criteria to assess competence have not won adherents given the considerable variation in clinical presentations. On the contrary, the law can vitiate what should be a clinically based encounter governed by ethical principles.

Ottosson (76), the doyen of ECT research in Europe, has addressed a range of ethical issues, drawing on data that show persuasively its 'very favourable' risk-benefit ratio, especially in severe depression and acute catatonia. He has also lamented the unfairness of ECT's patchy availability around the world and disparities in its use even in the same country—an obvious example of distributive injustice.

Ethical aspects of psychosurgery

Psychosurgery is rarely used in contemporary psychiatry, having been supplanted by treatments that are equally effective and much less invasive. However, lessons from the history of its deployment over more than half a century bear on ethical aspects of psychiatric treatment in general.

Mersky (77) highlighted problems that arise when psychosurgery is proposed and informed consent is not forthcoming because of a patient's disordered mental state. Unlike the case of ECT, psychosurgery should never be performed on patients 'who decline explicitly or are implicitly unwilling' for three main reasons: treatment involves permanent brain change, it is ethically impermissible to impose potentially permanent alterations in mental functioning, and it may lead to a change in personality and the source of all future judgements.

Valenstein (78, 79) offers a cautionary tale by carefully examining factors that lay behind the uncritical acceptance of psychosurgery; we may avoid doing the same with respect to other potentially hazardous treatments in the future. Kleinig (80) has also highlighted ethical perils inherent in embracing a treatment that permanently alters brain structure. He has considered such issues as the right to treatment, the right to refuse treatment, proxy consent in the face of the incompetent patient, and essential characteristics of valid consent. Like Valenstein, he has viewed psychosurgery as a suitable vantage point for a broader consideration of key aspects of medical ethics.

Ethical aspects of psychotherapy

The definition of psychotherapy is elusive: is it an art, a branch of science, a blend of both, or comparable to a trusting friendship? Psychotherapists do not belong to a unitary profession; they may be, *inter alia,* psychiatrists, psychologists, social workers, chaplains, lay analysts, psychiatric nurses, or counsellors. Moreover, each of these disciplines uses a certain set of premises. The goals for which they strive are frequently ill-defined, ranging from symptom relief to ambitious personality change. The multiplicity of objectives is matched by the number of 'schools', each with its own theory of what constitutes normal and abnormal mental health. Finally, the effectiveness of various modes of treatment is subject to much debate. Given all these factors, the practice of psychotherapy involves many decisions with ethical ramifications.

Who should be offered psychotherapy?

Although psychotherapy has a place in psychiatry, the question still arises whether a substantial proportion of people receiving it are, as Szasz puts it, simply wrestling with 'problems of living' (38). Some might argue that psychotherapy should only be 'prescribed' for those who have a clearly defined psychiatric disorder. An explicit form of therapy would then be selected from an established range of treatments and outcome measured in terms of specific, objective criteria. Thus, a satisfactory outcome for a person with depressive symptoms would be elevation of mood, for a bulimic patient cessation of bingeing and vomiting, and for a socially phobic student the ability to dine in the college canteen.

This scientific approach owes much to Freud, who developed a mode of treatment to deal with specific neurotic symptoms, among them hysterical conversion, obsessions, and anxiety. It rests in the medical model, however, which is constraining and not well-suited to the psychotherapeutic pursuit for several reasons. First, legitimate treatment goals may encompass much more than symptomatic relief. Moreover, pinpointing a diagnosis and plan of treatment is contrary to the notion of psychotherapy as a journey of personal exploration, with the opportunity for greater self-knowledge and self-realization. This broadening is not without ethical difficulty. Freud captured the dilemma in *Analysis Terminable and Interminable* (81) when arguing that the aim of psychoanalysis was 'not to rub off every peculiarity of human character for the sake of a schematic "normality", nor yet to demand that the person who has been "thoroughly analyzed" shall feel no passions and develop no internal conflicts.' (81, p. 250).

Ethical issues in the therapeutic process

Ethical issues arise as clinician and patient embark on the psychotherapeutic process. At the outset, they may be polarized; the patient is inevitably distressed, dependent, and vulnerable in the presence of a therapist often viewed as omniscient. Dependency increases the authority already vested in the therapist, and may be reinforced by his opting to divulge little about himself or the nature of treatment on the premise that disclosure would undermine the transference, and interfere with the unconstrained flow of free associations, regarded by dynamically oriented schools as central to therapy.

Informed consent is one means to dispel this air of mystery. An admirably clear model, provided by Carl Goldberg (82), invokes the concept of therapeutic partnership, its cornerstone a 'mutually agreed upon and explicitly articulated working plan' that is subject to regular review. Among its elements are identifying goals and methods to reach them, monitoring efficacy, and permitting either partner to voice any dissatisfaction. The partnership does not imply an equal share of power but rather an agreement about how the power inherent in the relationship will be allocated at various times. A patient in the throes of an intense crisis, for instance, may agree to a redistribution of responsibility to the therapist who assumes a more paternalistic role. As the crisis wanes, restoration of the patient's autonomy ensues.

In reviewing models pertinent to informed consent, Dyer and Bloch (83) proposed that a therapeutic relationship based on trust enduring over time is most apt; thus, the therapist continually works to earn the patient's confidence. The trust-based relationship also promotes a sense of responsibility in the therapist who seeks to respond to particular needs in the patient. Patient autonomy is always a pre-eminent goal, but the therapist may need to act paternalistically on occasion, comparable to the concern manifest by responsible parents for their child.

Values and psychotherapy

A partnership grounded in trust obviates many ethical pitfalls intrinsic to psychotherapy; it is a necessary but not sufficient condition for sound clinical practice. Permeation of treatment by values is another complication that warrants attention. Given that the problems for which patients seek help are inextricably bound up with the question of how they should live their lives, the therapist is inevitably at risk of imposing his values, intentionally or unwittingly (84).

Engelhardt (85) has posited that psychotherapy is not about ethics *per se* but about meta-ethics, that is, it paves the way for ethical decision-making by patients. The aim is not for them to adopt a particular set of values as a result of treatment but to reach a point where they can make their own choices unhindered by psychological conflict and unconscious influences. But in affirming the therapist's role to help patients map out their own values, Engelhardt has necessarily accepted an inescapable feature of psychotherapy; namely, that it is value-bound.

Freud was also intent on promoting value-free treatment. Indeed, he argued, '[t]he [therapist] should be opaque to his patients and, like a mirror, should show them nothing but what is shown to him' (86, p.118); he insisted that the task of therapy was limited to liberating the patient from symptoms, inhibitions, and abnormal characteristics by making the unconscious conscious. On the other hand, he also pointed out an educative role: '[the analyst] must possess some kind of superiority, so that in certain analytic situations he can act as a model for his patient and in others as a teacher' (86, p.248). It is difficult to regard this hybrid role of mirror, model, and teacher as value-free, even if the ultimate goal is to promote a sense of autonomy that is free of the influence of unconscious, irrational forces.

Many notable figures in psychotherapy agree that therapists do embrace values in their work. Strupp (87) asserted that moral values are always 'in the picture' and the therapist influences the patient's values. Crown (88) reminded us that this influence occurs at both verbal and non-verbal levels. While he may be aware of his utterances, 'his non-verbal communication through gesture, facial expression, nods of approval or disapproval, can be almost unconscious'. Erikson (89) extended these views when proposing that therapy is in its essence an ethical intervention. In his thoughtful paper he concluded, 'What the healing professionals advocate . . . is always part of the value struggle of the times and, whether 'avowed' or not, will be—therefore had better be— ethical intervention'.

If therapy must, to a degree, amount to ethical intervention, how should the therapist handle this? He could strive to minimize the ethical role, but the likelihood of success is slim since his 'unavowed' values will manifest non-verbally. Another option is to accept the inevitability of 'ethical interventionist' but recognize it as a 'problem' for the therapist, not the patient. The latter is not burdened by a dilemma that does not belong to him. The therapist by contrast has the responsibility to remain aware of his potential role as moral agent. He is sensitive to his own values and monitors any unconsciously derived impulses to influence the patient. A process of 'value testing' occurs constantly to ensure attention to possible intrusion of values is never neglected and to preclude their imposition unwittingly.

A third option is for the therapist to declare his own value system as a value in itself. The argument runs as follows: psychotherapy is a means of social influence; the therapist is more powerfully placed to influence his patients than vice versa; the therapist acknowledges this state of affairs; and is entirely 'transparent' regarding the values he espouses. Robert Jay Lifton (90) was an eloquent spokesman for this position in his work with US veterans of the Vietnam War. He elaborated a view in which the professional avoids the 'trap of pseudo-neutrality'; instead, he combines attitudes of advocacy (Lifton used the term 'affinity') and detachment. The process entails voicing 'moral advocacies' in tandem with 'maintaining sufficient detachment to apply the technical and scientific principles of one's discipline'. In helping the veterans, Lifton articulated his anti-war position explicitly to former soldiers who had shared the experience of fighting an allegedly unjust war and wished to make sense of it.

Other examples of 'affinity' have evolved, all typified by the therapist assuming the role of moral advocate. Certain homosexual therapists, for example, have aligned themselves with the gay movement when treating homosexual patients who are striving to adjust to their sexual identity. A distinguished therapist and committed Christian, Alan Bergin (91), evolved a school he called 'theistic realism' in which the therapist shares values derived from a Judeo-Christian tradition, including forgiveness, reconciliation, spiritual belief, supremacy of God, marital fidelity, and primacy of love. Some therapists who functioned in the context of apartheid South Africa declared their rejection of racism and demonstrated their support for traumatized black people, especially those who had been victims of detention and torture (92).

Particular constituencies are being served in these illustrations, but the therapist's explicit avowal of his values can be applied generally. A therapist may adopt an approach with *all* his patients in which he will be transparent about his ethical outlook in various clinical circumstances. He does this on the premise that values are central in assessing a problem, formulating goals, and selecting therapeutic options.

Jeremy Holmes provides a valuable contribution (84). As a long-standing scholar of psychotherapy ethics and a practitioner of psychodynamic therapy, he has been well placed to consider the interface between values and psychological treatment— historically, philosophically, and practically. Accepting that psychotherapy cannot be value-free, he has offered therapists a way of examining their 'ethical countertransference', highlighting the need for therapists to be aware of unconscious influences that might contradict what they espouse overtly.

Prospects

Though a nascent field, psychiatric ethics has developed impressively since the 1980s. Youth, however, is marked not only by strength but also by impediments and future challenges. We end this essay with a few thoughts about what the field requires to advance further.

Education

Given that awareness of accomplishments in, and current limitations of, psychiatric ethics has to be transferred to the next generation, a cogent starting point is the state of education of the subject. The evolution of teaching programmes has been patchy. As Bloch (93) noted in 1980, '. . . a dearth in systematic instruction' was conspicuous. He hoped that '. . . trainees (would) come to recognize the subject as an integral component of their professional education', but the record has not been as bright as desired. For example, a US-based study of 10 training programmes revealed that one-half of the respondents had received no instruction in ethics, while other trainees were critical of their educational experience (94, 95). These findings are troubling, given the requirements of professional associations and colleges that psychiatric ethics should be fully integrated into training programmes.

Bloch and Green (96) have described core problems with ethics education: initiatives have been intermittent, precluding sustained progress; training bodies have only generated embryonic programmes; and reports on innovative teaching projects have been scanty, and limited in their impact. A factor contributing to slow progress has been the vagueness of pedagogical objectives, largely due to the sheer diversity of goals: promoting moral character, developing skills in ethical reasoning, raising moral consciousness, and becoming familiar with what the psychiatric profession accepts as ethical norms. Attempting to achieve this plethora of goals is bound to confuse and discourage trainees.

The educational task could best be advanced by focusing on outcomes rather than goals. Three 'competencies' that graduates should demonstrate are: (1) appreciating ethical aspects of practice and according them the same cogency as the scientific dimension; (2) discerning the ethical features of a case that must be managed (e.g. enforcing treatment, breaching confidentiality); and (3) acquiring skills to deal with these sorts of issues (e.g. realizing when principles clash, understanding the nature of multiple loyalties). Future teaching efforts must help trainees to acquire these competencies. Certain measures have already proved facilitatory, including incorporation of the ethical dimension of practice into clinical rounds and case conferences, and exposing trainees to respected senior clinicians who exhibit sensitive and coherent ethical decision-making. More needs to be done, such as distributing didactic material about ethics at the outset of training (e.g. codes of ethics and position statements of professional organizations); introducing curricula that promote relevant knowledge; publishing articles on psychiatric ethics in established journals; and discussion of relevant ethical matters at scientific meetings.

Defining an ethical framework for psychiatry

The vagueness and range of pedagogical goals are related to another issue that should engage psychiatrists in the future, namely, refining a framework that provides a more objective reference point for ethical thinking. Ethical decision-making is a demanding task, compounded by radically divergent rationales and methods. Philosophers continually debate the merits of moral theories so variegated that they go as far as contradicting one another, thereby generating intellectual tension, if not scepticism. Competing theories may lead psychiatrists to devalue the need for ethical deliberation or so confound them that they become ambivalent about bringing reasoning to the situation and resort to personal preferences that may be emotionally based and ill-founded.

Psychiatrists encounter similar ethical quandaries as their medical colleagues. However, as Radden (97) points out, issues intrinsic to mental health care—competence, self-harm, harm to others, and involuntary treatment are but a few of them—suggest that ethical aspects of psychiatry differ in critical ways from those applicable to other fields of medicine. Moreover, the confluence of three core elements of psychiatric treatment—the therapeutic alliance in which the relationship is central, distinctive features of the patient (e.g. impaired reasoning, feeling stigmatized) and goals which can extend to fundamental personality change—define its special place in respect to the ethical demands it imposes on clinical practice.

For these reasons psychiatry perhaps has a need for a particular ethical framework. We have attempted to formulate one (98), but know that our contribution is a preliminary step in need of elaboration and refinement. In brief, we have reviewed competing moral theories and noted their strengths and limitations. This has led us to posit a complementarity between principle-based ethics and care ethics which suits the psychiatrist *qua* clinician and therapist.

Principle-based ethics (often called principlism) links ethical decision-making to a range of 'mid-level' principles that may be subject to change in the light of factors like scientific discoveries, as opposed to the absolutist constraints of classical moral theories encountered in Kantianism and utilitarianism. Principlism posits that well established and widely applied principles (first of all, do no harm; act to benefit others; respect a person's right to 'self-government'; and treat people fairly) in tandem with other illuminating information like relevant empirical data or consistent clinical observation, offer an approach to ethical deliberation that adheres to commonly agreed upon rules but permits flexibility in interpreting their intent.

Care ethics, a contemporary variant of virtue theory, draws on feminism and the role of emotion in moral deliberation. This blend affords primacy to character and interpersonal relationships rather than rules. Decision-making is grounded in the core value of humankind's capacity to extend care to people who are in need or vulnerable. Care ethics promotes greater sensitivity to the 'moral' emotions—compassion, friendship, love, and trustworthiness. The conventional family serves as the model for moral behaviour; for example, fidelity is interpreted as the type of feeling held by a parent towards a child in contrast to a more impersonal attachment between a professional and patient. In the clinical sphere, empathizing enables the therapist to understand patients' fears, wishes, and needs, and then mould treatment in the light of unique life narratives.

Although a place for a rule-based approach to determine ethical practice has been widely supported, the finely tuned interpretations required in the clinic prompt criticism of rules for their remoteness from the psychological context in which ethical decisions are made. Edmund Pellegrino (99), in response, has espoused an Aristotelian perspective grounded in the virtuous character of the doctor who is inclined to promote his patient's interests and hold them above his own. Virtue theory has a particular appeal in psychiatry, given its emphasis on relationships and, in turn, the salience of emotions, in moral deliberation. Morality is, after all, centred on what transpires between people, a reality that may well be overlooked when rules predominate. That said, virtue theory is subject to criticism, particularly for its elusiveness in defining the good to which one should aspire. Lacking objective criteria of that good, clinicians may be so influenced, wittingly or unwittingly, by their own values as to arrive at idiosyncratic judgements.

We believe an ethical framework for psychiatry should address the shortcomings of both rule- and character-based ethics by offering objective guidelines as well as flexibility in the face of unique clinical circumstances. Our approach resonates with the philosophy of David Hume (100) who argued that ethical behaviour derives primarily from sentiment, not reason, and that the natural motivation of human beings is to act benevolently, albeit within social constraints, the latter prompting a need to establish principles of justice. Therefore, ethical guidelines derive from matters of the heart and are adopted eventually as societal norms. Reason enables us to understand an ethical dilemma but sentiment determines what is fair and unfair. In this way Humean theory allows for a balance between rule- and character-based theories by granting significance to 'moral' emotions that are then applied to derive or modify moral rules.

Care ethics, as articulated by the philosopher Annette Baier (101), is a contemporary framework that echoes Hume. She emphasized the intimate connection between moral and psychological development, because emotional sensitivity 'positively reinforces our responses to the good of cooperation, trust, mutual aid, friendship, and love, as well as regulating responses to the risk of evil'. We see great merit in Baier's care ethic but do not believe that it stands on its own. We feel it needs to be complemented by a more structured framework that allows the psychiatrist to resort to a set of *guiding*, as opposed to wholly *binding*, rules; principlism fulfils this requirement most appropriately because of its inherent flexibility and pragmatism.

Conclusion

As we mentioned in the introduction, the long-held notion of ethics resting comfortably in the paternalistic arms of Hippocrates has been projected into a rapidly evolving world of technological, moral, and societal change. Yet, at its core, ethics has to retain its humanism and guard against influences that try to make it a set of rules, thereby negating the uniqueness of patients. Moreover, new ethical pressures on clinical practice will undoubtedly arise. Our historical foray of identifying key existing dilemmas may assist in their early recognition so that psychiatrists can be forearmed to face them with skill and confidence.

References

1 Edelstein, L. (1967). The Hippocratic Oath, text, translation and interpretation. In: *Ancient medicine*, ed. O. Temkin and C. L. Temkin. Baltimore, MD: Johns Hopkins University Press, pp. 17–18.

2 Pargiter, R. and Bloch S. (2002). A history of psychiatric ethics. *Psychiatric Clinics of North America* **25**, 509–24.

3 Tuke, S. (1813/1964). *Description of the Retreat, an institution near York for insane persons.* London: Process.

4 Percival, T. (1985). *Codes of institutes and precepts adapted to the professional conduct of physicians and surgeons.* Birmingham, AL: Classics of Medicine Library.

5 American Psychiatric Association (2001). *Principles of medical ethics with annotations especially applicable to psychiatry.* Washington, DC: American Psychiatric Association.

6 Braceland, F. (1969). Historical perspectives of the ethical practice of psychiatry. *American Journal of Psychiatry* **126**, 230–6.

7 Redlich, F. and Mollica, R. (1976). Overview: Ethical issues in contemporary psychiatry. *American Journal of Psychiatry* **133**, 125–36.

8 Moore, R. (1978). Ethics in the practice of psychiatry: origins, functions, models and enforcement. *American Journal of Psychiatry* **135**, 157–63.

9 Szasz, T. (1970). *Ideology and insanity.* Syracuse, NY: Syracuse University Press.

10 Clare, A. (1967). *Psychiatry in dissent: controversial issues in thought and practice.* London: Tavistock.

11 Bloch, S. and Chodoff, P. (eds.) (1981). *Psychiatric ethics.* Oxford: Oxford University Press.

12 Bloch, S. and Green, S. (eds.) (2009). *Psychiatric ethics* (4th edn). Oxford: Oxford University Press.

13 Green, S. and Bloch, S. (eds.) (2006). *An anthology of psychiatric ethics.* Oxford: Oxford University Press.

14 Busse E. (1969). APA's role in influencing the evolution of a health care delivery system. *American Journal of Psychiatry* **126**, 739–44.

15 Waggoner, I. R. (1970). Cultural dissonance and psychiatry. *American Journal of Psychiatry* **127**, 1–8.

16 Peele, R. and Chodoff, P. (1999). The ethics of involuntary treatment and deinstitutionalization. In: Bloch, S., Chodoff, P., and Green, S. (eds.) *Psychiatric ethics* (3rd edn). Oxford: Oxford University Press, pp. 423–40.

17 Gutheil, T. H. and Gabbard, G. O. (1998). Misuses and misunderstandings of boundary theory in clinical and regulatory settings. *American Journal of Psychiatry* **155**, 409–14.

18 Fullinwider, R. (1996). Professional codes and moral understanding. In: Coady, M. and Bloch, S. (eds.) *Codes of ethics and the professions.* Melbourne: Melbourne University Press.

19 Katz, J. (1984). *The silent world of doctor and patient.* New York: Free Press.

20 Stone, A. (1990). Law, science, and psychiatric malpractice: a response to Klerman's indictment of psychoanalytic psychiatry. *American Journal of Psychiatry* **147**, 419–27.

21 Klerman, G. (1990). The psychiatric patient's right to effective treatment: implications of Osheroff v. Chestnut Lodge. *American Journal of Psychiatry* **147**, 409–18.

22 Hastings Center (1978). In the service of the state: the psychiatrist as double agent. *Hastings Center Reports, Special Supplement*, S1–23.

23 Chodoff, P. (1972). The effect of third-party payment on the practice of psychotherapy. *American Journal of Psychiatry* **129**, 540–5.

24 Wells, K., Hays, R., Burnam, M., et al. (1989). Detection of depressive disorder for patients receiving prepaid or fee-for-service care: results from the medical outcomes study. *JAMA* **262**, 3298–302.

25 Eisenberg, L. (1992). Treating depression and anxiety in the primary care setting. *Health Affairs* **11**, 149–56.

26 Lazarus, J. and Sharfstein, S. (1994). Changes in the economics and ethics of health and mental health. In: Oldham, J. and Riba, M. (eds.) *Review of psychiatry*, vol. 13. Washington, DC: American Psychiatric Press, pp. 389–413.

27 Proctor, R. (1988): *Racial hygiene*. Cambridge, MA: Harvard University Press.

28 Cocks, G. (1985). *Psychotherapy in the Third Reich: the Göring institute*. New York: Oxford University Press.

29 Dyer, A. (1999). Psychiatry as a profession. In: Bloch, S., Chodoff, P., and Green, S. (eds.) *Psychiatric ethics* (3rd edn) Oxford: Oxford University Press, pp. 67–79.

30 Bok, S. (1996). *Secrets*. Oxford: Oxford University Press, pp. 116–35.

31 Stone, A. (1984). The Tarasoff case and some of its progeny: suing psychotherapists to safeguard society. In: *Law, psychiatry and society*. Washington D.C., American Psychiatric Press, pp. 161–90.

32 Kelly, K. (1987). AIDS and ethics: an overview. *General Hospital Psychiatry* **9**, 331–40.

33 Commission on AIDS. (1993). AIDS policy: Position statement on confidentiality disclosure and protection of others. *American Journal of Psychiatry* **150**, 852.

34 Williams, R., Singh, T., Naish, J. et al. (1987). Medical confidentiality and multidisciplinary work: child sexual abuse and mental handicap registers. *BMJ* **295**, 1315–19.

35 Szmukler, G. and Bloch, S. (1997). Family involvement in the care of people with psychoses. *British Journal of Psychiatry* **171**, 401–5.

36 Gabbard, G. (2000). Disguise or consent. *International Journal of Psychoanalysis* **81**, 1071–86.

37 Kaplan, M. (1983). A woman's view of DSM-III. *American Psychologist* **38**, 786–92.

38 Szasz, T. (1960). The myth of mental illness. *American Psychologist* **15**, 113–18.

39 Laing, R. (1970). *Sanity, madness and the family*. Harmondsworth: Penguin. 40 Laing, R. (1969). *The divided self*. New York: Pantheon Books.

41 Snezhnevsky, A. (1971). The symptomatology, clinical forms and nosology of schizophrenia. In: Howells, J. (ed.) *Modern perspectives in world psychiatry*. New York: Brunner-Mazel, pp. 423–47.

42 Kendell, R. (1975). The concept of disease and its implications for psychiatry. *British Journal of Psychiatry* **127**, 305–15.

43 Boorse, C. (1976). What a theory of mental health should be. *Journal for the Theory of Social Behaviour* **6**, 61–84.

44 Wakefield, J. (1992). The concept of mental disorder: on the boundary between biological facts and social values. *American Psychologist* **47**, 373–88.

45 Fulford, K. W. (1998). Mental illness, concept of. In Chadwick, R. (ed.) *Encyclopaedia of applied ethics*, Volume 3. San Diego, CA: Academic Press, pp. 213–33.

46 Aboujaoude, E., Gamel, N., and Koran, L. (2004). A case of kleptomania correlating with premenstrual dysphasia. *Journal of Clinical Psychiatry* **65**, 725–6.

47 Halasz, G. (2002). A symposium of attention deficit hyperactivity disorder (ADHD): an ethical perspective. *Australian and New Zealand Journal of Psychiatry* **36**, 472–5.

48 Healing vs. honesty: for doctors, managed care's cost controls pose moral dilemma. *The Washington Post*, 15 March 1998, H-1.

49 Novack, D., Deterring, B., Arnold, R. et al. (1989). Physicians attitudes toward using deception to resolve difficult ethical problems. *JAMA* **261**, 2980–5.

50 Wallace, E. (1994). Psychiatry and its nosology: a historico-philosophical overview. In: Sadler, J., Wiggins, O., and Schwartz, M. (eds.) *Philosophical perspectives on psychiatric diagnostic classification*. Baltimore: Johns Hopkins University Press, pp. 16–86. 51 Leff, J. (1988). *Psychiatry around the globe: a transcultural view*. London: Royal College of Psychiatrists.

52 Roberts, L. (2002). Informed consent and the capacity for voluntarism. *American Journal of Psychiatry* **159**, 705–12.

53 Mill, J. (1976). On liberty. In: *Three essays*. Oxford: Oxford University Press, p. 15.

54 Chodoff, P. (1984). Involuntary hospitalisation of the mentally ill as a moral issue. *American Journal of Psychiatry* **141**, 384–9.

55 Szasz, T. (1986). The case against suicide prevention. *American Psychologist* **41**, 806–12.

56 Heyd, D. and Bloch, S. (1999). The ethics of suicide. In: Bloch, S. and Green S. (eds.) *Psychiatric ethics* (4th edn). Oxford: Oxford University Press.

57 Munetz, M., Galon, P. and Frese, F. (2003). The ethics of mandatory community treatment. *Journal of the American Academy of Psychiatry and the Law* **31**, 173–83.

58 Appelbaum, P. (1988). The right to refuse treatment with antipsychotic medications: retrospect and prospect. *American Journal of Psychiatry* **145**, 413–19.

59 Henderson, C., Flood, C., Leese, M. et al. (2004). Effect of joint crisis plans on the use of compulsory treatment in psychiatry: single blind randomized controlled trial. *British Medical Journal* **329**, 136–8.

60 Jensen, P. (1998). Ethical and pragmatic issues in the use of psychotropic agents in young children. *Canadian Journal of Psychiatry* **43**, 585–8.

61 Eisenberg, L. (1971). Principles of drug therapy in child psychiatry with special reference to stimulant drugs. *American Journal of Orthopsychiatry* **41**, 371–9.

62 Diller, L. (1996). The run on Ritalin. Attention deficit disorder and stimulant treatment in the 1990s. *Hastings Centre Report* **26**, 12–18.

63 Diller, L. (2003). Prescription stimulant use in America: Ethical issues. *President's Council on Bioethics*, 24 January 2003. See http://bioethicsprint.bioethics.gov.

64 Angold, A., Erkanli, A., Egger, H., and Costello, J. (2000). Stimulant treatment for children: a community perspective. *Journal of the American Academy of Child and Adolescent Psychiatry* **39**, 975–84.

65 Klerman, G. (1972). Psychotropic hedonism vs. pharmacological Calvinism. *Hastings Centre Report* **2**, 1–3.

66 Carstairs, G. (1969). A land of lotus eaters? *American Journal of Psychiatry* **125**, 1576–80.

67 Kramer, P. (1994). *Listening to Prozac*. London: Fourth Estate.

68 Elliott, C. (2000). Pursued by happiness and beaten senseless. *Hastings Centre Report* **30**, 7–12.

69 Fink, M. (1991). Impact of the antipsychiatry movement on the revival of electroconvulsive therapy in the United States. *Psychiatric Clinics of North America* **14**, 793–801. 70 Fink, M. (1977). Myths of 'shock therapy'. *American Journal of Psychiatry* **134**, 991–6.

71 Fink, M. and Ottosson, J.-O. (2004). Ethics in convulsive therapy. New York: Brunner-Routledge. 72 Salzman, C. (1977). ECT and ethical psychiatry. *American Journal of Psychiatry* **134**, 1006–9. 73 Reiter-Theil, S. (1992). Autonomy and beneficence: Ethical issues in electroconvulsive therapy. *Convulsive Therapy* **8**, 237–44. 74 Leong, G. B. and Eth, S. (1991). Legal and ethical issues in electroconvulsive therapy. *Psychiatric Clinics of North America* **14**, 1007–19.

75 Culver, C. M., Ferrell, R. B., and Green, R. M. (1980). ECT and special problems of informed consent. *American Journal of Psychiatry* **137**, 586–91.

76 **Ottosson, J.-O.** (1995). Ethical aspects of research and practice of ECT. *Convulsive Therapy* **11**, 288–99.

77 **Merskey, H.** (1999). Ethical aspects of the physical manipulation of the brain. In: Bloch, S., Chodoff, P., and Green, S. (eds.) *Psychiatric ethics* (3rd edn). Oxford: Oxford University Press.

78 **Valenstein, E.** (1986). *Great and desperate cures: The rise and decline of psychosurgery and other radical treatments for mental illness*. New York: Basic Books.

79 **Valenstein, E.** (ed.) (1980). *The psychosurgery debate*. San Francisco: W. H.Freeman.

80 **Kleinig, J.** (1985). *Ethical issues in psychosurgery*. London: Allen and Unwin.

81 **Freud, S.** (1937). *Analysis terminable and interminable*. Standard edition, 23. London: Hogarth Press, pp. 211–53.

82 **Goldberg, C.** (1977). *Therapeutic partnership: ethical concerns in psychotherapy*. New York: Springer.

83 **Dyer, A. and Bloch, S.** (1987). Informed consent and the psychiatric patient. *Journal of Medical Ethics* **13**, 12–16.

84 **Holmes, J.** (1996). Values in psychotherapy. *American Journal of Psychotherapy* **50**, 259–73.

85 **Engelhardt, H. T.** (1973). Psychotherapy as meta-ethics. *Psychiatry* **36**, 440–5.

86 **Freud, S.** (1924). *Recommendations to physicians practising psychoanalysis*. Standard Edition, 12. London: Hogarth Press, pp. 111–20.

87 **Strupp, H.** (1990). Observation on the fallacy of value-free psychotherapy and the empty organism. *Journal of Abnormal Psychology* **20**, 11–15.

88 **Crown, S.** (1977). Psychotherapy. In: Duncan, A. S., Dunstan, G. R., and Wellbourn, R. B. (eds.) *Dictionary of medical ethics*. London: Darton, Longman and Todd, pp. 264–8.

89 **Erikson, E.** (1976). Psychoanalysis and ethics-avowed and unavowed. *International Review of Psychoanalysis* **3**, 409–15.

90 **Lifton, R. J.** (1976). Advocacy and corruption in the healing professions. *International Review of Psychoanalysis* **3**, 385–98.

91 **Bergin, A.** (1980). Psychotherapy and religious values. *Journal of Consulting and Clinical Psychology* **48**, 95–105.

92 **Steere, J. and Dowdall, T.** (1990). On being ethical in unethical places. The dilemma of South African clinical psychologists. *Hastings Centre Report* **20**, 11–15.

93 **Bloch, S.** (1980). Teaching psychiatric ethics. *British Journal of Psychiatry* **136**, 300–1.

94 **Roberts, L., Lyketsos, C., Jacobson, J,. et al.** (1996). What and how psychiatry residents at ten training programs wish to learn about ethics. *Academic Psychiatry* **20**, 131–43.

95 **Roberts, L., Hammond, K., Geppert, C., et al.** (2005). The positive role of professionalism and ethics training in medical education: A comparison of medical student and resident perspectives. *Academic Psychiatry* **29**, 301–9.

96 **Bloch, S. and Green, S.** (2009). Promoting the teaching of psychiatric ethics. *Academic Psychiatry* **33**, 89–90.

97 **Radden J.** (2003). Forced medication, patients' rights and values conflicts. *Psychiatry, Psychology and Law* **10**, 1–11.

98 **Bloch, S. and Green, S.** (2006). An ethical framework for psychiatry. *British Journal of Psychiatry* **188**, 7–13.

99 **Pellegrino, E.** (1985). The virtuous physician, and the ethics of medicine. In: Shelp, E. (ed.) *Virtue and medicine*. Dordrecht: Reidel, pp. 237–55.

100 **Hume, D.** (1983). *An enquiry concerning the principles of morals*. Indianapolis: Hackett.

101 **Baier, A.** (1985). *Postures of the mind*. Minneapolis: University of Minnesota Press.

Essay 10

Defining and classifying mental illness

German E. Berrios

Introduction

The adjective 'mental' and the noun 'illness' refer to constructs and not to qualities or objects existing *sub specie aeternitatis*. This means that the referent of the phrase 'mental illness' can only be explored in relation to a specific conceptual and historical frame (1). By the same token, the taxonomic enterprise is based on the assumption that the objects to be grouped be stable at least during the classificatory process. It follows that an essay dedicated to current definitions and classifications of mental illness will need to be preceded by an account of the successive historical contexts within which the 'objects' of alienism (later renamed psychiatry) were constructed and classified (2).

The current concept of 'mental disorder' was constructed during the 19th century based on the then newly constituted notion of 'disease'. Likewise, alienism was moulded upon the general epistemology and social structures of post-Enlightenment medicine (3). In this sense, the period 1780–1830 provides the appropriate frame to study the origins of the current concept of 'mental illness'. A large body of work has accumulated on the definitions of health and disease (4). Continental writers such as Riese (5), Canguilhem (6), Taylor (7), and Gadamer (8) have excelled in this regard. Following a different approach, Anglo-American analytical philosophers have sought to define the said concepts without their cultural context (9). At best, these inventories rehash the broader issues extant in the history and sociology of knowledge but are unable to explain why, for example, 'objectivist' definitions (according to which disease is purportedly defined in terms of specific descriptions and causes—e.g. they prefer to conceive of mental and somatic illness as being the 'same' concept) are more popular among biologically oriented psychiatrists than 'constructivist' ones (their definitions of abnormality are always prescriptive, normative, and intra-epistemic; they are also preferred by sociologists and non-medical health professionals).

In this essay I will propose the view that, on account of its deep hybrid epistemological structure, mental illness is a concept *sui generis*. An adequate epistemological analysis of the problem in hand must: (a) take into account the historical fact that psychiatry has been a part of medicine only since the 19th century and that far more evidence is needed before this (contingent) association is consecrated as a 'fact of nature'; (b) create a native philosophy rather than import off-the shelf philosophies or burden psychiatry with (generic) problems borrowed from the philosophy of mind (10); (c) abandon the view that defining 'physical illness' is a *sine qua non* condition for defining mental illness; (d) make sure that the exploratory techniques to be used combine history and philosophy; and (e) develop alternative conceptualizations of mental afflictions if it is thought that the current ones are not going to help sufferers much, this because the first duty of the mental health professional is to the mentally ill and not to the fashions of psychiatry.

The conceptual components of 'mental illness'

Mind

Due to the time-lag that often separates inception from adoption of philosophical ideas, the concepts of 'mind' available to early 19th-century alienists were not contemporary (i.e. those entertained by, among others, Kant, Fichte, Hegel, and Maine de Biran) but earlier ones (11). French alienists, the first in Europe to adopt the new anatomo-clinical model, made use of two models of the mind (12): one developed by the Scottish philosophers of common sense (as sponsored by the philosopher Pierre Paul Royer-Collard (13)) and another by John Locke. The former conceived of the mind as a cluster of innate separable active and passive powers and the latter, inspired in Newtonian atomism, proposed that the mind was a *tabula rasa* and a passive receptor of primary ideas originated from the world at large, and secondarily put together by the laws of association. Both models were able to link the two components of the anatomo-clinical model of disease, namely, the putative brain lesion and its related symptomatology (madness).

Until the early 19th century, the view was still influential that the mind (soul, *l'âme*, spirit) could not become decomposed or diseased. That the mind could fragment was only possible after the development of phrenology, with its notion that mental functions were regionally represented in the brain (14). This provided grounds for the theoretical inference, still central to thinking in neuropsychology and neuropsychiatry (15), that causal chains can be established by working backwards from impaired faculty of the mind (as expressed in the content of the symptom) to impaired region of the brain (where the faculty is putatively located) (16).

Illness

In regards to the idea of illness we need to distinguish between the history of words (historical etymology), concepts (conceptual history), and referents (history of objects or behaviours) (17). In popular 18th-century parlance: 'disease' meant distemper, uneasiness, malady; 'illness' meant badness or inconvenience of any kind, sickness, malady, disorder or health, and wickedness; and 'disorder' meant want of regular disposition, irregularity, confusion, tumult, disturbance, bustle, sickness, distemper, neglect of rule, discomposure of mind, and turbulence of passions (18). This suggests that they constituted a family whose members relied upon one another for their definition.

Since the 17th century, the ontological stability of a disease was made to depend upon the interaction between (putative) internal causal forces and stereotyped somatic responses. According to the *more botanico* view, developed during the 18th century, diseases were considered similar to plants; indeed, most of the great nosologists of the period were also botanists. To classify *per genus et more botanico* taxonomists needed to privilege certain features of each species; sexual organs in the case of plants and certain symptoms in the case of diseases (19). With only a minor change, the 19th century adopted the same model of disease: the forces that kept the disease true to form (i.e. looking more or less the same irrespective of the patient affected) were to be the tissular structures and functions pertaining to the 'diseased' organ. In other words, the definition of disease was to be sought in the specificity of its substratum and aetiology (20).

After having offered some information on the history of the word, concept and referent, it is now possible to analyse the construction of the concept of 'mental illness' during the first half of the 19th century.

The concept of 'mental illness'

The so-called anatomo-clinical model of disease was based on the belief that there is a cause–effect link between body and the signs and symptoms of disease. During the early 19th century the concepts of 'sign' and 'symptom' become redefined as units of analysis and markers of disease; this grew into a new medical discipline called 'semiology'. The old concept of madness—that had until then been defined as a metaphysical entity—was broken up into fragments and each of these became a 'mental symptom'. *Pari passu*, the body was reconceptualized as a mosaic of specialized organs and tissues each of which might be held responsible for certain symptoms and signs. The final stage in this epistemological change was the appearance of 'medical physiology' (the study of function) which in the realm of general medicine made it possible to fill the explanatory gap between tissues and symptoms.

The medicalization of alienism encouraged the direct application to madness of the anatomo-clinical model of disease. Indeed, every aspect of alienism was reconceived as being part of a 'medicine', including the professionalization of its practitioners, the creation of rites of passage (examinations, degrees), social networking (associations, guilds, meetings), databases (journals, books), and the building of specific venues of care (mental asylums). From then on the generic category 'madness' together with alienation, lunacy, insanity, and dementia were *in toto* replaced by the new generic concept of mental disease or illness. Alienism became, *de facto*, a branch of medicine, which it has remained to this day.

Vis-à-vis these historical facts, two explanatory narratives present themselves to the epistemologist of psychiatry. According to the first, the process consisted in an enlightened 'discovery' made in response to the ineluctable progress of science towards the truth; it is in this sense that many consider the view that madness is a 'disease' as a 'fact of nature'. According to the second narrative, the medicalization of madness must be considered as a 'contingent' event, a social response to a particular problem. Hence, its success should depend less on its intrinsic 'truth' than on its social usefulness and on the fact that it fits in well with the socio-economic needs of capitalistic Europe.

In regards to the analysis of 'mental illness' and of its classification these two narratives lead to different consequences. According to the 'fact of nature' view it would be idle (or perverse) to conceive madness in any other way. According to the 'contingency' view, and given that the 'fact of nature' approach does not seem to be working well, seeking alternative conceptualizations of madness becomes the duty of the professional career. For reasons which remain unclear, the 'contingency' view has been dismissed as yet another manifestation of the so-called 'anti-psychiatry' movement. This is wrong and needs clarifying.

The claim that madness is only (and can only be) a physically based phenomenon does away with the possibility of understanding it (or at least some of its forms) as purely semantic, symbolic acts susceptible to interpretation and to hermeneutic management. *Ab initio*, this blindness to meaning characterizing the biological view of madness is likely to have been accepted as a small price to pay for the enormous potential benefits of achieving total and rapid medical cure. That this promise has not been fulfilled in the real world of psychiatry needs accounting for. The stock answer remains that finding 'the cause of' is only matter of more time and more research funding. This answer is no longer acceptable. Analysis of the problem suggests that the idea of a 'full naturalization' of madness is fundamentally misconceived and needs to be replaced.

The difficulty is that any new narrative proposed to replace the medical view will raise all manner of scientific, medical, social, and professional hackles. This is because the rhetoric of the biological view has been so successful that often enough patients themselves and their supporting associations (e.g. those related to the so-called 'chronic fatigue syndrome') would not countenance any explanation of their symptoms that is not absolutely biological.

This is a pity, for the 'contingency' view is able to provide adequate conceptual space for both biological and hermeneutic accounts of madness, or combinations thereof. The biological view has failed because it has been indiscriminately applied to all forms of mental illness. The hybrid model that I shall propose in this essay advocates for the creation of subgroups of afflictions, each susceptible to a different conceptualization and management. Given that psychiatry is not a contemplative but a modificatory discipline, the crucial questions are: (a) whether there may be other ways of conceptualizing madness that can give rise to more efficient, ethical, dignified, and affordable routines than those currently in place; and (b) if these conceptualizations were to be shown to be superior to what we have now, what would be the arguments against their adoption?

The hybrid model

Objects of psychiatry

One of the tasks of the epistemology of psychiatry is to explore the nature of psychiatric objects (i.e. mental symptoms and disorders). On account of their ontological stability, mental symptoms are to be considered as the units of analysis or fundamental building bricks of psychopathology (21). What we consider as psychiatric diseases or disorders are but higher-level, contingent, abstract clusters of mental symptoms. On account of their historically contingent origin, categories such as schizophrenia, general anxiety disorder, obsessive-compulsive disorder, and personality disorder must be regarded as temporal heuristic devices with little ontological stability. Whatever enduring power these 'disorders' may exhibit is likely to be parasitical upon: (a) the ontological stability of the mental symptoms whose cluster they are, and (b) the role they play in society and continuing culture. Ontological stability refers here to the capacity of certain objects to show 'transtemporal' and 'transcultural' persistence. Most current mental symptoms owe their stability to the fact that they are likely to be linked to some neurobiological kernel. Mental disorders, on the other hand, owe their stability to the mental symptoms they name and the cultural and social forces that created them in the first place.

The 'contingency view' therefore has little to do with the anti-psychiatry movement because it fully accepts that mental symptoms do exist and are hybrid entities resulting from biological signals modified by cultural forces. What it calls into question is the view that mental disorders *per se* are anything more than the cluster of individual mental symptoms that constitute them. The hybrid model also proposes that 'mental symptoms' are heterogeneous phenomena each of which needs to be studied independently.

Mental symptoms

According to the Cambridge model, formatting may change not only the form or intensity of the neurobiological signal but also its content and specificity (22). The process of symptom-formation starts when a dysfunctional or distressed brain issues signals that upon entering the patient's awareness create entirely novel subjective experiences in him. This means that he has no templates to compare, describe, and name them; hence, the experiences are *ab initio* ineffable, prelinguistic, and preconceptual. In order to be communicated they need to be configured into mental and speech acts.

Patients are led to construct mental symptoms (e.g. hallucination, delusion, obsession, depersonalization) to manage and report the experiences caused by the intrusion into their awareness of neurobiological signals of distress. These 'experiences' (the 'primordial soup') are inchoate, preconceptual, and prelinguistic and not yet differentiated as thoughts, images, or emotions. To integrate them into the concert of their minds, patients give these experiences meaning by configuring them in terms of personal, familial, and cultural templates. Translating them into words and embedding them into speech acts are parts of this process. The final result can be described as a 'configured' experience; that is, an experience ready to be communicated via an utterance or a behavioural gesture. The depth of the configuration is such that the 'content' of the reported symptom may have little to do with the functional signature of the brain site that originated the intruding signal. Thus, the same biological signal may be configured into different mental symptoms, or alternatively two different signals may be configured as the same mental symptom. Once the mental symptom has been configured, the person may decide to complain; that is, to report it to someone else (e.g. a clinician). The dialogical interaction in the context of which the person complains is often characterized by haggling and negotiation and this adds another stage to the process of configuration. In the context of a shared culture and often enough influenced by the clinician's diagnostic hypothesis, each report by the patient is renegotiated into the final 'mental symptom' (as recorded in the case notes). This also means that mental symptoms are not just members of a uniform class but differ in origin, nature, history, and meaning (3,23).

The brain inscription of mental symptoms

According to one of the tenets of biological psychiatry, the 'validity' of psychiatric knowledge depends upon the strength of the relationship between mental disorders and the brain. If so, issues pertaining to brain localization must also be of interest to the epistemology of psychiatry. The current view of localization is based on (24): (a) the cultural belief that behaviour in general and the mind in particular must be a function of the brain alone; (b) the observation that persons suffering from traumatic brain lesions may show alterations of behaviour or mind redolent of conventional 'mental symptoms'; (c) empirical research showing that mechanical, chemical or electrical manipulation of regions of the brain may induce predictable changes in behaviour (in animals and humans); and (d) finding that changes in proxy variables representing mental activities changes proxy variables representing brain activity correlates (e.g. as detected by neuroimaging).

The assumptions listed above need to be explored: motor and sensory functions and mental symptoms are different type of phenomena; hence, from the fact that the former are hard-wired it cannot be inferred that the latter are equally located in the brain. From the fact that subjects with brain lesions show mental symptoms it cannot be inferred that they are localized in the regions affected by the traumatic lesion. It is not clear that mental symptoms occurring in the context of brain lesions and in patients with psychiatric diagnoses such as schizophrenia or obsessive-compulsive disorder are to be considered as the same phenomena, for example that organic and psychiatric hallucinations have the same structure and provenance. It is very difficult to transform correlational information provided by neuroimaging or neurophysiological stimulation into a cause–effect relationship.

Therefore, the question of the brain 'localization' of mental symptoms is not about the mapping or determination of an 'ontological fact' but rather about how a historical construct (i.e. the report of a configured 'subjective experience') relates to another construct represented by proxy variables (body). Throughout history both 'subjective experience' and 'body' have received varied definitions. For example, until the 19th century the former included organs other than the brain (e.g. the stomach) (25). The current narratives about the 'brain localization' of mental symptoms bank on the strength of statistical correlations between proxy variables representing both terms of the putative association.

As stated earlier, mental symptoms are hybrid constructs and their brain localization (by neuroimaging or other technique) poses an epistemological problem. In this essay two forms of brain representation are proposed. First, there are hard-wired forms of inscription (e.g. perception, memory) where the nature of the relationship between mental function and anatomical substratum is such that: (a) a lesion of the latter will affect the former, generating, when appropriate, a symptom; and (b) therapeutic manipulation of a primary brain inscription may alleviate the disturbance associated with the concomitant mental function (as may occur in neurological disorders, e.g. a brain tumour causing hallucinations and certain manifestations of epilepsy).

Secondary brain inscriptions refer here to the manner in which complex symbolic mental states generated in the medium of language relate to the brain. Symbolic mental states are defined as states whose content and causal force no longer depend on a neuro-biological substratum (whether cognitive, emotional, or volitional) but on the specific meaning they have within a dialogical interaction. What matters is not that they can be thoughts, emotions, or volitions (and hence the expression of neurobiological activity) but that: (a) the contents of those mental acts have been translated into symbols, allegories, metaphors, and the like; and (b) it is these connotational meanings, not the original neuropsychological actions, that carry the motivational force making the person act or feel in a particular way.

These connotational or supervenient meanings originate in the interpersonal semantic space formed during social exchange. If recorded or remembered they may endure but often enough they are transient and fade away with the disappearance of the semantic space. Nonetheless, while present they may induce strong feelings and behaviours. An interesting feature of supervenient meanings is that they are no longer 'inside the head' but inhabit interpersonal space. Thus explained, the question is how they relate to the brain.

Given the neurobiological postulate that all behaviour must be represented in the brain, it would be appropriate to expect that the original mental symptom and the configurative process itself should be supported by a neural substrate. The issue is whether connotational meanings are (or need to be) inscribed in the brain. It is proposed that such meanings may become 'secondarily' inscribed on the brain, particularly when they need to be recalled. Such secondary representation must, however, be conceived as differing from the primary one. First, it would not be fixed (in the sense of hard-wired) but fleeting and dynamic. Secondly, there would be no 'mental function' with which it would be associated. Supervenient meanings might be temporarily inscribed wherever there is an idle region of the brain but they would not have a specific relationship with that region.

Obvious consequences of this process are that: (a) it would still be possible to find correlations between supervenient meanings and a brain region (e.g. through neuro-imaging); but (b) given that that region is not the primary originator of the mental state, therapeutic manipulation of the region will not lead to any behavioural change and clinical improvement.

An example of a supervenient meaning is provided by the function of speech that conveys psychological consequences. If one were to ask whether 'speech acts' (as defined by Austin, 26) are inscribed in the brain, the answer should be that it depends to which of the Austinian components one is referring. Given that language is hard-wired, the performance of speech (an utterance) should be primarily inscribed. Therefore, when a priest tells a couple 'I declare you husband and wife' or the Queen utters 'I name this ship Queen Elizabeth the Second. May God bless her and all who sail in her', the fact that it would be perfectly possible to localize by neuroimaging in their brains neural activity corresponding to the pronunciation of their words and their general intention is irrelevant to the specific status and meaning of the act itself (because these are localized not in their brains but in the semantic collective space). The same neural activity would occur whether they are rehearsing at home or performing in the appropriate social context. However, in the latter context, a connotational meaning will supervene that is cogent to the newlyweds or to those embarking on the voyage.

I propose that certain mental symptoms are structurally and symbolically similar to these performative meanings in that they are secondarily inscribed in the brain. In such cases, interference with the correlated brain region would not alter the symbolic force of the performative meaning; the latter could only be managed by manipulating reasons as opposed to causes. If it is the case that primary inscriptions identify 'causes' and secondary inscriptions relate to 'reasons' then it becomes imperative that psychiatrists develop conceptual and empirical criteria to differentiate between the two.

Classifying mental illness

Classifications can only succeed when there are stable objects to categorize. I dealt with one way of defining and circumscribing these objects above and will now deal with the way in which the objects of psychiatry may be grouped.

Conceptual tools and meta-language

Since the 18th century, classifications have been divided into 'natural' and 'artificial'. According to a 'weak' version, objects can be classified in terms of 'essential' or 'man-made features' (e.g. flowers grouped according to their sexual organs or their use: funerals, weddings, and the like). In a 'strong' version, 'natural' must mean 'natural kind' (27–29) and 'artificial' man-made (30, 31). Based on the view that psychiatric objects are constructs (32) it has been argued that psychiatric classifications must be considered as 'artificial'. This may also explain why 'proxy' variables have continued to be used to steady up the ontology of psychiatric objects since the 19th century; brain inscriptions, neuropathology, encephalography, neuropsychological networks, psychophysiological variables, genetics, among others, have all been used in their day. Apart from the fact that in psychiatry there is not yet a good theory of proxyhood, there is the danger that the ignorant may confuse it with 'naturalization'.

The 'list versus structured' dichotomy refers to the manner in which classes relate to each other. Examples of 'listings' are the International Classification of Diseases (ICD) of the World Health Organization (WHO) and the *Diagnostic and Statistical Manual* (DSM) of the American Psychiatric Association (33). Social and economic factors are important to a listing membership. This is not a problem in itself as long as the classification is not exported from the country in which it was constructed. In 'structured' classifications classes constitute a hierarchy and purport to map a given universe (e.g. like the periodic table of elements). No one has seriously put forward a structured psychiatric classification during the 20th century but one could easily concoct one. Hierarchical (multilayered) classifications consist in structures where high-level classes embed lower-level ones and can be used as decisional trees. 'Exhaustive versus partial' refers to the compass of a classification. Exhaustive classifications purport to include all the entities in a given universe; for example, some 19th century classifications of mental disorders assumed that the entire realm of mental functions could be classified into intellectual, emotional, and volitional. It was further assumed that each of these functional packages could be independently affected by disease leading to intellectual, emotional, and volitional 'mental disorders'. In fact, this approach constitutes the epistemological basis of current classifications: schizophrenia and paranoia (first group);

mania, depression, anxiety, phobias, etc. (second group); and character and personality disorders (third group). To deal with cases where more than one function seemed involved, rules were created to decide which was primary (34).

Lastly, idiographic versus nomothetic is occasionally mentioned. Its origin has nothing to do with psychology or psychiatry although it concerns efforts made at the turn of the 20th century to differentiate between the natural and social sciences. In his 1894 inaugural lecture as vice-chancellor of Strasburg University, Wilhelm Windelband stated:

> We can therefore say that in approaching reality the empirical sciences search for either of two things: the general in the form of natural laws or the special, as a specific event of history. They thus contemplate the permanent and immutable or the transitory as contained into real life happenings. The former sciences concern laws, the latter events; the former teach what has always been, the latter what has happened once. In the first case, scientific thinking is—if we were allowed to coin new technical terms—*nomothetic*, in the second case *idiographic* (35).

What are classifications for?

Of all the potential benefits of a classification the most important is prediction—the capacity to release additional knowledge about the sorted objects. The fact that this epistemological fruitfulness is rarely present in psychiatry needs to be accounted for. One explanation may be that the classification must start from a clear theoretical basis (like the periodic table of elements). There is little hope that this can be achieved in psychiatry. Such pessimism led some years ago to resorting to old notions of 'prototype' or 'ideal type'. As Hampton has stated:

> It is claimed that uncertainty about classification is a result of people's inadequate knowledge of the categories that exist in the real world. The prototype view is directed, however, at a characterization of exactly this inadequate knowledge—it is a model of the beliefs people have. Whether or not the real world is best described with a classical conceptual framework or not is an interesting and important question, but irrelevant to this psychological goal of the prototype model (36).

Are the notions of 'clearest case', 'best example', and 'procedural criteria' applicable to psychiatry? Can prototypes for all mental disorders be generated? What might their sources be? All that we have in our discipline are periodic recalibrations valid within specific timespans. As is the case with convergences, 'prototypes' do not form a progressive series either which may eventually culminate in the identification of a final Platonic idea (the definite phenotype). Prototypes simply capture, as Hampton put it, the extension of our 'current beliefs' about the object (disease) in question.

The 20th century and beyond

Since the 19th century, the drive to define and classify the objects of psychiatry in terms of the 'received view' of mental disorders has continued unabated and fruitlessly, in spite of the availability of new neurobiological and statistical data-gathering techniques. In all probability this failure is due to unwillingness or inability to replace the received view.

The 19th-century classificatory enterprise was fundamentally driven by personal and national needs. Composing a new classification of mental disorders was considered central to academic or professional achievement. Classifications soon became markers of national prestige and dominance. For example, after the Franco-Prussian war, German classifications went through a period of supremacy in Europe.

After World War II, new factors came into play. In certain countries, the pharmaceutical and medical insurance industries became powerful lobbyists. For example, compromises were reached in the United States (e.g. in the third and later editions of DSM) to counterbalance these intervening forces (37). In spite of its socio-economic topicality the DSM system was soon exported and its use extended to most countries.

The question of whether it is best for psychiatric patients worldwide to be managed according to one or to multiple classificatory systems has not yet been fully answered. The fact that no direct empirical evidence has been marshalled so far in favour of a unitary option (resulting from a dedicated trial comparing the two options in relation, for example, to therapeutic outcome) suggests that the reasons for accepting it are of a sociopolitical rather than of a scientific nature.

The epistemology of the 20th-century classificatory enterprise is also characterized by internal shifts, for example, in its 'truth-making' structure, the way in which candidate groupings are legitimated (38). *Ab initio* (say in the 1810s) classifications were exclusively based on observation. As quantification entered medicine during the second half of the 19th century, percentages and other basic numerical devices began to be used to differentiate random from clinically meaningful groupings. The introduction during the 20th century of factor and cluster analysis and of other pattern recognition techniques (e.g. numerical taxonomy) (39) marked the culmination of this process. From then on, discrepancies between groupings drawn clinically or statistically were resolved in favour of the latter. This shift has also been accompanied by the gradual replacement of the time-honoured narrative, qualitative diagnosis (the original source of groupings and boundaries) by structured, criterial, quantitative forms of 'case-identification'. This process has now been completed to the point where no 'major' professional journal accepts manuscripts in which cases have not been identified by means of criterial, quantitative techniques. From an epistemological point of view, the worry is that this form of identification and statistical groupings have been made to form closed loops which in practice impede the entry of much-needed corrective informational variance. Hence, as things stand presently, it could be argued that statistical analysis 'confirms' official classifications not on account of the 'truth' or 'validity' of groupings but because information collected by the structured systems is already biased in the direction of confirmation.

Overlapping or intersection of group boundaries can affect lists, orders, and classifications. Only good-quality classifications possess mechanisms to lessen such confusions. Because their simplistic lists and orderings lack such mechanisms, DSM (the 4th, revised edition) for example seems to have given rise to an inordinate number of overlappings (40). Made into a putative new class of clinical phenomena grandly called 'comorbidity' (also coexistence, co-occurrence, dual diagnosis, double diagnosis, mixed diagnosis, blended diagnosis, double jeopardy, combined disorders, codisorders), these overlappings have become the object of yet another research industry (41).

What we seem to need are criteria to decide which overlappings are clinically meaningful and which artefactual, and also to specify when the word and concept of comorbidity is being used as descriptive or explanatory. The absence of stable causal explanations in psychiatry also means that whether or not a 'comorbid' pair is considered to contain a relationship of potential clinical interest cannot be easily decided, particularly using 'statistical significance' criteria.

Clinical overlappings (putative comorbidities) can be analysed in space and time and in relation to systems of expression (42). Since the 19th century, there have been changes in the type of container within which mental disorders are believed to exist. For example, by the 1880s Meynert (and later Wernicke under Meynert's influence) proposed the existence of sets of virtual spaces where diseases could be 'located'. In Meynert's model of the brain, these spaces were mappable as regions or networks (43). Because cerebral (psychiatric) diseases were located in different brain spaces, they did not interfere with each other. As against this mosaic model, Freud believed that mental disorders originated and expressed themselves within only one integrated psychological space. Disorders needed to be differentiated on the basis of the level of regression that caused them in the first place. In this sense, comorbidity was not possible, for a person could not have regressed to two stages at the same time.

Even when not overlapping in space, clinical objects can 'overlap' within given time frames (what can be called serial as opposed to parallel comorbidity). In these cases the duration of the time frame (i.e. the length of time allowed between the comorbid pairs), needs to be clinically determined. Overlappings in time remain under-researched. Parallel overlappings can also occur, for example, when it is believed that one of the comorbid pair (e.g. schizophrenia) never quite abandons the individual even if it is in remission.

The third relational mode corresponds to what is called 'systems of expression'. Regardless of whether one or multiple spaces are allocated to a mental disorder, it could be postulated that human beings have either one or many systems of expression for their mental disorders. For example, the concept of 'mixed state' in Kraepelin (44) can be interpreted according to each option. If there is only one system of expression, then the person cannot be sad and euphoric at the same time and will have to express each of these emotions intermittently. If there are various systems of expression then parallel expression will be possible and the 'perceived' result (by the clinician) would be some sort of mixed mood in which both emotions have 'blended'.

Little attention has been given to the nature and characteristics of the clinical objects that are to become members of a comorbid pair. According to current (broad) psychiatric use, pairs can result from overlappings of classes of disorders (e.g. neuroses versus psychoses), disorders, syndromes, symptoms, signs, traits, and deficits. Thus, in theory there could be homotypical and heterotypical pairings according to whether the 'comorbid' clinical objects have the same (say two diseases or two syndromes) or different level of organization and complexity (say a disease and a syndrome)—schizophrenia and substance misuse as an example of the former and depression and morbid jealousy as an example of the latter. Originally, comorbidity was used to refer only to the coexistence of two distinct disorders. Current use, however, often includes pairings with trivial clinical meaning; for example, some authors call the association of traumatic brain damage with the deficits identified in its wake comorbid (45).

Lastly, there is the issue of a comorbid hierarchy. In his original study, Feinstein (46) allocated different weights to the components of the comorbid pair: one was the index disease, the other the secondary disease. Such an approach has been lost in the psychiatric application and it looks as if the members of the pair are given the same weight.

One of the few theoretical aspects of comorbidity that has been studied in some depth concerns its relationship to nosological theory. It appears that categorical systems of disease, that is, those that consider diseases to be autonomous, independent, stable, and properly bounded categories, are more likely to be affected by the comorbidity problem. The dimensional nosological model, on the other hand, is less likely to be open to the threat of comorbidity. Indeed, as Meehl (47) has claimed, the concept itself does not apply to dimensional systems.

Objects such as tables, flowers, dogs, clouds, and diseases exhibit two types of properties—intrinsic and extrinsic. Intrinsic, non-relational properties such as colour, form, smell, and the material of which it is made may contribute to the very definition of the object to which they are attached. Extrinsic, relational properties such as 'larger than', 'equal to', 'caused by', and 'linked to' only crystallize when objects are considered in *relation* to something else (48). Since at least the time of Aristotle there have been disagreements as to the nature of properties and on their reality, objectivity, and independence from the object itself (i.e. their ontology). Over the centuries conceptual instruments have been devised to deal with the ontology and epistemology of properties and relations.

Given that there is no epistemological framework to place comorbidity, it could be usefully considered as an instance of a 'relational property'. Comorbidity pairs could thus be classified according to whether the nature of their relationship is intrinsic or extrinsic (genotypic or phenotypic respectively), with only the latter considered as genuine comorbid pairs.

Discussion and conclusions

The concept of mental illness can only be explored in relation to specific historical frames. Since the association between the alienism (now psychiatry) and general medicine has been historically determined, there is little reason to consider it as a 'fact of nature'. If the current association is not working well, those charged with helping the mentally ill are duty-bound to seek alternative conceptualizations.

While evidence exists that mental symptoms do have ontological stability, mental illnesses are high-level historical constructs parasitical upon the symptoms they name. I have presented a hybrid model of the structure and objects of psychiatry. The model conforms to the view that mental symptoms have a neurobiological origin, but emphasizes the role of cultural factors so that on occasions the same biological signal may give rise to different mental symptoms, and biological signals of a different origin may be formatted into the same symptom. This model also suggests that current views on the brain localization of mental symptoms must be revised. Only those mental symptoms related to hard-wired functions are likely to be primarily inscribed in the brain and allow for the prediction that biological modification of the substratum may lead to their alleviation. Symptoms are symbolic representations, adianoetas generated in the transient semantic space created through language and intersubjective exchange. Although this information may also be inscribed in the brain it provides no therapeutic purchase, that is, biological modification of the transient inscription will not affect the symptoms.

The psychiatric epistemologist can study classifications in two ways: (a) accept the 'received view' that the rules of classifying are inherent to nature and the human mind and that they fit perfectly into the eternal ontology of all psychiatric objects; or (b) consider psychiatric classifications as cultural products. This essay follows the second approach. After mapping the history of classification and its meta-language, it was shown that it is essential to differentiate between taxonomy, classification, and its object domain. The ontological and epistemological nature of the psychiatric object is far more important in developing a meaningful classification than any statistical or empirical procedure applied to objects which are far from understood. There is a real danger that proxy variables which originally have been chosen as mere handles or correlational terms end up replacing the disease itself by a process that the 20th century has for some obscure reason chosen to call 'naturalization'.

During the 19th century alienism borrowed from general medicine the so-called 'anatomo-clinical' model of disease. This epistemological device has enjoined psychiatrists to anchor both the psychiatric object and its putative classification in neurobiology. Looking for a 'biological invariant' responsible for symptoms still seems a task worth pursuing but has led to a neglect of the mechanism of psychological causation and of the way in which accepting this principle may lead to an entirely different way of classifying mental disorders.

During the last few years, it has been proposed that many mental disorders are not natural kinds and therefore do not survive well when translocated from one historical period to the next; mental symptoms may in fact be more appropriate units of neurobiological and epistemological analysis (35). This view has different taxonomic consequences, since classifying symptoms then becomes a different epistemological enterprise (38).

In general terms, taxonomy and its associated classificatory activity constitute a self-contained and more or less exhaustive conceptual system. Within a given historical period, thinking about and crafting classifications is like playing a game of chess in that everything will occur within strict boundaries and according to explicit or implicit rules. For example, not all possible moves will be made, some because they are forbidden by the rules, others because they are patently nonsensical, and yet others because they are unfashionable. Up to the 19th century most of the classificatory game was played within biology and concerned natural kinds. Within this domain classifications are important for they can generate knowledge. Classifications of artificial objects, common as they may be, have only an actuarial function and everyone recognizes that. The issue here is what the nature of psychiatric classifications is. Certainly, it would be nonsensical to believe that they are like plant taxonomies and that one day we will be able to classify mental disorders by using a sort of *per genus et differentia* technique or, even worse, creating a sort of neuropsychological periodic table of elements on the basis of which we could predict the existence of new forms of mental disorder which have not yet been reported.

In summary, 17th-century taxonomic theory was constructed to make possible the classification of plants, animals, and minerals, and hopefully to predict new information about the nature of the members of a given class (49, 50). Whether classifications are based on privileged features or countenance the possibility of a numerical taxonomy, they work at their best when the objects to be classified are ontologically stable (e.g. are natural kinds) and epistemologically accessible (defined by capturable attributes). When applied to abstract objects (e.g. virtues), artefacts (e.g. poems), or constructs (e.g. mental symptoms or disorders), such classificatory approaches are no longer on safe territory and require ad hoc epistemological aids for their functioning. When applied outside of their field of competence and validity, it is not possible to predict what modifications classificatory systems require. Much research, both conceptual and empirical, needs to be done to decide which are required by each type of object to be classified. The inchoate nature of current knowledge on the epistemological and ontological status of psychiatric objects makes it particularly difficult to decide what modifications in the classificatory system are required and on what expectations should classificators have in respect to the usefulness of classifying mental disorders.

When talking about classifications, we should take the word seriously. They are more than lists, glossaries, or inventories. Instead, they are structured and commonly hierarchical clusters of objects having a relationship with one another. The more one thinks about their application to mental disorders the more one realizes that the problem here is not only our lack of knowledge about taxonomy but the possibility that psychiatric objects may not be susceptible to classification at all.

References and endnotes

1 Sendrail, M. (1980). *Histoire culturelle de la maladie.* Paris: Privat.
2 Watts, S. (2003). *Disease and medicine in world history.* London: Routledge.
3 Berrios, G. E. (1996). *The history of mental symptoms.* Cambridge: Cambridge University Press.
4 Caplan, A. L., Engelhardt, H. T., and McCartney, J. J. (eds.) (1981). *Concepts of health and disease.* London: Addison-Wesley.
5 Riese, W. (1953). *The Conception of Disease.* New York: Philosophical Library.
6 Canguilhem, G. (1966). *Le normal et le pathologique.* Paris: PUF.
7 Taylor, F. K. (1979). *The concepts of illness, disease, and morbus.* Cambridge: Cambridge University Press.
8 Gadamer, H. G. (1996). *The enigma of health.* Cambridge: Polity Press.
9 Boorse, C. (1975). On the distinction between disease and illness. *Philosophy and Public Affairs* 5, 40–68.
10 Berrios, G. E. (2006) Mind in general and Sir A. Crichton. *History of Psychiatry* 17, 469–86.
11 On the general philosophical background in France during the 19th century see: Brooks III, J. I. (1998). *The eclectic legacy: academic philosophy and the human sciences in nineteenth-century France.* London: Associated University Presses.
12 Berrios, G.E. (1988). Historical background to abnormal psychology. In Miller E. and Cooper J (eds.) *Adult abnormal psychology*, Edinburgh: Churchill Livingstone, pp. 26–51.
13 His biographer, De Barante, tells how Royer-Collard found in a bookstall a copy of the French translation of Thomas Reid's 'Essays' and this provided him with the purview he

was looking for to oppose Condillac, at the time the predominant philosophical influence in France (p. 108 in de Barante, M. (1861). *La vie politique de M. Royer-Collard. Ses discours et ses écrits.* Vol. 1, Paris: Didier).

14 Gall, F. J. and Spurzheim, G. (1811). *Des dispositions innées de l'âme et de l'esprit.*Paris: Schoell.

15 Uttal, W. R. (2001). *The new phrenology. The limits of localizing cognitive processes in the brain.* Cambridge, MA: MIT Press.

16 Riese, W. (1950) *La pensée causale en médecine.* Paris: PUF.

17 Berrios, G. E. (1994). Historiography of mental symptoms and diseases. *History of Psychiatry* 5, 175–90.

18 Johnson, S. (1756/1994). *Dictionary of the English language*, Chalmers, A. (ed). London: Studio Editions.

19 In this regard, Linné's epigram is also well known: '*Symptomata se habent ad morbum ut folia et fulcra ad plantam*'; on this Pinel commented: 'The revolution brought about by Linné in natural history, together with the introduction of a method to offer descriptions that be short and exact, could not but greatly influence medicine' (see **Pinel** (1813) *Nosographie Philosophique* (5th edn), Paris: Brosson, Vol 1, p. lxxxiv).

20 Chamberet, J. B. (1818). Maladie. In: *Dictionaire des sciences médicales*, Vol. 30. Paris: Panckoucke, pp. 172–203.

21 Marková, I. S. and Berrios, G. E. (2009). Epistemology of mental symptoms. *Psychopathology* 42, 343–9.

22 Berrios, G. E. and Marková, I. S. (2006). Symptoms—historical perspectives and effect on diagnosis. In: Blumenfiels, M. and Strain, J. J. (eds.) *Psychosomatic medicine*. Philadelphia, PA: Lippincott Williams & Wilkins, pp. 27–38.

23 Marková, I. S. and Berrios, G. E. (1995). Mental symptoms: are they similar phenomena? The problem of symptom heterogeneity. *Psychopathology* 28, 147–57.

24 Hécaen, H. and Lanteri-Laura, G. (1978). *Evolution des connaissances et des doctrines sur les localizations cérébrales.* Paris: Desclée de Brouwer.

25 Broussais, F. J. V. (1828). *De l'irritation et de la folie.* Paris: Delaunay.

26 Austin, J. L. (1962). *How to do things with words.* Oxford: Clarendon Press.

27 See: Granger, H. (1985). The scala naturae and the continuity of kinds. *Phronesis* 30, 181–200.

28 Dupré, J. (1981). Natural kinds and biological taxa. *Philosophical Review* 90, 66–90.

29 Wilkerson, T. (1993). Species, essences, and the names of natural kinds. *Philosophical Quarterly* 43, 1–19.

30 Dagognet, F. (1970). *Le catalogue de la vie.* Paris: Presses Universitaires de France.

31 For an example of a proposal for an artificial classification, i.e. one that emphasizes certain features or 'questions', see **Mellergård, M.** (1987). Psychiatric classifications as a reflection of uncertainties. *Acta Psychiatrica Scandinavica* 76, 106–11.

32 Ellenberger, H. (1963). Les illusions de la classification psychiatrique. *L'Evolution Psychiatrique* 28, 221–48.

33 Cooper, R. (2005). *Classifying madness.* Dordrecht: Springer.

34 In this regard, Jaspers's views are well known: 'The principle of medical diagnosis is that all the disease phenomena should be characterized within a single diagnosis. Where a number of different phenomena co-exist the question arises which of them should be preferred for diagnostic purposes so that the remaining phenomena can be considered secondary or

accidental.' (in **Jaspers, K.** (1963) *General psychopathology,* translated by J. Hoenig and M. W. Hamilton, Manchester: Manchester University Press, pp. 611–12.

35   p. 317 in **Windelband, W.** (1949). Historia y ciencia de la naturaleza. In: *Preludios Filosó-ficos,* translated by W. Roces, Buenos Aires: Santiago Rueda. pp. 311–28 (original German edition 1903).

36   **Hampton, J.** (1993). Prototype models of concept representation. In: Mechelen, I. van, Hampton, J., Muchalski, R.S., and Theuns, P. (eds.) *Categories and concepts.* London: Academic Press, 70.

37   **Cooper, R.** (2005). *Classifying madness.* Heidelberg: Springer.

38   **Kendler, K. and Parnas, J.** (eds.) (2012). *Philosophical issues in psychiatry II: Nosology.* Oxford: Oxford University Press.

39   **Sokal, R. R. and Sneath, P. H .A.** (1963). *Principles of numerical taxonomy.* San Francisco, CA: W. H. Freeman.

40   **Maj, M.** (2005). 'Psychiatric comorbidity': an artefact of current diagnostic systems? *British Journal of Psychiatry* **186**, 181–4.

41   **Vella, G., Aragona, M., and Alliani, D.** (2002). The complexity of psychiatric comorbidity: a conceptual and methodological discussion. *Psychopathology* **33**, 25–30.

42   **Berrios, G. E.** (2011). *Hacia una nueva epistemología de la psiquiatría.* Buenos Aires : Polemos.

43   **Meynert, Th.** (1884). *Psychiatrie. Klinik der Erkrankungen des Vorderhirns.* Wien, Braumüller.

44   **Kraepelin, E.** (1913). Mischzustände. In: *XI. Das Manisch-depressive Irresein. Psychiatrie. Ein Lehrbuch für Studierende und Arzte* (8th edn), Vol. III, *Klinische Psychiatrie.* Leipzig: Barth, pp. 1284–303.

45   **Scherer, M. R. and Schubert, M. C.** (2009). Traumatic brain injury and vestibular pathology as a comorbidity after blast exposure. *Physical Therapy* **89**, 980–92.

46   **Feinstein, A. R.** (1970). The pre-therapeutic classification of co-morbidity in chronic disease. *Journal of Chronic Diseases* **23**, 455–568.

47   **Meehl, P. E.** (2001). Comorbidity and taximetrics. *Clinical Psychology Science Practice* **8**, 507–19.

48   **Mellor, D. H. and Oliver, A.** (eds.) (1997). *Properties.* Oxford: Oxford University Press.

49   **Winston, J. E.** (1999). *Describing species.* New York: Columbia University Press.

50   **Bowker, G. C. and Star, S. L.** (1999). *Sorting things out.* Cambridge, MA: MIT Press.

Essay 11

From alienist to collaborator: the twisting road to consultation–liaison psychiatry

Don R. Lipsitt

Among scientists are collectors, classifiers, and compulsive tidiers-up; many are detectives by temperament and many are explorers; some are artists and others artisans. There are poet-scientists and philosopher-scientists and even a few mystics.
—*The Art of the Soluble,* Sir Peter Medawar, 1967 (1)

Introduction

For many years, philosopher-physicians and then general physicians were hospitable to the notion that mind and body were inseparable. Mind and body were thought to be related, no matter how primitively. The ancient Greek philosophers were hardly the first to ponder the issue. Prehistoric tribes believed that bodily 'possession' could be 'treated' by drilling holes in the skull to get at the presumptive source of the 'problem.' Even ecclesiasts believed that the residence of the soul was most likely in the brain, although influential throughout the body. The advent of specialization was very likely the enemy of the integrated wholeness of mind-body relations.

To counteract reductionist trends of medicine, efforts to reassemble the mind–body composition have been vigorous throughout history. An avalanche of endeavours to pull mind and body back together have punctuated the literature (2), clinic efforts, and certain avenues of research. At least since the beginning of the 20th century, these efforts to put the 'Humpty-Dumpty' of mind and body, psychiatry and medicine, back together again, have struggled against the impediment of Cartesian dualism. In this endeavour, the growth of consultation–liaison (C-L) psychiatry, as one aspect of the profession, has perhaps shown the greatest promise.

A meandering history

Currently, C-L psychiatry is defined as that branch of psychiatry and psychosomatic medicine that provides psychiatric consultation at the borderland or 'interface' of medicine and psychiatry; it also encompasses teaching and research that focuses on an integrated mind body approach to the understanding and treatment of complex medical illness and its social ramifications in all areas of medicine that otherwise are generally considered 'non-psychiatric.' Originally formulated and developed in the United States, it has since found application, to varying degrees, in virtually every developed country in the world.

C-L psychiatry has a long and meandering history. Contributions to its end-product are attributed to a catalogue of individuals who most likely did not prophesy what that evolution would be. But all in some measure had a passion for wanting to see psychiatry and medicine functioning harmoniously for the good of the patient. And one might say that C-L, with all its lurchings and impediments, has to a large degree addressed that objective.

In an endeavour to 'tidy up' that history, we look largely at the early turning of the 20th century, but with preambling reference to relevant highlights in earlier times. This essay traces the development of C-L psychiatry, its possible antecedents, affiliations, tributaries and ancillary byways, and its place—present and future—in psychiatry in the 21st century. The designation 'consultation–liaison' generally will be used throughout although that hyphenated form gradually evolved only by the 1980s; when relevant to the field's evolution, the historically correct terms 'consultation psychiatry' or 'liaison psychiatry' will be used. This essay is not intended as a thorough historical account of all contributing sources to C-L psychiatry; many excellent texts provide that perspective (3–6).

An evolutionary process

Searching for the roots of C-L psychiatry is an elusive endeavour. Where in the history of psychiatry do we fix the practice of psychiatric consultation? Who was the first to acknowledge and apply the value of psychiatric consultation? The location of such activity will most likely thwart earnest scholars, for emergent ideas in almost any field of exploration are more likely the product of slow evolution than identifiable occurrences, whether temporally specific or epochal.

Psychiatry and medicine divided

Psychiatry's relationship with its progenitor, medicine, has been one of approach-avoidance for eons. Before Johann Christian Reil, a German physician, coined the term 'psychiatry' in 1808, matters of mind (soul) and body were the clinical province of all general physicians; there were no 'psychiatrists' to address the problems of 'insanity,' or 'lunacy,' or 'feeble-mindedness.' Patients with 'mental diseases' were, for the most part, sequestered away in almshouses, poorhouses, and eventually asylums where treatment was virtually non-existent.

Warehousing mental patients, both in the United States and Europe, was a large factor in segregating psychiatry from the rest of medicine. It was perhaps only by separating mental patients from others that physicians began to define themselves, or be defined by others, as 'alienists' (from the French word meaning 'strange'). Physicians working in institutions were seen as peculiar, largely due to the isolated environment in which they worked. Their patients' condition was one of 'alienation' not only from their communities, but also from their families and other patients 'entitled' to be treated differently.

Seeing psychiatry and its practitioners from this perspective may have contributed greatly to the rise of stigma against mental patients, their treatment and their treaters. The launching in 1879 of a professional journal called '*The Alienist and Neurologist: A Journal of Neurology and Psychology, Psychiatry and Neuriatry* [*sic*]', probably did little to reduce stigma or to help reintegrate medicine and psychiatry. Perhaps in its search for 'cures', psychiatry, as it existed, alienated itself further from the rest of medicine by seeking remedies in mesmerism, animal magnetism, Emmanuelism (a blend of hypnosis, suggestion, and 'moral persuasion') and other pursuits of dubious scientific validity. Against these divisive forces, counterforces arose.

Mending *medicina mentis* and *medicina corporis*

As early as 1854, Dr Forbes Winslow, the British physician perhaps best known for his interest in the famous Jack the Ripper case in London in the 1880s, gave a special academic lecture to the Medical Society of London entitled 'The psychological vocation of the physician' (7). Republished in the same year that Freud acquainted America with his theories, its intent was to counteract the '. . . substitutes [like mesmerism—au.] for rational medical thinking . . .' that pervaded medicine at the time. Appearing in 1909 in the *Alienist and Neurologist,* it set out to claim for physicians (the 'cultivators of medical science') 'higher and more exalted functions than those usually assigned to them, to consider the physician . . . having at his command, and under his control, a *medicina mentis* as well as a *medicina corporis*—agents of great power and magnitude—which have not been sufficiently recognized or appreciated' (7, p. 1). It was Winslow's bold objective '. . . to establish the close connection between the SCIENCE OF MIND, and the SCIENCE AND PRACTICE OF MEDICINE [caps in original text], and to illustrate the true philosophic character of the professors of the healing art' (7, p. 2), a remarkably progressive notion for a man whose early history was as a child living on the grounds of asylums where his father had been superintendent. As voiced by Winslow, 'It may be within the compass of the medico-psychologist, aided by discoveries in physiological and other collateral sciences, to unravel that *mysterious union existing between mind and matter* [italics added]; and to trace the origin and source of the emotions, and the mode in which spirit and matter reciprocally act upon each other.' (7, p. 12). Winslow was one of many who sought greater integration of the domains of psyche and soma.

Psychoanalytic influence

Halfway around the world, a Viennese neurologist, Sigmund Freud, was attempting to 'unravel that mysterious union existing between mind and matter', exploring new ways to unite mind and body. The results of these explorations were first revealed in America in 1909 at Clark University in Worcester, Massachusetts. Following Freud's famous visit, psychoanalysis virtually took America by storm, extolling the wholeness of the individual and the recognition and appreciation of personality and character, not merely the illness of the person with mental disorder. That notion, Freud later wrote, was more favourably received in America than in Europe.

The emigration of European psychoanalysts to America during World War II found a strong kinship with psychiatry of the early 1900s. Psychoanalyst psychiatrists became the pre-eminent directors of psychiatric services as well as teachers of psychiatry in medical schools and general hospitals. This was a trend that brought psychiatry into closer proximity to medicine and would last for several decades. Indeed, psychodynamic techniques, derived from psychoanalysis, became the prevailing model in psychiatric training and education, and the notion that medical symptoms had meaning beyond mere bodily disturbance became a salient concept in C-L psychiatry.

At first, Freud's studies on hysteria, conversion, and dissociation seemed a giant step towards reintegrating mind and body, understanding the 'mysterious leap from mind to body'. Both psychoanalysts and non-psychiatrists exalted in the promise of a 'new medicine'. But Freud's interest in pursuing such connections lagged, and he preferred to leave to others the exploration of psychophysiological aspects of illness, including those of hypochondriasis, which he briefly discussed in the Schreber case. His entire corpus of work makes no reference to 'psychosomatic', although his earliest cases (e.g. Anna O., Dora) all presented with 'physical' or 'psychosomatic' symptoms. By focusing more exclusively on the mentalistic side of the equation, psychoanalysis actually may have widened rather than narrowed the gap between medicine and psychiatry. Nonetheless, its influence on the practice of C-L psychiatry, through an appreciation of psychodynamics, transference and countertransference, and defence mechanisms was considerable; all brought greater awareness of the powerful influence of mind over body.

The evolution of 'liaison'

Introduction of 'liaison': Albert M. Barrett

Liaison psychiatry, with a defined objective, did not emerge until the 1930s. The importance of 'psychological medicine' as part of patient care and a medical curriculum was not a new idea, but Dr Albert M. Barrett may have been the first to conceive of a 'liaison' function for psychiatry. His presidential address to the American Psychiatric Association in 1922 (8) declared a new period wherein psychiatry 'has shaped for itself a definite position as a branch of medicine . . . a new epoch in which its interests are extended to all that concerns mental disorders in their widest relationships, as problems of disease and their social effects' (8, p. 13). Barrett anticipated the importance of 'liaison' for psychiatry in establishing collaboration between itself and the rest of medicine, its general practitioners, hospitals, and communities.

Coming as they did shortly after World War I, Barrett's remarks took account of the psychiatrist's suitability for treating soldiers with battle fatigue and 'soldier's heart', as well as other stressful medical-psychological consequences of war. Barrett's exposition had sown the seeds of liaison, collaboration, and education as essential components of C-L psychiatry, as well as effective and humane care of the sick.

Thirty years earlier, in 1894, in efforts to restore mental care to physical care, neurologist S. Weir Mitchell had vociferously berated his listeners at the 50th annual meeting of the American Medico-Psychological Association for having severely distanced themselves from medicine, belying the title of their organization. He said they failed to deliver any new scientific knowledge, produced flawed records, and exercised little educational effort among its members to remedy the situation. Although Mitchell's remarks did not have the imprimatur of a recognized professional organization, they eloquently stressed the importance of the psychological aspects and requirements of medical practice. Such exhortation has surfaced in virtually every decade since; many besides Barrett and Mitchell were restlessly determined to improve the status of psychiatry's affiliation with medicine.

Psychiatry a 'liaison agent': George K. Pratt

Another important contributor to the development of C-L psychiatry was George K. Pratt, a physician who wrote prophetically in the *American Journal of Psychiatry* in 1926 that psychiatry, acting as a 'liaison agent', would eventually 'become the integrator that unifies, clarifies and resolves all available medical knowledge concerning that human being who is the patient, into one great force of healing power' (9, p. 408). Although he did not see this lofty aspiration realized in his lifetime, he became one of America's most influential psychiatrists. In his own practice and as a member of the National Committee for Mental Hygiene, he called for an integration of medicine and psychiatry. He was a staunch advocate for the collaboration of medical and psychiatric practitioners, and all members of the caretaking team for the benefit of the mentally ill.

Emergence of 'liaison psychiatry': George W. Henry

It took another decade, during the Great Depression, before the concept, if not the name, of liaison psychiatry was articulated by Dr George W. Henry, Director of the Research Laboratory at Bloomingdale Hospital in New York, where he had already initiated close collaborative relations with non-psychiatrist physicians and nurses. He proposed guidelines for such collaboration, elaborating them in his 1929 paper, 'Some modern aspects of psychiatry in general hospital practice' (10). He later collaborated with Gregory Zilboorg on the seminal work *A History of Medical Psychology* (11).

Henry is generally credited with defining the essential skills and functions of the C-L psychiatrist in practice, research, and teaching. He wrote that the staff of every general hospital should include a psychiatrist who would 'make visits to the wards, who would direct a psychiatric outpatient clinic, who would continue the instruction and organize the psychiatric work of interns and who would attend staff conferences so that there might be a mutual exchange of medical experience and a frank discussion of the more complicated cases' (10, p. 494).

The ambience of Bloomingdale Hospital, through the influence of Pliny Earle, may have enhanced Henry's push for a more psychological medicine. Pliny Earle had been superintendent of that institution 70 years earlier; he wrote in the *American Journal of Insanity* (forerunner from 1844 to 1921 of the *American Journal of Psychiatry*) that psychological medicine should be a part of every medical student's and physician's training and expertise, in order to promote more humanitarian treatment of the mentally ill. He helped psychiatry make the transition from an Association of Medical Superintendents to the American Medico-Psychological Association in 1892 and finally to the American Psychiatric Association in 1921, a founding member of each group.

First liaison psychiatry department: Edward G. Billings

Almost a decade after Henry's writing, the full term 'liaison psychiatry' was coined by Dr Edward G. Billings (12). With Dr Franklin Ebaugh, chair of the Department of Psychiatry at the University of Colorado, Billings founded in 1939 what was probably the first 'psychiatric liaison department' in the United States. Its aims, outlined by Billings, were to (1): sensitize physicians and students to apply a psychiatric approach 'for the betterment of the patient's condition' (2); encourage physicians and students of all branches of medicine to make psychobiology (after Adolf Meyer) an integral part of their professional thinking; and (3) correct misconceptions, distortions, misunderstandings, and taboos among the public that hampered their capacity to make use of the help available from physicians with a psychobiological approach.

Ebaugh and Billings had been avid students of Adolf Meyer before inaugurating their own liaison programme in Colorado. Meyer, who came to the United States from Switzerland in 1892 to be a neuropathologist, became one of America's most influential psychiatrists. His teachings were highly regarded and application of his therapeutic methods was extensive. Meyer attended Freud's lectures at Clark University and was not opposed to psychoanalysis, but believed that it needed broader application to general medicine and gave it the name 'psychobiology'. In 1910, he was installed as professor of psychiatry at Johns Hopkins' Phipps Clinic and founded one of the earliest 'psychosomatic' clinics in the United States. In 1915 he developed his 'common sense' psychiatry that took account of important psychosocial factors he found lacking in Freud's psychoanalytic postulates and had broader application to general medicine. Meyer's influence greatly expanded American psychiatry, especially through his disciples in psychosomatic medicine, such as Flanders Dunbar and other prominent advocates of psychosomatic medicine.

What role for 'liaison'?

The word 'liaison' itself is originally defined as an illicit affair, or used to describe wartime communication. As an agent of psychiatry it has an engaging superfluity of associations, variously applicable to the practice of C-L psychiatry: the psychiatrist as a 'go-between' of diverse parties, a facilitator of communication, is indisputable; some C-L psychiatrists see their function as a 'battle' in having their ideas and recommendations accepted; the connotation of an illicit affair, romance, or 'hookup' has tongue-in-cheek implications for the grab-bag of devices sometimes required of the C-L psychiatrist to accomplish a marriage between medicine and psychiatry. Whatever its connotations, the word 'liaison,' defining what a C-L psychiatrist does, has adhered to the name of the specialty; only later was its usefulness challenged in the context of reimbursement, an activity thought by insurers to not be a 'medically necessary' intervention. Even some psychiatrists regarded it as a form of leisurely 'gossip'.

For the most part, early contributors to the concept of 'liaison psychiatry' fostered a pedagogical rather than clinical consultative function of the psychiatrist; only with the evolution of psychosomatic medicine did a consultative clinical approach begin to be applied.

A confluence of tributaries

The late 1920s and early 1930s brought great scientific excitement in psychoanalysis, psychosomatic medicine, and psychophysiological research, tributaries with multiple intertwining facets of development. General hospital psychiatry had also begun to emerge. C-L psychiatry was indeed the benefactor, flourishing in the matrix of these various trends in American psychiatry. Various authors hold that C-L psychiatry is essentially an outgrowth of psychosomatic medicine, while others as adamantly consider it born of general hospital psychiatric units. In truth and retrospect, it is historically too foggy to make accurate attribution.

Psychosomatic medicine and psychoanalysis

Psychosomatic medicine in America essentially evolved in tandem with psychoanalysis. It attracted great attention in psychiatry—and to some extent in medicine—with its promise of bridging the gap between medicine and psychiatry, mind and body, psyche and soma. Said to have originated in Germany with Heinroth in 1818 in describing clinical aspects of insomnia, British literature of the mid-1860s declared '. . . the psycho-somatic [sic] theory is here, as elsewhere, in the ascendant . . .' (13, p. 324). Psychosomatic medicine flourished in the United States, where it became a major building block of C-L psychiatry. Dubbed by some as the 'clinical arm of psychosomatic medicine,' C-L made practical application of the research findings of psychosomatic medicine to the real quotidian needs of patients.

Psychoanalysis was incomprehensible to most non-psychiatrist physicians and seen as divorced from medicine. The 'psychosomatic' ideas of Adolf Meyer were more acceptable in general practice and an alternative to psychoanalysis. Additionally, Flanders Dunbar found Meyer's biologically based concepts compatible with her own psychosomatic ideas. As founding editor of the esteemed research journal *Psychosomatic Medicine*, and a founding member of the American Psychosomatic Society in the late 1930s and early 1940s, she helped propagate the prolific psychoanalytic and psychophysiological researches for many years to come.

During this early phase of psychosomatic medicine, Dunbar had firmly planted the seeds of interest in psychosomatic medicine, familiarizing both professional and lay audiences with the 'psychosomatic approach' to illness articulated in her book *Psychiatry in the Medical Specialties*. She and her associates made the bold prediction that 'the time should not be too long delayed when psychiatrists are required on all our medical and surgical wards, and in all our general and surgical clinics,' (14, p. 679), a fervent hope of psychosomaticians then and yet.

Even before World War II, considerable interest in psychosomatic medicine had been generated by the American psychoanalyst William Alanson White, a charismatic psychiatrist, highly respected by his peers and the public. An excellent teacher, writer, and humanitarian, he was perceived as one who could 'speak the language' of diverse professional communities. Through presidencies of the American Psychopathological Society, the American Psychiatric Association, and the American Psychoanalytic Society during the 1920s, he was probably more influential than any other psychoanalyst of his time in promoting acceptance of psychiatry by non-psychiatrist physicians as well as the public.

White had been appointed Superintendent of the Government Hospital for the Insane (later St Elizabeth's Hospital) in 1903 by President Theodore Roosevelt. His avid interest in training social workers, psychologists, nurses, and others as team members in the care of the mentally ill probably anticipated subsequent growth of community mental health programmes as well as the team approach of C-L psychiatry. His non-jargonistic communicative style became a model for future C-L psychiatrists consulting to non-psychiatrist physicians.

Psychosomatic researchers like Franz Alexander, perhaps one of the most productive of the émigré psychoanalysts in America, initially focused on 'the holy seven' illnesses—rheumatoid arthritis, thyrotoxicosis, peptic ulcer, neurodermatitis, ulcerative colitis, essential hypertension, and asthma. The 'Chicago Group' of the Chicago Psychoanalytic Institute, led by Alexander, initially believed that psychogenic factors or personality traits caused these diseases. This gave rise to the 'specificity theory' of disease, discredited several decades later as too narrow and limited in its application to most disease states. Some feared that psychosomatic medicine might defeat its own avowed mission of integrating medicine and psychiatry because of its limited focus on only a few specific diseases, its overspecialized purview, and its reliance on psychoanalysis for its theoretical framework. Ultimately, convention held that there were no specific psychosomatic disorders, only illness with psychosomatic attributes.

Nonetheless, early psychosomatic inquiries served a catalytic function to expand the field to include broader investigation into and understanding of the vast panoply of factors that impinged on individuals to create a broad spectrum of mind–body illness and disease. Hope for a reconciliation of medicine and psychiatry abounded. Émigré psychoanalyst Felix Deutsch, in 1922, is said to have coined the term 'psychosomatic medicine' and proclaimed confidently that medicine was on the threshold of a new revolutionary approach to understanding all disease.

Eventually inhabiting many medical schools around the country, psychoanalytic psychosomaticians promoted the contribution of psychoanalysis and psychosomatic medicine to psychiatric education and practice. Alexander's own book on psychosomatic medicine and that of O. Spurgeon English and Edward Weiss, *Emotional Problems of Living: Avoiding the Neurotic Pattern*, were read widely as interest in psychosomatic medicine surged in the 1950s. In 1955, the exhilaration managed to infuse the production of the Broadway musical *Guys and Dolls* with its popular number 'Adelaide's Lament.' The catchy tune proclaimed that

> The average unmarried female
> Basically insecure
> Due to some long frustration
> May react

With psychosomatic symptoms
Difficult to endure
. . .
You can feed her all day with the vitamin A
And the Bromo Fizz,
But the medicine never
Gets anywhere near
Where the trouble is.

This singable ditty was a harbinger of the large category of somatoform disorders that would engage the psychiatrist working in medical settings, trying to understand and treat 'medically unexplainable symptoms'.

Psychophysiology

No less important in bringing together advances in psychosomatic medicine, psychology, psychoanalysis, and psychiatry was the growing field of psychophysiology. Arising in Germany in the late 1800s, this specialized field became a fundamental aspect of psychosomatic research.

Wilhelm Wundt

Wundt was perhaps the first 'official' psychologist in history. He arguably created the first-ever psychophysiology laboratory at Leipzig University in 1879, having first taught a course there on the 'new science' of physiological psychology in 1867. Embracing introspection as a legitimate subject of investigation that provided a lattice upon which subsequent researchers and clinicians could build, he was held in low regard for his 'unusual' practices. His ideas were nonetheless vindicated by others. Freud credits Wundt with having provided the basis for the use of word-association in the exploration of 'complexes'. He also acknowledged that Bleuler and Carl Jung, working with Wilhelm Wundt at Burgholzli Asylum in Zurich, had built the 'first bridge from experimental psychology to psycho-analysis [sic]' (15, p. 109). Referred to variously as psychologist, philosopher, and physiologist, Wundt was, in fact, a teacher of prominent American psychologists like G. Stanley Hall, the 'father of developmental psychology' in America, who introduced Freud to America.

William James

History is confounded to some extent as to who founded the first American psychology (psychophysiology) laboratory—whether it was Hall, while at Johns Hopkins before moving to Clark University, or William James at Harvard. James and Wundt both allegedly began their rudimentary labs in 1875; James, however, disdained the work of the laboratory and recruited Hugo Munsterburg, a student of Wundt, to inaugurate a more dedicated undertaking of psychophysiological research. Wundt, Munsterburg, and James all shared a common interest in psychophysical parallelism, wherein all physical processes were thought to be accompanied by parallel brain processes. James co-authored the James–Lange theory of emotions, attempting to clarify which was 'chicken' and which 'egg' in the interaction of mental and physical processes; it hypothesized that emotions were triggered by the response of internal organs to external stimuli.

Walter Cannon

Exposed to James and Munsterburg at Harvard in 1900, Walter B. Cannon, as a student, investigated the effects of emotions on gastrointestinal function in animals. Later, as physician and chairman of Harvard's physiology department in 1906, he explored the 'wisdom of the body' in his own laboratories. With select students he studied the effects of internal organs on one another through a mechanism of internal secretions, later described as 'chemical messengers'—we know them as hormones.

Cannon was especially interested in the adrenal gland and its secretion, adrenaline, that fuelled the 'fighting instinct.' Soon followed a description of the all-important 'fight or flight response' of survivorship so relevant to understanding much of illness behaviour. By 1914, he had published his classic book *Bodily Changes in Pain, Hunger, Fear, and Rage: An Account of Recent Researches into the Function of Emotional Excitement.* In addition to stating that '. . . we are organized as a psycho-organismic unity' (16, p. 140) maintained by homeostasis, Cannon also challenged the James–Lange theory of emotions, proposing that emotions were first mediated through the neural system (rather than internal organs) before being experienced as bodily sensations. Cannon's work was highly referenced by Hans Selye of McGill University in 1936, who introduced the important concept of stress and the 'general adaptation syndrome'. The consequences of biological and emotional stress are of central interest to the C-L psychiatrist.

Ivan Pavlov

While Cannon was pursuing his ideas, Ivan Pavlov in Russia was expounding on conditioned (and unconditioned) responses, primarily in animals. By observing the negative effects of stress on some animals, he described a reaction he called 'experimental neurosis'. Pavlov was less receptive to psychology than Cannon, but together they provided the basics for an understanding of the autonomic nervous system and how it functioned in disease and health; it was a prominent scientific underpinning of C-L psychiatry and psychosomatic medicine. Cannon wrote appreciatively of Pavlov's contributions as having transformed '. . . our knowledge of the functions of the digestive glands and the more complex processes of the nervous system. . . .' (16, p. 137). The discovery that autonomic functions once thought to be totally involuntary were subject to voluntary control opened a whole new field of research and clinical application (e.g. biofeedback and other forms of self-regulation) and provided a fundamental tenet of medical psychotherapy.

General hospital psychiatry

Patients with 'mental diseases' were generally placed 'out of sight' if not 'out of mind' in asylums. Reformists like Tuke, Pinel, and Esquirol, observing the primitive conditions in such settings, had proposed treatment of mentally diseased patients in general hospitals, a prospect not readily accepted. By the mid-to-late 18th century, a few large general hospitals like Pennsylvania Hospital (founded 1751) and New York Hospital (opened in 1791) did admit occasional 'psychiatric' patients to their medical wards, but this was a rarity.

At Pennsylvania Hospital, Benjamin Rush, as professor of medicine (not psychiatry), hoped to 'modernize' care of the mentally ill. His book of 1812, *Medical Inquiries and Observations upon Diseases of the Mind*, was the first 'psychiatric' text in America; it strongly advocated a humanized medicine that simultaneously took account of perturbations of the mind as well as the body. It was readily apparent, however, that neither the staff nor the accommodations of traditional asylums were prepared to offer appropriate or adequate care.

On 16 October 1844, more than 30 years after Rush's death, 13 physician directors of insane asylums met in Philadelphia and endorsed Rush's ideas about care of the mentally ill. They established psychiatry as the first American specialty and embraced humane care of the mentally ill with the implementation of 'moral treatment'. This assemblage, as the Association of Medical Superintendents of American Institutions for the Insane, became the springboard for the transition from the overburdened, ineffective, disagreeable asylums to the growth of general hospital psychiatry programmes where C-L services later found a home.

However, the wheels of progress turn slowly. In another 50 years, the benefit of including psychiatric treatment in general hospitals was still feverishly debated. In his presidential address in 1890 (17) before the Medico-Psychological Association of Great Britain and Ireland, Dr David Yellowlees, superintendent of Glasgow Asylum in Scotland, discussed a report of the Committee of the London County Council that strongly endorsed '... placing the insane under the care of physicians and surgeons of general hospitals' (17, p. 483). Alleging that the report slandered 'inept' asylum superintendents, Yellowlees summarily dismissed it. He argued that such a move would yield no better results than already existed in asylums, since '... in the principal medical schools of Europe the insane have long been treated in general hospitals' (17, p. 484) without superior results (to asylums)—an assertion that is difficult to affirm. The German psychiatrist Wilhelm Griesinger, founder of 'university psychiatry' as professor of psychiatry and neurology at Berlin University, encountered similar enmity of asylum superintendents in the 1860s with his vigorous proposal to establish psychiatric wards in general hospitals.

First psychiatric unit: J.M. Mosher

By the turn of the 20th century, the establishment of psychiatric units in general hospitals began to look more likely. In 1902, Dr J. Montgomery Mosher at Albany Hospital (New York) (18) designed and implemented the first such unit. Although structurally part of the general hospital, 'Pavilion F' was segregated from other hospital wards and functioned like future med-psych units. Nevertheless, this unit marked the historical beginning of a movement.

By the 1950s, deinstitutionalization of the mentally ill finally became a reality, as 'warehoused' mentally ill began their migration back to their communities and the medical hospitals that serviced them. In the 1970s, there were well over 1000 inpatient units in general hospitals in the United States. The trend soon followed in Europe, especially in the United Kingdom where transfer of patients from asylums to general hospitals was well under way by 1950. In 1971, the government put forth a policy in England and Wales for integrated community and hospital psychiatric services 'to meet the needs of populations within defined geographic areas, and based on departments of psychiatry within district general hospitals' (19, p. ix). By the 1980s, Japan organized an Association of General Hospital Psychiatrists with its own journal, modelled after the American Association of General Hospital Psychiatrists and the journal *General Hospital Psychiatry*.

Uneasy acceptance

Assimilation, however, was not easy. The immersion of psychiatry within the general hospital milieu, even as psychiatry and medicine appeared to achieve some intimacy, did not necessarily assure smooth interprofessional relations. Psychiatrist teachers in the 1960s were still writing of the resistance to, and distortion about, psychiatry and the animosity towards psychiatrists.

In some instances psychiatric units were experienced as out of the flow of usual hospital commerce, or their democratic method of milieu or team treatment appeared alien in a general medical setting where a formal medical model prevailed. Thus, the alliance of psychiatry and medicine seemed more an uneasy coexistence than a true integration of service. One prominent commentator noted that 'despite the very successful attempts to bring about an ever-closer rapprochement between psychiatry and medicine . . . there are still many defects in the synthesis' (20, p. 182). To counteract the tendency to view the patient with a separate body and a separate psyche, he said ' . . . requires a coordination of all the king's horses and all the king's men if it is hoped to put the patient together again. And few have the temerity even to try' (20, p. 183).

To face the challenge of assimilation, psychiatrists in the general hospital have had to acquire good diplomatic and communicative skills as requirements of effective, developing 'liaison' programmes. As expected, negative attitudes and beliefs persist in some quarters and it is likely that no amount of expert pedagogy will alter this state of affairs. In the 1950s, the Hungarian–British psychoanalyst Michael Balint, who taught groups of general practitioners (GPs), predicted it might be another 100 years before GPs would be able to accept psychological aspects of medical treatment—more than 50 years have already passed.

Despite obstacles from the world of general medicine, psychiatry's rightful place in community and university general hospitals seemed assured, perhaps enhanced by the inclusion during the 1950s of psychopharmacology in the treatment of serious mental illness. Not only did newer drugs help former asylum patients become more 'manageable' in general hospitals, but they expanded the armamentarium of the C-L psychiatrist. A more concrete management of medical/psychiatric comorbidities brought new respect for the psychiatrist who could offer such 'medical' advice to his or her colleagues. The door to collaborative care of the patient was opened, even while sacrificing some of the more lofty objectives of psychiatric liaison like extended history-taking, active listening to patients, and empathic counselling.

By 1981, a bicentennial assessment of psychiatry's status noted that 'one of the most far-reaching developments in [its] history' was the evolution of psychiatry in the general hospital (21, p. 893). Opportunity existed for receptive non-psychiatrists to interact and exchange views with psychiatrists, to facilitate the growth of liaison services, and to build interprofessional referral networks for the growth of psychotherapeutic practice. According to Lipowski, the general hospital psychiatric programmes 'helped raise the standards of psychiatric patient care, training and research and to reduce the isolation of psychiatry from progress in the rest of medicine' greater than any other single organizational change (21, p. 894).

C-L psychiatry faces the challenge

Between the late 1930s and mid-1940s, interest and activity in consultation psychiatry had slowed, but the seeds that had been planted for the growth of C-L psychiatry began to germinate robustly after World War II. Psychiatry's potential to help address morale and humanistic issues that generally emerge after war was incontrovertible. The National Institute of Mental Health (NIMH) and the Group for the Advancement of Psychiatry (GAP) in 1947 were founded in this climate, helping to promote the trend towards an integration of psychiatry and medicine.

By 1945, medical institutions appeared receptive to the kind of collaborative care practiced during the war. And C-L psychiatrists were ready to accept the challenge of 'putting Humpty-Dumpty together again'. Physicians returning from the military in 1945 brought with them an appreciation of collaborative triage and treatment, crisis intervention, and rehabilitation. During the war, physicians and surgeons of all specialties worked arm in arm with psychiatrists to provide support for the troops and treatment for those who suffered the stresses and injuries of war. On their return, a great surge of interest in, and respect for, psychiatry prompted many GPs, internists, and surgeons to apply for psychiatric training. With increased need and improved attitudes towards mental illness and treatment, federal funds were made available through the recently-established NIMH to underwrite courses and training for returning physicians.

The American Psychiatric Association established a liaison committee with the Academy of General Practice to launch a Physician Education Project, directed by Dr Howard Kern, that designed courses of instruction for returning physicians. Renamed the Committee on Psychiatry and Medical Practice, it continued to offer 'Colloquia for Postgraduate Teaching of Psychiatry' to satisfy the interest of physicians wishing to broaden their understanding and to develop a more comprehensive style of medical practice (22). A cadre of psychiatrically trained physicians took positions in general hospital settings, where their newly acquired skills could be applied not only to returning veterans but also to patients with a diversity of medical/surgical conditions. Triage, crisis intervention, and rehabilitation became important building blocks of C-L psychiatry and took their place among psychiatric interventions in the general hospital setting. Psychosomatic medicine was now more readily accepted as well. The psychiatric treatment units within the general hospital, utilizing milieu and team treatment methods, assured greater availability of psychiatrist consultants for the beginnings of 'consultation services'. Non-psychiatrist physicians began to recognize a need for and acceptance of C-L psychiatrists to properly manage and care for their hospitalized patients.

Rockefeller money: an essential ingredient

Although the fundamental tenets of C-L psychiatry were in place in the early part of the 20th century, there was little assurance of survival without adequate funding. As serendipity would have it, a young student named Alan Gregg was greatly impressed by Freud's presentation of new ideas about mental illness at Clark University in 1909. After graduation from medical school, Gregg became director of the Medical Sciences Division of the Rockefeller Foundation. Observing the 'deplorable state of psychiatry' of the 1920s and 1930s, he leveraged his authority and long-standing interest in psychiatry and psychoanalysis to assign copious Foundation funds (over $11 million) to nascent programmes in psychiatry in American medical schools and hospitals. Thus, Rockefeller largesse fuelled the economic engine of improvement in the quality of psychiatric education, research, and training. Psychiatric units, C-L services, and psychosomatic research proliferated through the 1930s. Gregg's supervision of Rockefeller funding facilitated the work of such titans of American psychiatry as Stanley Cobb, Franz Alexander, Franklin Ebaugh, and others, all of whom promoted the role of psychiatry in general hospital settings. The work of Hans Selye in Canada and a few psychophysiology laboratories in Europe were likewise beneficiaries. This great improvement in psychiatry's profile attracted increased numbers of medical school graduates to choose training and ultimately careers in general hospital settings. There they interacted with non-psychiatrist colleagues and developed enthusiasm for teaching, defined as a prominent part of 'liaison.' If C-L psychiatry was not actually born in this setting it was at least baptized and relatively assured of a promising future.

NIMH support

Of course, Rockefeller support was not endless and, indeed, the NIMH picked up where the Rockefeller Foundation left off. James Eaton, director of the Division of Medical Education in NIMH, skilfully spread the concept of C-L psychiatry by recruiting some of the country's pre-eminent C-L psychiatrists to visit, assess and make recommendations for programs to receive federal funds—$5.3 million supported 130 C-L programs, 60 stipends, and fellowships for approximately 300 psychiatrists. Their quality and quantity benefitted accordingly, but again faltered when federal monies were cut in the 1980s. Recognizing their services were at risk, C-L psychiatrists had a strong incentive to explore other funding mechanisms. Research reports describing the significant cost-effectiveness of C-L interventions began to appear, with evident justification for adequate reimbursement and funding.

Growth of C-L programmes

Model C-L programs sprang up in academic medical centres like Cincinnati; Rochester (New York); Beth Israel Hospital and Massachusetts General Hospital in Boston; Henry Ford Hospital in Detroit; Mount Sinai Hospital and the Einstein Medical Center in New York; and Allen Memorial Hospital in Canada.

Cincinnati

The University of Cincinnati programme, under Dr Maurice Levine's direction from 1942, created a virtual diaspora of psychoanalytically trained psychosomaticians (Milton Rosenbaum, John Romano, Morton Reiser, Ralph Kahana, George Engel, and others) who migrated to many of the institutions mentioned, and established psychiatry departments as well as C-L services. The wish for a functional collaboration between psychiatrists and other physicians seemed, at long last, achievable.

Rochester

A programme of true cross-disciplinary alliance existed at Rochester University. John Romano, professor of psychiatry, joined with George Engel, an internist with interest and experience in psychoanalysis, to establish a unique medical liaison programme. Internal medicine fellows rather than psychiatric residents were trained as 'second messengers', to bring psychiatric and psychological principles of medical care to their own non-psychiatrist colleagues. The 'Rochester Group' consisted of several psychiatrists, psychologists, and other prodigious contributors to the corpus of American psychosomatic research. The 'interface of psychiatry and medicine', as it came to be called in C-L psychiatry, achieved a major boost from collaborative studies of this group.

Mount Sinai Hospital and Beth Israel Hospital

Two programmes that created the 'dedicated' model of C-L psychiatry were at Mount Sinai Hospital in New York, under the direction of psychoanalyst M. Ralph Kaufman, and the Beth Israel Hospital in Boston, directed by the psychoanalyst Grete L. Bibring, a student of Freud. Beginning as chair of a nascent department at Beth Israel, Kaufman abandoned the programme when he joined the military. On his return, he was recruited by Mount Sinai where he developed a rich, influential C-L programme, with an outpouring of instructional papers on the organization of such facilities. Psychiatric consultants in both programmes were assigned continuously to specific wards and services, offering sustained visibility and availability, performing regular rounds with non-psychiatrist trainees, medical students, and attendings.

Kaufman's model stressed collaborative relations between an inpatient unit and a consultation service, but not all consultation programmes relied entirely on inpatient wards. The Liaison Department of Colorado General Hospital, for example, was basically a free-standing non-bed programme. Bibring also chose to go 'bedless'. Her decision reflected the wish to strengthen the teaching relation between psychiatrist and non-psychiatrist by discouraging the transfer of 'troublesome' patients away from medical and surgical wards. In later years the pressures of 'managed care' and economic stringencies forced creation of a small inpatient unit, with the concomitant weakening of the previous strong liaison teaching focus.

Bibring's classic article in the *New England Journal of Medicine* (23) generated greater awareness of the role of psychiatry in the care of patients in general hospitals through use of a more 'psychotherapeutic medicine'. Enhancing treatment and outcome of medical and surgical illness without imposing the stigma of 'psychiatric disease', it helped physicians optimize their engagement in the patient–physician relationship, an approach that became the bedrock of C-L activity.

Massachusetts General Hospital

A Rockefeller beneficiary and prominent neuropsychiatrist, Dr Stanley Cobb, developed a new department and psychiatric research program at Boston's Massachusetts General Hospital (MGH) in 1934. Trained primarily as a neurologist and inspired by Meyer's views of psychiatry, he had nonetheless been very sympathetic to psychoanalytic ideas and approaches and recruited psychoanalysts with psychosomatic interests such as Felix Deutsch, Avery Weisman, and Jacob Finesinger to his staff.

Weisman, with Thomas Hackett, founded a prominent C-L service, modestly pre-empted by another professor of neurology, James Jackson Putnam. Having attended Freud's 1909 lecture in Worcester and engaged in extensive correspondence with him, Putnam was intrigued with the possibilities of application of psychoanalysis to general medical conditions. He was instrumental in promoting psychoanalytic ideas in America, and helped establish the first psychoanalytic training programmes in the United States. At the MGH, in the early 1900s, neurologist Putnam is said to have launched a 'psychiatric consultation' service from his small quarters adjacent to an electricity closet, for which he was scurrilously dubbed by doubters the 'electrician' and his office the 'cloaca' of the hospital.

MGH became a major centre of liaison psychiatry under Cobb's leadership, succeeded in 1955 by psychoanalyst Dr Erich Lindemann, whose studies of bereavement contributed significantly to the consulting psychiatrist's repertoire of interventions. Other psychoanalytic psychosomaticians who emerged from the programme were John Nemiah and Peter Sifneos, authors of the first papers on alexithymia.

With several excellent models of C-L psychiatry programmes in place by the 1950s, other institutions soon followed by example. Consultation was refined into patient-oriented, crisis-oriented, consultee-oriented, and situation-oriented. Specialty rounds that included the psychiatric consultant promoted more comfortable interaction. A trend towards superspecialization defined areas of interest like psychooncology, inaugurated by Dr Jimmie Holland, and psychonephrology, founded by Dr Norman B. Levy. Other areas of special interest included transplantation, palliative care, dermatology, and obstetrics/gynaecology. By the 1980s, significant international interest, programmatic development, and research in the field was seen in Europe, Japan, Australia, New Zealand, the United Kingdom, and Latin America (24). Emergence of the European Consultation-Liaison Workgroup (ECLW) in 1987 was a major catalyst in this growth. In the Netherlands, an admission screening test was approved by the government to detect patients who could benefit from psychiatric consultation (25).

The successes of inpatient C-L psychiatry were extended to outpatient settings. The Integration Clinic (26) at the Beth Israel Hospital in Boston in the 1960s, for example, invited physicians in other outpatient clinics to refer their 'troublesome' patients for an 'integrated' consultation about management. Results showed attendance by patients who would otherwise not attend psychiatry clinic, a centralizing of patients' chronically fragmented care, and in some cases decreased emergency room use and hospitalization (27). Success with 'somatizing' patients, those most often defiant of medical explanation, generated a marked increase in referrals from other clinics. The category of somatoform disorders (formerly referred to as psychophysiological disorders in the official diagnosis classification) became a prominent teaching focus for C-L psychiatrists in the Integration Clinic.

Identity and the politics of change

By the 1970s, departments of psychiatry, inpatient psychiatric units, and C-L services were quite securely installed in most academic and some non-academic institutions. From the formative classic articles of Zbigniew Lipowski (28–30) and the first

Handbook of Psychiatric Consultation of John Schwab (31) in 1968, all tributaries had coalesced in the special branch of psychiatry called consultation-liaison.

The American Psychiatric Association's Committee on Medical Practice had morphed into the Committee on Consultation-Liaison Psychiatry. The American Board of Psychiatry and Neurology (ABPN) had made residency training in C-L psychiatry a requirement. A new spirit infused programme expansion in clinical research and teaching, heralded by George Engel's assessment in his 1977 paper in *Science* (32) that medicine was in a need of a new model of patient evaluation and treatment; his biopsychosocial approach generated widespread discussion, deliberation, and no little controversy. Publications multiplied, the journal *Psychiatry in Medicine* was founded to accommodate increasing numbers of C-L articles, and a spate of texts on psychiatry in primary care, psychosomatic medicine, and C-L psychiatry inhabited physicians' bookshelves.

Identity crisis?

Nevertheless, even with accumulating evidence that C-L psychiatry had successfully challenged medicine's reductionistic dualism, consolidation of its identity and role were perceived as unsettled. This sense of vulnerability was the product of several factors.

C-L psychiatrists felt snubbed when their services were not engaged to fulfil the 15% 'behavioural science' component of primary care training programmes mandated to qualify for federal funding; C-L psychiatrists were bypassed as the presumptive benefactors of the primary care movement in favour of psychologists, social workers, sociologists, anthropologists, and other non-physician 'behaviourists.' The emergence of 'health psychologists' appeared to invade a domain previously considered proprietary by C-L psychiatry.

Assuming that the name of the field of activity accounted for its troubles, and seeking greater visibility and utilization, C-L psychiatrists floated a plethora of name changes for the field: medical psychiatry, medical-surgical psychiatry, psychiatric medicine, psychosocial medicine, biopsychosocial medicine, psychosomatic psychiatry, and other more cumbersome terms. Curiously, psychosomatic medicine was not considered until much later when certification for the field as a specialty was sought. Similar confusion of terminology prevailed in Europe. Psychosomatic medicine had a centuries-old foothold in countries like Germany and consultation was offered by family doctors, internists, and psychologists or nurses in other countries like Japan and the United Kingdom. Such history gave rise to questions of who 'owned' C-L services and how they should be called, a dilemma that delayed the formation of national organizations for C-L psychiatry in those countries.

Other developments seemed to plague the field. The community mental health movement catalysed by President Kennedy's Community Mental Health Centers Construction Act of 1963 democratized the administration of such programmes, with less expensive mental health professionals recruited to leadership positions in preference to psychiatrists.

Furthermore, rapid advancements in the pharmaceutical domain encouraged primary care physicians, even without adequate training, to usurp the recently acquired role of C-L psychiatrists in psychopharmacological treatment. A focus on drug treatment by referring physicians tended to supplant psychodynamic issues in the management of patients' comorbid illness. And just at a point where psychiatric consultation was beginning to establish its usefulness, the American Psychiatric Association paradoxically suggested 'sunsetting' its Committee on Consultation-Liaison Psychiatry.

Further confusing matters, the ABPN suggested that perhaps medical training was not essential for psychiatrists. Responding with outrage, John Romano wrote: "To reduce the dimensions of the role of the psychiatrist as physician would seriously reduce our contributions to the rest of medicine . . .' and compromise ' . . . advantageous liaison teaching programs for medical students and house staff. . . . It is a degradation of quality' (33, pp. 1565 and 1575). Fortunately, Romano and others prevailed; the suggestion was dropped, and psychiatry's identity as a medical specialty was reassured.

Some of the woes of C-L psychiatry could be traced to budgetary and administrative concerns; even some chairs of psychiatry were reluctant to 'invest' in C-L services lacking adequate reimbursement. By the 1980s, C-L psychiatrists as a group began to see a need for greater strength, funding, visibility, and understanding of their specialty; financial support required thoughtful pursuit. Impatient with the slowness with which medicine changed, a growing restlessness arose among its C-L practitioners.

Application for specialty certification

A C-L Consortium was convened in 1982 to plan a strategy. It was reasoned that certification as a specialty and establishment of training programmes would invite greater utilization, quality-standardized training, and justifiable requests for funding. Competition with other professional groups like health psychologists and behavioural medicine practitioners was beginning to cloud the field with questions of definition and identity.

Plans emerged from two meetings of the Consortium for submission of an application to the ABPN for official subspecialty certification of C-L psychiatry. First attempts were rejected on the grounds that no specific class of patients could be identified for C-L services (an ironic side-effect of C-L's applicability to all patients).

Alterations were made: the name of the specialty was changed to psychosomatic medicine and the patient population defined as 'the complex medically ill'. The process may have been a case of terminological acrobatics, but the application was successful and in 2003 psychosomatic medicine became the seventh accredited subspecialty recognized by the ABPN, with widespread endorsement by various organizations, such as the APA and American Medical Association.

A significant membership component of the American Psychosomatic Society (APS) consisted of C-L psychiatrists. Curiously, however, a growing number of C-L psychiatrists felt that their interests and objectives differed from those of psychosomatic medicine. The APS, with its diverse membership of psychophysiological and psychosomatic researchers and C-L psychiatrists began to see programmatic splits, with one Society president lamenting the possibility that the popular image of psychosomatic medicine would be that 'C-L psychiatry is all there is [to psychosomatic medicine]' (34, p. 359).

Special interest groups began to form within other organizations, like the Association for Academic Psychiatry (AAP), the American Association of General Hospital

Psychiatry (AAGHP) (now dissolved), and the APA. The Academy of Psychosomatic Medicine (APM) appropriated the mantle of an 'official' C-L organization and began to develop training guidelines, reimbursement surveys, and other areas of special interest to C-L psychiatrists. There began a slow migration of C-L psychiatrists from the APS to the APM.

Following successful approval for specialty status, guidelines for training in psychosomatic medicine (née C-L psychiatry) have been established and a certifying examination has been offered under the auspices of the APM. Considering that the word 'psychosomatic' was virtually expunged from medical language after the 1950s, its reinstatement has continued to foster some confusion about how it relates to C-L psychiatry. Some leaders in the field continue to vacillate over what to call their services, some have questioned whether psychosomatics belongs more appropriately under the umbrella of psychiatry or medicine. Interestingly, Germany long ago avoided this problem by designating psychosomatic medicine a totally separate specialty, 'belonging' to neither psychiatry nor medicine. The definitions of 'consultation-liaison psychiatry' and 'psychosomatic medicine' in Campbell's *Psychiatric Dictionary* are virtually indistinguishable (35).

Looking to the 21st century: the future

In the 21st century C-L psychiatry appears to have sustainability around the world. With a defined identity and scope of operation, it has been most effective in helping non-psychiatrist physicians and medical students understand the value of detecting psychological aspects of illness early enough to promote quality health care without wastage of time, effort, and money. It can reduce suffering, promote healing, and assist in rehabilitation. Effective consultation is able to prevent unnecessary hospital admission and excessive utilization of other health care services. By applying special skills, it helps shorten hospital stays, assure medical adherence, and relieve affective disorders that complicate and worsen organic disease. The psychiatrist consultant can also help to differentiate between disease of the mind, brain, and body; assist in management of patients with addictive disorders; assess competency; and begin the process of helping patients with terminal illness face impending death. This provides therapeutic assistance for survivors of the deceased to mourn, grieve, and adapt to loss. Psychopharmacology, a specialty often shunned by many physicians, is part of the consulting psychiatrist's skill.

Regular referrals to a consulting service include suicidal patients, individuals with eating disorders, factitious disorders, and symptoms that are medically unexplainable. Ultimately, the objective of C-L psychiatry is to promote a comprehensive, integrated medicine that can address biological, psychological, social, spiritual, and other aspects of illness in the patient. If, in the process, consultation helps to enhance the patient–doctor relationship, the liaison function of C-L psychiatry is accomplished.

Summary and conclusion

We arrive at the 21st century with a good comprehension of where we come from (36). Our journey has taken us through the use and description of the word 'liaison'; program development in psychiatric consultation and inpatient psychiatry in the general hospital; the influence of psychosomatic medicine, psychoanalysis, and psychophysiology; funding by the Rockefeller Foundation and NIMH; development of specialized services to disciplines like cardiology, oncology, and nephrology; expansion to outpatient programmes; a period of restless searching for a strong identity, scientific rigour through clinical research, and assessment of opportunities for fiscal sustainability; and recognition as a defined specialty of psychiatry. Applicability and support is demonstrated both locally and abroad, with American certification bolstering development in other countries.

The evolution of consultative psychiatry into a subspecialty of C-L psychiatry and psychosomatic medicine also reflects the history of efforts to establish the inseparability of mental and physical processes. Survival is almost certainly predictable, but we must heed the many failed predictions by our forebears about the fate of psychoanalysis and psychosomatic medicine on the future direction of general medicine; how often was a 'new medicine' predicted by such pioneers as Dunbar, Deutsch, and Engel?

What form C-L psychiatry takes in the future depends on the same travails that face health care in general and medicine in particular. Lack of funding in the past has been known to cause closure of some respectable programmes. Future funding is always at the whim of political forces, economic trends, and the goodwill of philanthropies. The direction taken by science or life itself is inevitably determined by social events like wars, natural disasters, even the waves of public response to a published book.

We can confidently say that modern life will continue to be technologized and while that often represents progress for good, how it will affect patient–physician relations of the future can only be speculated. The avidity for neuroscience is greatly in vogue, intensified by exciting derivatives of the genome project and the utility of neuroimaging. (One hopes that the search for new localized bits of brain matter to explain all illness and behaviour does not become the new phrenology.)

Changes in hospital structure, staffing, and form will define the C-L psychiatrist's locus in those institutions. Will the advent of hospitalists, for example, influence the way C-L psychiatrists interact (or don't) with patients, their primary care doctors, and their temporary carers?

The changing population of hospitalized patients will also define the use of the C-L psychiatrist's skills, as a growing number of aged patients with chronic medical problems additionally suffer from dementing illnesses that greatly complicate their ability to communicate to all carers the distress, wishes, and fears they are experiencing.

The insurance industry, already controlling the way medicine is practised in some parts of the world, is not likely to reward empathy, compassion, listening, talking and the 'healing arts', unless innovative 'cost-effective' research can demonstrate their 'added value'. More regulation of all kinds is probably in the offing.

With increasing time pressures on all aspects of medical care and mountains of knowledge to be mastered, will psychiatry and its subsets be squeezed out of the busy curriculums of medical schools? Will 'evidence-based' medicine overshadow the 'experience-based' individuality and spontaneity of physicians and their patients?

No doubt C-L psychiatrists will continue to exercise their pedagogical instincts even if the liaison function atrophies. Questions about ethics and forensic issues will undoubtedly become more compelling as the complexity and mechanization of patient care escalates.

Medicine's struggle with somatizing conditions and their drain on facilities, services, funding, and tolerance will continue to enlist psychiatry's help as a 'last resort.' The tragic sequelae of war and other atrocities will surely require psychiatric assistance in some form. Research must of necessity become more productive and relevant if C-L psychiatry and psychosomatic medicine are to fulfil their promise of a more humanized subspecialty.

Whatever twists and turns occur in the road ahead, it will require the 'art of the soluble' to adapt. In 30 years, C-L psychiatry may have a very different look. The road from alienist to collaborator in efforts to bridge the gap between psyche and soma, medicine and psychiatry, has taken over 100 years, and psychosomatic medicine has survived the barriers and impediments of that journey. Constant vigilance, innovation and sensitive adaptability to the vicissitudes of working relationships between psychiatry and its non-psychiatry elements in medicine will redound to the benefit of the patient. C-L psychiatry, in blending psychiatry and medicine, may well be the safeguard of humanism in medicine of the future.

Acknowledgement

'Adelaide's Lament'.
Words & Music by Frank Loesser.
© Copyright 1950 (Renewed 1978) Frank Music Corporation, USA.
MPL Communications Limited.
All Rights Reserved. International Copyright Secured.
Used by Permission of Music Sales Limited.

References

1 Medawar, P. B. (1967). *The art of the soluble*. London: Methuen.

2 Lipsitt, D. R. (2000). Psyche and soma: struggles to close the gap. In: Menninger, R.W. and Nemiah, J.C. (eds.) *American Psychiatry after World War II (1944–94)*. Washington, DC: American Psychiatric Press.

3 Alexander, F. (1950). *Psychosomatic medicine*. New York: Norton.

4 Kaufman, M. R. (1965). *The psychiatric unit in a general hospital. its current and future role*. New York: International Universities Press.

5 Taylor, G. (1987). *Psychosomatic medicine and contemporary psychoanalysis*. Madison, CT: International Universities Press.

6 McGuigan, F. J., Ban, T. A. (1987). *Critical issues in psychology, psychiatry and physiology*. Amsterdam: Gordon and Breach.

7 Winslow, F. (1909). The psychological vocation of the physician. *Alienist and Neurologist* 30, 1–17.

8 Barrett, A. M. (1922). The broadened interests of psychiatry. *American Journal of Psychiatry* 2, 1–13.

9 Pratt, G. K. (1926). Psychiatric departments in general hospitals. *American Journal of Psychiatry* 82, 403–10.

10 Henry, G. W. (1929–30). Some modern aspects of psychiatry in general hospital practice. *American Journal of Psychiatry* 86, 481–99.

11 **Zilboorg, G.** (with G.H. Henry) (1941). *A history of medical psychology*. New York: W.W. Norton.

12 **Billings, E. G.** (1939). Liaison psychiatry and intern instruction. *Journal of the Association of American Medical Colleges* **14**, 376–85.

13 **Browne, W. A. F.** (1866). On medico-psychology. *Journal of Mental Science* **12**, 309–27.

14 **Dunbar, H. F., Wolfe, T. P., and Rioch, J. McK.** (1936). Psychiatric aspects of medical problems. *American Journal of Psychiatry* **93**, 649–79.

15 **Freud, S.** (1916). The premises and technique of interpretation. *Standard Edition of the Complete Psychological Works of Sigmund Freud* **15**, 100–12.

16 **Yerkes, R. M.** (1946). Walter Bradford Cannon 1871–945. *Psychological Review* **53**, 137–46.

17 **Yellowlees, D.** (1890). Proposals for general hospital treatment of insanity. *Journal of Mental Science* **36**, 473–89.

18 **Mosher, J. M.** (1900). The insane in general hospitals. *American Journal of Insanity* **57**, 325–9.

19 **Little, J. C.** (1974). *Psychiatry in a general hospital*. London: Butterworths.

20 **Rome, H. P.** (1965). The psychotherapies: the sociology of psychiatric practice in a general hospital. In: Kaufman, M. R. (ed.) *The psychiatric unit in a general hospital: its current and future role*. New York: International Universities Press, pp. 177–92.

21 **Lipowski, Z. J.** (1981). Holistic-medical foundations of American psychiatry: a bicentennial. *American Journal of Psychiatry* **138**, 888–95.

22 **American Psychiatric Association Committee on Psychiatry and Medical Practice** (1961). *Proceedings of the first colloquium for postgraduate teaching in psychiatry*. Washington, DC: American Psychiatric Association.

23 **Bibring, G. L.** (1956). Psychiatry and medical practice in a general hospital. *New England Journal of Medicine* **254**, 366–72.

24 **Huyse, F., Saravay, S. M., and Smith, G.** (2008). Internationalization and integration of the C-L psychiatry field. *Journal of Psychosomatic Research* **64**, 557–8.

25 **Stiefel, F. C., Huyse, F. J., Sollner, W. et al.** (2006). Operationalizing integrated care on a clinical level: the INTERMED project. *Medical Clinics of North America* **90**, 713–58.

26 **Lipsitt, D. R.** (1964). Integration clinic: an approach to the teaching and practice of medical psychology in an outpatient setting. In: Zinberg, N. E. (ed.). *Psychiatry and medical practice in a general hospital*. New York: International Universities Press, pp. 231–49.

27 **Fox, F., Kuhns, N., Monto, M., Nordhaus, B., and Weisberg, C.** (1966). A study of 31 patients seen in the first year of operation of the Integration Clinic. Thesis in support of master's degree in Social Work (unpublished). Simmons School of Social Work, Boston, MA.

28 **Lipowski, Z. J.** (1967). Review of consultation psychiatry and psychosomatic medicine. I. General principles. *Psychosomatic Medicine* **29**, 153–71.

29 **Lipowski, Z. J.** (1967). Review of consultation psychiatry and psychosomatic medicine. II. Clinical aspects. *Psychosomatic Medicine* **29**, 201–24.

30 **Lipowski, Z. J.** (1968). Review of consultation psychiatry and psychosomatic medicine. III. Theoretical issues. *Psychosomatic Medicine* **30**, 395–422.

31 **Schwab, J. J.** (1968). *Handbook of psychiatric consultation*. New York: Appleton-Century-Crofts.

32 **Engel, G. L.** (1977). The need for a new medical model: a challenge for biomedicine. *Science* **196**, 129–36.

33 **Romano, J.** (1970). The elimination of the internship—an action of regression. *American Journal of Psychiatry* **126**, 1565–76.

34 **Graham, D. T.** (1979). Presidential address: What place in medicine for psychosomatic medicine? *Psychosomatic Medicine* **41**, 357–67.

35 **Campbell, R. J.** (ed.) (1996). *Psychiatric dictionary* (7th edn). New York: Oxford University Press.

36 **Lipsitt, D. R.** (2006). Psychosomatic medicine: history of a 'new' specialty. In: Strain, J. J. and Blumenthal, M. (eds.) *Psychosomatic medicine*. Philadelphia, pa: Lippincott, Williams & Wilkins, pp. 1–20.

Child and adolescent psychopathology: past scientific achievements and future challenges

Michael Rutter

Mid-20th-century landmarks

This essay considers the worldwide scientific achievements from the mid-20th century onwards that have relevance for the revolutionary changes that have taken place in child and adolescent psychopathology, and which are likely to be important in the future. Deliberately, achievements are considered without attention to whether they came from child psychiatrists, provided they are relevant for child and adolescent psychopathology. It does not, however, deal with developments in clinical services. Only a limited set of key references are provided but fuller referencing is available in the published article on which this essay is based (1).

Although there were important roots in the 19th century and earlier, child and adolescent psychiatry only came of age as a recognized specialty in the 20th century (2). Its origins lay in the mental hygiene movement in the United States, one characterized by a multidisciplinary emphasis, a child-welfare approach, and a focus on environmental causes. The term 'child psychiatry' was probably first used at the Paris congress of 1934, but it had been preceded by the child psychiatry clinic in Heidelberg in 1926. Leo Kanner's 1935 textbook provided the first English-language systematic account of child psychiatry, although several earlier German texts had preceded it; Kanner credited them as a major influence. Psychometrics as exemplified in the work of Alfred Binet (1857–1911) and the growth of child psychoanalysis were influential, the latter accompanied by bitter infighting between Melanie Klein and Anna Freud and their respective groups (3).

Numerous important scientific contributions were made in the mid-20th century. Their diversity may be illustrated by simply noting several examples. In many ways the most significant of these was John Bowlby's report (4) for the World Health Organization (WHO) of the effects of maternal deprivation. While not all his claims have stood the test of time, it was a revolutionary document that changed forever people's realization of the salience of children's experiences, and it led to radical changes in the patterns of care provided for them in hospital (including the option of parents staying overnight, and encouraging them to visit frequently). This led to Bowlby's trilogy on attachment (5) which was influential in several respects. To begin with, it was remarkable in bringing together diverse sources of evidence, both human and animal, as well as a range of theoretical perspectives. It alerted the world to the key role of children's selective attachments in early life and the ways in which they formed the basis for later social relationships of all kinds. Also it led to key methodological advances by pioneers such as Mary Ainsworth and Mary Main (6). Although Bowlby was the leading conceptualizer, the films made by James and Joyce Robertson (7) on children's behaviour following admission to hospital made a huge impact and played a major role in altering hospital practices.

David Levy's (8) study of maternal overprotection was outstanding in its analysis of what was involved in this form of parental behaviour—particularly his identification of key features both in child and parent that led to overprotection—and its psychological consequences for the child.

Many of the clinical studies undertaken at that time were of indifferent quality, but there were also some good examples of high-quality research—such as Lionel Hersov's study of the syndrome of school refusal and James Anthony's studies of encopresis and of infantile psychoses. Kanner's delineation of the syndrome of infantile autism in 1943 forever changed people's thinking, and constitutes a splendid example of the insights provided by the careful observations of an unusually astute clinician (9). The follow-up studies taken up jointly by Leon Eisenberg and Kanner (10) did much to increase understanding of the nature and qualities of this behavioural pattern.

The first randomized controlled trial (RCT) was undertaken in the United Kingdom in 1948, investigating the use of streptomycin to treat tuberculosis. However, Eisenberg and Keith Conners in the United States were pioneers in the 1960s in the use of RCTs to study the effects of treatments in the field of child and adolescent psychiatry (11).

In the first half of the 20th century, most clinicians and researchers paid little attention to the importance of diagnostic distinctions, but this was changed by Lester Hewitt and Richard Jenkins' (12) important factor-analytic study of patterns of emotional and behavioural disturbance (which they termed 'maladjustment'). This led to an acceptance of the need to differentiate between emotional disturbances on the one hand and disorders of disruptive behaviour on the other hand.

Value of longitudinal studies

The first of the several birth cohort studies in the United Kingdom was established in 1946 by James Douglas, later led by Michael Wadsworth. Among other things, it charted the continuities and discontinuities over time in patterns of psychopathology. Taken in conjunction with the later birth cohorts established in 1958 and 1970, it also established the possibility of examining changes over time in patterns of development and in the operation of risk factors.

The most important longitudinal study, however, was undoubtedly Lee Robins' (13) classic study, *Deviant Children Grown Up*. This introduced high-quality concepts and measures that set the standard for all longitudinal studies over the next half-century. This showed the links between conduct problems in childhood and antisocial personality disorder in adult life as well as between childhood psychopathology in childhood and exposure to adverse environments in adult life. It was not the first long-term longitudinal study because there had been several predecessors—most notably the several Californian studies. Each of these made important contributions in their own right, but Robins' study revived an interest in the use of longitudinal studies by demonstrating powerfully the ways in which such studies could tackle vital questions about both nosology and the operation of risk and protective factors. This led to the establishment of the international Life History Research Society in the 1950s which brought together some of the key researchers using longitudinal strategies who sought to learn from one another about matters of both methodology and substance.

Many more longitudinal studies were undertaken around the world in the years that followed. The two in New Zealand—namely in Dunedin (14) and in Christchurch (15)–are probably the best in the world because of their innovativeness in using longitudinal data to tackle crucial and diverse questions. However, equal credit must go to the quite different follow-up study by Robert Sampson and John Laub of Glueck and Glueck's sample of seriously delinquent boys. The research is unique in the duration of follow-up to age 70 years (16) and is notable for its skilled combination of quantitative and qualitative approaches, its methodological innovations, and the light that it has shed on both causes of psychopathology and protective factors operating in adult life through 'turning point' (meaning alteration in life trajectory) effects.

A third set of longitudinal research strategies is provided by the various Scandinavian register-based follow-ups (17) which have capitalized on the availability of systematic national registers, and the means to link them. Again, their use has been informative about risk and protective factors.

Along with the introduction of crucial design features in longitudinal studies, there has been the development of many statistical devices. Specific mention must be made of multivariate regression techniques, especially multilevel modelling. These have been most useful in dealing with issues implicit in nested studies (meaning that individual differences are embedded in family factors, community factors, and so forth). Growth-curve statistical models have been important in enabling comparisons of different growth-curve patterns and using the differences to draw conclusions about how risk and protective factors operate. Finally, RCTs warrant special mention. These have become the 'gold standard' way of assessing the efficacy of various interventions. Although not developed primarily for psychiatry, they have served the field exceptionally well. While they are not free of limitations (particularly uncertainties about external validity—in contrast to their strength, which lies in internal validity) (18) RCTs have had a major impact on assessing evidence regarding which treatments work and for which conditions.

Key developments since the 1960s

Diagnostic distinctions

Until the 1960s, most psychiatrists paid little attention to diagnostic distinctions. This changed completely under the impetus of the Washington University group in St. Louis led by Eli Robins (19). They showed how phenomenology could be used to distinguish between diagnoses, they set standards for determining the validity of these distinctions, and they showed that diagnosis mattered. Their work led to what came to be described as the 'Feighner' criteria, the basis of the classification used in the third edition of the American Psychiatric Association's *Diagnostic and Statistical Manual* (DSM-III, 1980). During the 1960s and early 1970s, WHO held a series of international, interdisciplinary seminars to develop the 9th edition of the International Classification of Diseases (ICD). These not only delineated areas of agreement and disagreement but also revealed that substantial disagreements were derived from the ways in which clinicians used features to fit their theoretical preconceptions rather than from different perceptions of clinical features. In child psychiatry this led to the creation of a multiaxial classification of disorders that separated clinical features from associated risk and protective factors. This approach served the field well in having much in common with the way that most clinicians liked to operate.

Recognition of the importance of diagnosis was followed by the identification of several new conditions. For example, the fetal alcohol syndrome was described in 1973, bulimia nervosa 10 years later, and attachment disorders were first introduced into DSM-III in 1980. Rett's syndrome was first described in 1966, but only had an impact some years later when it was put on the map by Bengt Hagberg and his colleagues, and is now recognized to be a distinct condition caused by a single mutant gene and associated with an unfortunate progressive course. Post-traumatic stress disorder (PTSD) had been reported on in the early 20th century, but was only clearly conceptualized in veterans of the Vietnam War and then applied to children in 1987. Quasi-autism as a syndrome associated with profound institutional deprivation was described first in 1999. It is noteworthy that these newly described syndromes derived from clinical observations and not from the application of laboratory research findings. Although there is now interest in seeking to translate basic science into clinical practice, there is two-way interplay between the two (20).

Epidemiology to plan services and study risk factors

The Isle of Wight epidemiological studies led by Jack Tizard, Kingsley Whitmore, and Rutter in the late 1960s and early 1970s were associated with crucial innovations (21–23). To begin with, the research was planned with the twin objectives of planning services and studying causal risk factors. The studies established the value of systematic interviewing of children, which had been rejected hitherto as a waste of time. They established the frequency of co-occurring patterns—so-called 'comorbidity'. They established the causal role of organic brain dysfunction in mental disorders in childhood, they demonstrated marked school variations in rates of disorder, they showed the important psychopathological risks associated with family dysfunction, they showed marked area differences in rates of disorder, and they indicated the problems in the widespread concept of so-called 'adolescent turmoil'. More generally, they showed the importance of systematic, standardized methods and measurement.

The Isle of Wight studies were followed by the Waltham Forest study which was instrumental in showing that preschool psychopathology was often a precursor of later disorders. This was important because, hitherto, preschool problems had been rather dismissed as being of little long-term significance. The Isle of Wight findings on school variations and rates of disorders led on to the systematic studies undertaken by Rutter, Barbara Maughan, Peter Mortimore, and Janet Ouston in inner London of school effectiveness (these used epidemiological/longitudinal research strategies and were innovative in showing the importance of studying variations in patterns of intake to schools) in order to identify the influence of schools on pupil outcomes (24).

Measures of psychopathology

Although not constituting a scientific advance in their own right, the development of structured interviews—both respondent-based and investigator-based (meaning reliance on the ratings of respondents and those relying on the ratings made by the investigators using specific rules) have been crucial in providing the instruments for scientific advances. There has also been the development of screening questionnaires, of which the Child Behavior Check List (CBCL) is the best developed. These have been used in many epidemiological studies but are not suitable for individual diagnosis.

The value of developmental psychopathology

It might be thought that developmental perspectives had always been a prominent part of conceptual thinking in relation to child and adolescent psychopathology, but, in reality, this was far from the case before the 1970s. The value of considering psychopathology from a developmental perspective was argued persuasively in key papers by Norman Garmezy, Alan Sroufe, and Dante Cicchetti as well as by Rutter (25). Each of these approached the issues in a somewhat different way, but they came together in an agreement that it was necessary to consider both continuities and discontinuities over behavioural variation (i.e. similarities and differences between normal development and psychiatric disorder), and continuities and discontinuities over the course of development (recognizing that it could not be assumed that either continuity or discontinuity was normative).

Several rather distinct bodies of research played key roles in conceptualization of developmental psychopathology. Thus, longitudinal studies had shown the neurodevelopmental origins of both autism (26) and schizophrenia (27). Adult psychiatrists had originally conceptualized schizophrenia as an adult psychosis for which development in childhood was utterly irrelevant. It is now very clear that this is very far from the case. Individuals who later develop schizophrenia have been found to show impairments in the early development of both language and motor functions. Similarly, autism was found to be followed in about 20% of cases by the development of epileptic seizures, usually in adolescence or early adult life. In addition, basic cognitive deficits were found to be part of the core problem.

Judith Rapoport and her colleagues (28) showed age differences in young people's response to drugs, both as prescribed medications and for illicit recreational use. Surprisingly, this observation has been little investigated and remains a key research priority. Age differences in children's responses to lateralized brain injury affecting parts of the brain concerned with language has alerted people to the importance of plasticity in development (29). The effects of brain injury in early life were previously thought to be less damaging than those in later life, but that proved to be a mistaken notion. It is not that the effects of brain damage vary in severity by age, but rather that their patterns differ. Moreover, the main difference is between the early years of child-hood and later, rather than between childhood and adolescence. During the same time period, basic research by Hubel and Wiesel was showing the importance of sensory input to the development of the visual cortex during a sensitive period confined to early childhood.

The work of George Brown and Tirril Harris (30) was pivotal in identifying the impact of early life vulnerability factors in influencing children's response to later life stressors. Clinical studies pointed to the possible role of early life experiences in relation to the risk for later mental disorders, but a major step forward was taken by the use of 'natural experiments' to test rigorously any causal inference (31). The work of Kenneth Kendler and Carol Prescott stands out in this connection with its focus on the long-term sequelae of sexual abuse (32). The Dunedin longitudinal study was influential in showing that a majority of mental disorders leading to treatment in early adult life had already been manifest in childhood (33). Maughan used a follow-up of the Isle of Wight sample to show that reading problems in childhood were followed by a markedly increased rate of spelling difficulties.

Temperament, personality and personality disorder

An interest in temperament features extends back to the 19th century, especially in the Germanic literature. The application to child psychiatry, however, was pioneered by Alexander Thomas and colleagues (34). The study of the biology of temperament was particularly taken forward by Jerome Kagan and Mary Rothbart but numerous other investigators made important contributions. Both developed an important four-dimensional questionnaire measure of temperament and conceptualized temperament as inherited traits that appeared early in the first year and remained stable over time. Neither of these concepts has proved fully correct but they served to put temperament on the map. Research during the last few decades has focused on four key issues. First, there is the evidence on the longitudinal course of temperament—showing very low predictive power from the infancy period, substantial stability from age 3 years, but continuing changes even in adult life. Second, prompted by Richard Bell's (35) challenge on the role of child effects in socialization studies, there has been investigation of the effects of children's behaviour on eliciting responses from other people. Third, there was a recognition of the need to consider the connections between personality and personality disorders with an appreciation that some personality disorders, such as schizotypy, are best conceptualized as a variant of a psychiatric condition (in this case schizophrenia) rather than a variant of temperament or personality (36). Finally, there has been research showing that psychopathic features are identifiable in childhood and that they are highly heritable.

Development of focused psychological therapies using problem-solving strategies

The first important study was that undertaken by William Reid and Ann Shyne (37) in which they examined the relative value of time-limited focused approaches, and more open-ended long-term methods. The findings were striking in showing the advantages of a focused approach. Similar findings came a few years later from the research undertaken by Israel Kolvin and his colleagues in the United Kingdom. Brief psychotherapy, as used with adults, was pioneered by Malan (38), and problem-solving methods as used with children by Myrna Shure and George Spivack (39). Aaron Beck (40) was the key pioneer in the development of cognitive-behaviour therapies (CBT) in adults, and Donald Meichenbaum and Joseph Goodman (41) were the pioneers in developing CBT with children. Focused parenting programmes were developed by both Carol Webster-Stratton and Gerald Patterson, applying a range of innovative techniques, accompanied by systematic evaluations of efficacy.

Historically, psychoanalytically influenced, long-term interventions differed markedly from highly focused behavioural interventions as developed mainly by psychologists. Although substantial differences in psychological therapies remain, there has been a considerable coming together. Psychodynamic psychotherapists have recognized the importance of real-life experiences, and behaviour therapists have recognized the importance of cognitive processes. Both groups have come to appreciate the potential benefits of short-term focused approaches governed by clear objectives.

Over the same period of time, multiple family therapies were developed. These suffered substantially from ideological commitments and disagreements among the various schools of family therapy. Nevertheless, the development of family methods was important in an explicit focus on real-life family interactions and the expectation that families would undertake problem-solving tasks during the intervals between therapeutic sessions. In recent years, too, there has been the development of various attachment therapies that share some of the qualities outlined above (42). For example, they focus on real-life interactions and there is a focused approach in time-limited interventions.

Use of pharmacological treatments and randomized controlled trials

There are several rather different aspects of the advances that have taken place in the evaluation of pharmacological treatments. The recognition of the importance of using RCTs has already been mentioned, but there are several other important advances that made a difference in conceptualization. Thus, at one time, the therapeutic benefit brought about by the use of stimulant medication in the treatment of attention-deficit hyperactivity disorder (ADHD) in children was assumed to represent a paradoxical response. That is to say, it was assumed that the response was qualitatively different from that found in normal individuals. The research undertaken by Rapoport and her colleagues (28) was crucial in indicating that this was not so. Stimulants did indeed have an effect in improving attention in children with ADHD, but similar effects were also found in normal children. This did not mean, of course, that stimulants should be used in normal children (because they did not have the problems of inattention that warranted pharmacological intervention), but the findings did force people to consider the mediating mechanisms.

Longitudinal studies showed strong continuities between depression in childhood/adolescence and depressive disorders in adulthood (43). It was therefore surprising that childhood depression was not responsive to the tricyclic antidepressants that brought substantial benefits in adults. On the other hand, the selective serotonin reuptake inhibitor group of antidepressants (SSRIs) did seem to be effective for depression in young people (although subsequent concerns have been raised about a possible increased risk of suicidal behaviour).

Three issues have received increasing attention in the field of neuropharmacology. First, the question has arisen as to why people differ so markedly in their response to the same medication—in terms of both drug efficacy and side effects. One possible answer may lie in the realm of molecular pharmacogenomics (44). Replicated findings concern individual differences in drug metabolism, but genetic differences in response to different drugs could prove even more clinically useful. However, the hurdles in making 'individualized medicine' a practicality in the case of multifactorial psychiatric disorders are numerous and may prove unachievable. Second, the question of which drug action is responsible for efficacy is a major challenge in that nearly all drugs tend to act on multiple neurotransmitters. The third, related, query is why there are such minor differences in the clinical efficacy of different psychotropic drugs. The breakthrough has come through the use of positron emission tomography (PET scans), using radiolabelled ligands to examine the degree of neurotransmitter receptor occupancy. The work of both Shitij Kapur and colleagues and Nora Volkow and colleagues well illustrate the strategy as a means of providing a better understanding of drug efficacy.

At a more general level, there has been a widespread recognition that small-scale treatment studies are not going to provide adequate answers. Multisite collaborative research is essential, and has been undertaken with respect to the treatment of both depression and ADHD. Such studies, of course, require not only cooperation between academic centres, but also careful planning and monitoring to ensure that similar methods of measurement are used.

The importance of genetic influences and of gene–environment interdependence

This has been one of the major growth areas in research since the 1970s, and it is possible only to pick out a few highlights. The first systematic twin study of autism by Susan Folstein and Rutter (45) warrants mention, not just because it indicated for the first time that genetic influences were very important in the liability to autism (which many previously considered a psychogenic disorder), but more particularly because the findings showed that these influences applied to a broader phenotype than that presented by the traditional severe, handicapping form of autism, and that the genetic influences operated in a multifactorial, probabilistic fashion rather than the determinative way in which single-gene Mendelian influences operate. At the time, some geneticists resisted the departure from Mendelian assumptions, and the focus on a broader phenotype. Both are now accepted, not only in relation to autism, but much more broadly in the field of psychopathology.

During the latter part of the 20th century, a huge number of twin and adoptee (as well as family) studies showed that genetic influences operated on virtually all forms of mental disorder, albeit to differing degrees. In addition, attention moved away from the assumption of determinative direct effects on mental disorder to the recognition of the role of indirect genetic influences. Thus, Robert Plomin and Cindy Bergeman

(46) used quantitative findings on gene–environment correlations (rGE) to argue that a proportion of the risk effects of environmental features were actually genetically, rather than environmentally, mediated. It took a little while for psychosocial researchers to accept the reality of this issue, but it has become generally accepted. Quantitative genetics had also pointed to the likely operation of gene–environment interactions (G×E) (47). Researchers and clinicians became aware that genetic influences often operated through genetic effects on environmental risk exposure (through G×E) and differences in environmental susceptibility (operating through G×E).

The study of G×E was revolutionized, however, when molecular genetic methods were used to identify individual susceptibility genes and when there were good measures of environmental features. A series of seminal papers based on the Dunedin study published by Avshalom Caspi, Terrie Moffitt, and their colleagues (48,49) showed the importance of such effects and also outlined the strategic approach needed to investigate G×E. There are three other advances that were crucial in providing some better understanding of gene–environment interdependence. First, there was the use of animal models which were useful in demonstrating in primates that similar G×E effects were operative. Second, there was the experimental study of the neural effects of G×E in humans, led by Daniel Weinberger, Andreas Meyer-Lindenberg, and Ahmad Hariri (50). Structural and functional brain imaging techniques were used in conjunction with molecular genetics for this purpose. Interestingly, and importantly, these studies focused on effects in individuals without evidence of psychopathology. The fact that the neural effects were found in these participants was crucial in showing that the biological pathways had to be ones that operated more generally than just in individuals with significant disorders. The third advance was provided by the research of Michael Meaney and his colleagues (51) in demonstrating the epigenetic mediation of environmental effects. Epigenetic mechanisms involve an alteration in DNA methylation at specific sites on the genome, with consequent effects on gene expression, without any change in nucleotide sequence. As such, they serve to mediate the effects of environments (both social and physical) on the operation of genetic influences—such as on physiological and psychological responses to stress. This realization opened the way to a study of environmental moderation of genetic effects—thereby highlighting a rather different form of gene–environment interdependence.

Role of cognitive processes in social functioning

The pioneers in the sphere of cognitive processes and social functioning were undoubtedly Beate Hermelin and Neil O'Connor (52) through their research on autistic children's use of meaning in memory. They clearly identified mentalizing problems (in terms of not using meaning in memory), but were limited by the difficulty in indicating how this might operate in the liability to autism. The next step was demonstrating so-called 'theory of mind' deficits in autism by Simon Baron-Cohen, Uta Frith, and colleagues (53), who based their work on studies of the role of 'theory of mind' in normal children; as in the earlier research of Hermelin and O'Connor, the findings pointed to important parallels between normal and abnormal development (54). The benefits of studying of normal development to cast light on processes in mental disorders, and its converse, became firmly established. One limitation of this work was that, at least as measured at the time, the emergence of 'theory of mind' was too late to explain the social abnormalities in autism evident before the age of two. Research turned to eye gaze and joint attention as features that might be important, and indeed proved to be so. Whether or not these are precursors of 'theory of mind' or whether they represent a rather different cognitive pathway is not yet entirely clear.

Another strategy focused on similar issues was using siblings to investigate early manifestations of autism. Its rationale was that siblings of autistic children were themselves likely to develop an autism-spectrum disorder in 5–10% of cases.

Functional brain imaging techniques proved crucial in studying brain–mind interconnections. In the field of autism, these showed that the disorder did not lie in a localized abnormality in one part of the brain but, rather, a lack of normal connectivity across brain systems (55). In addition, imaging methods have enabled a wide range of ways in which brain–mind relationships can be studied.

Finally, mention must be made of Giacomo Rizzolatti's discovery of mirror neurons. These neurons respond to an individual's perceptions of what another person is doing or might be doing. Their salience lies in the possibility that their impaired function might constitute the neural basis of autism. A difficulty in testing this notion is the wide distribution of mirror neurons in the brain. However, steps have been taken to link mirror neuron activity with social functioning.

The role of social context

At one time, most discussion of the role of lack of social influences on the liability to psychopathology concentrated on family interaction with the implicit assumption that these family effects operated independently of the broader social environment. Urie Bronfenbrenner (56) was the pioneer who changed all of that in his discussion of ecological concepts of the ways in which environments were nested within broader arenas. Thus, there was the role of the individual, which was nested within the family, which in turn was nested within the community, and so forth. This appreciation had an influence on the concepts of how psychosocial influences operated, but also had crucial implications on the use of multilevel modelling to investigate such influences.

The demonstration of geographical variations in rates of crime and psychopathology goes back to the mid-20th century but progress was sluggish until Sampson and his colleagues in Chicago (57) suggested that the effects derived less from qualities that pushed people towards crime than social disorganization that failed to inhibit antisocial behaviour. The Moynihan report highlighted the role of ghettos in predisposing individuals to criminal behaviour. It got a very negative reception from many commentators who read into the report all sorts of values that actually were not present. A re-evaluation of the report served to confirm the validity of many of Moynihan's arguments.

Research into the effects on children of differences among schools in their effectiveness was put on the map by Rutter and his colleagues (24,58). Two key features were especially important. First, the use of longitudinal data made it possible to determine whether the variations among schools in pupil outcomes were simply an artefact of differences in pupil intake; it was found that they were not. Second, systematic measures of how the school functioned made it possible to identify the distinctive school features associated with greater effectiveness. Somewhat similar methodological issues applied to the possible role of antisocial gang membership in fostering increases in criminal behaviour. The work of Terry Thornberry and colleagues (59) stands out with respect to the use of longitudinal data to sort out selection effects and social influence effects. Both were found to be operative but it is the demonstration of within-individual changes over time that provided the first convincing evidence of a causal effect.

Clinicians and researchers have been aware for a long time that there are quite strong ethnic variations in rates of psychopathology and psychological functioning more generally. Unfortunately, most of the earlier research was based on the misguided assumption that comparisons had to be made with a normative, 'Caucasian' situation. It is now appreciated that this is a prejudicial approach and also that it gets in the way of understanding the mediating mechanisms. Rutter and Marta Tienda brought together a set of interdisciplinary, international essays, all of which served to show that the study of ethnic variations need not be prejudicial; indeed to the contrary they could be very informative in leading to the identification of the influences that mediated variations and, moreover, that findings could well be informative with respect to the broader population and not just to the particular ethnic minority group being studied.

'Natural experiments' to examine environmental mediation

Donald Campbell was the pioneer in outlining the range of different forms of 'quasi-experiment' that could be used to test hypotheses on environmental mediation of causal influences. The need for such approaches derives from the fact that there are several key threats to the causal inference, such as those deriving from genetic mediation, from social selection, from reverse causation, and from unmeasured confounding variables (18). A range of twin, adoptee, and migration strategies have been used to exclude genetic mediation, with Kendler (32), Caspi (60), and Plomin being among the pioneers here. There are then a variety of designs that may be used to contrast different types of environmental mediation, so enabling avoidance of the misidentification of causal effects (32). Designs using universal exposure are valuable in controlling for social selection (61). The use of these 'natural experiments' served to pull apart variables that ordinarily go together, and they have been effective in confirming some postulated causal effects and excluding other causal claims.

For example, the study of discordant twin pairs showed that the twin exposed to sexual abuse had a greatly increased risk of later mental disorder—thus showing the environmentally mediated causal effect stemming from sexual abuse (32). Multivariate twin analyses showed that physical abuse had an environmentally mediated causal effect on mental disorder, whereas corporal punishment did not (62). A range of natural experiment designs have confirmed the prenatal effect of maternal smoking on birth weight but cast doubt on the claimed prenatal effect in causing either antisocial behaviour or ADHD. The study of institution-reared children from Romania adopted into United Kingdom families showed that the initial developmental deficits were indeed due to the deprivation (because they remitted after removal from the institution) and that deprivation led to persisting disorders of an unusual kind, such as quasi-autistic patterns or disinhibited attachment (63).

The rise of anti-science ideologies, and the misleading claims of biological determinism

For quite some time, psychoanalysis acted like a religion with claims assessed in terms of ideological tenets, rather than either logic or empirical evidence (3). Because of this, psychoanalysis was to psychiatry what creationism is to biology. The issue is not whether their particular claims were or were not correct, but rather that the ideological approach took psychoanalysis outside the boundaries of science. This was accompanied by Donald Winnicott's (64) claim that clinical psychiatric training was irrelevant and that research was damaging. At about the same time, Bruno Bettelheim's 'blame the parent' agenda meant that many parents were wrongly charged with being responsible for their child's autistic problems (65). Somewhat similar ideological features were sometimes evident in the early days of family therapy, and in some of the current claims on attachment. All of this was followed by the equally misleading claims of biological, or genetic, determinism.

It is necessary, in order to avoid misunderstandings, to make explicit that individual psychoanalysts made important contributions to the development of psychological therapies and, also, that some of the claims of psychoanalysis (such as the existence of mental mechanisms) have proved valid. The damage came from treating a theory as a religion in which there was rejection of any use of non-psychoanalytic methods to test psychoanalytic claims, an insistence that practitioners had to undergo a personal analysis in order to be accepted, and that disputes regarding psychoanalytic theory had to be resolved by reference to the 'high priests' of the psychoanalytic world rather than by any form of dispassionate assessment.

Moving on in concepts and therapeutic approaches

We need to pay attention to Eisenberg's (66) warning that we should not replace a 'brainless' psychiatry with a 'mindless' psychiatry. The point he was making was that in the era when psychoanalysis dominated, everything was assumed to operate in terms of mental operations that had got nothing to do with the biology of brain functioning. Quite rightly, that narrow-minded approach has been rejected, but he was warning that there is now a parallel danger that we are running the risk of focusing exclusively on neural functioning without appreciating that we have evolved to have a mind that allows us to look back, to plan, and to look ahead. For all their faults, psychodynamic therapies led therapists to listen to patients and to appreciate that role of mental mechanisms. Initially, the emphasis was entirely in terms of patient's thinking and not in terms of their real-life experiences; however, as I have tried to indicate, the advances in psychological therapies have incorporated much more in the way of paying attention to actual experiences (both in the past and in the present) and to take problem-solving approaches of a systematic kind. There has been a relative coming together of different types of psychotherapy, together with a greater attention to evidence and the need to evaluate the efficacy of preventive and therapeutic interventions (67).

While there is every reason to suppose that a developmental perspective is important (as indicated by the evidence from developmental psychopathology), we also have to agree with Bowlby's (68) assessment that psychoanalysis was never more wrong than in its theory of child development. That is not its important contribution, and it is time to put aside those aspects of psychoanalysis.

Following on from the recognition in the 1970s of the importance of diagnostic distinctions, there came the development of many forms of standardized interviews relying on different forms of structure. There can be no doubt about the value of these systematic interviewing methods in both research and in clinical work, as discussed earlier in the essay. On the other hand, there is a very real danger that a blinkered adoption of structured diagnostic interviews will interfere with attention to patients' concerns and needs, to assessing strengths and weaknesses in the family and broader social situation, and in planning approaches to treatment. Diagnostic assessment should not be confined to just coming up with the 'correct' diagnostic label. This is not just a private value judgement because systematic studies of different approaches to interviewing have shown the frequency with which there are clinically important pieces of unexpected information that fall outside the scope of the structured interview.

Key opportunities in child and adolescent psychiatry

In this historical overview of the worldwide scientific achievements of the last 50 years relevant to an understanding of the causes, course, or treatment of mental disorders, it is evident that an enormous amount has been achieved. It is also clear that many of the major steps forward came from psychologists, sociologists, geneticists, and others from non-psychiatric disciplines. Moreover, even when focusing on child psychopathology the contributions of adult psychiatrists are at least as great as those of child and adolescent psychiatrists. Finally, the major advances have come from many different countries. We need to ask ourselves whether, given that the best modern clinical and basic sciences are both international and interdisciplinary, it is still appropriate to have single-discipline, regional organizations. There may be value if these are predominantly aimed towards self-help, but we need to look outwards and not inwards.

With respect to training in child and adolescent psychiatry, it is good that this has become both more systematic and evidence-based. Nevertheless, where there are exams in psychiatry to be passed, we need to query the increasingly exclusive focus on 'facts', with little or no attention to concepts and ideas. This has come about because of the greater convenience of marking correct or wrong answers in tick-boxes. Of course, there are crucial facts that must be mastered but we need to remind ourselves that history teaches us that of the 'facts' learned by the completion of training, about one-third will later prove to be correct, another one-third will have been found to be wrong, and a further one-third correct but not very relevant. The dilemma is that, at any one point in time, we do not know which facts fall in each third. A change of approach is needed if we are to foster continuing learning over the course of a person's professional career. With these features in mind, we need to consider the challenges still before us.

Genetic evidence is consistent in showing that there are major environmental effects on the liability to mental disorders, as in adult life. The excitement of the important technologies that are now available to use in research must not blind us to the appreciation that the environment has very important effects. On the other hand, there is the need to take seriously the testing for environmental mediation. This will continue to involve 'natural experiments' as well as employing laboratory manipulations (31).

In particular, there is a need to determine the biological basis of environmental effects that persist beyond the period of exposure to stress/adversity. That is, we have to undertake the appropriate research to determine how environments 'get under the skin'. In seeking to understand this biological basis, we will need to contrast epigenetic, neuroendocrine, and mental model mechanisms (meaning the processes that stem from the individual's mind-set about the meaning of his/her experiences and his/her role in them) to mention just three out of a broader range of alternatives. It is much too early to take decisions that any one of these is going to prove to be the predominant mediating mechanism.

Equally, there is a need to delineate the biological mediating mechanisms involved in gene–environment correlations and interactions (69). In other words, we need to study the indirect effects of genes, a process that is sometimes expressed in terms of how genes get 'outside the skin'. This will involve understanding how the behaviour of individuals acts to select and shape environments. Such research needs to have a focus on the role of these individual behaviours, with the determination of the extent of genetic influences as a secondary, rather than a primary, consideration. By contrast, the study of genetic effects on susceptibility to environmental causes requires genetic research strategies. As discussed, these need to use molecular genetic strategies to identify individual genes and to have good quality measures of relevant environments. If we are to understand the neural basis of G×E, it will be necessary to undertake experimental brain imaging studies using specific genes and intermediate phenotypes (i.e. behavioural features that are intermediate on the biological pathway from the genes to the disorder). The latter are important in order to study the immediate effects of G×E without waiting decades for psychopathology to develop (70). The way ahead in this connection has already been demonstrated (50), but more research of this kind is needed.

There is also a need for the development and use of animal models. Up until now, these have played rather a small role in child and adolescent psychiatric research, but they have an important place. Of course, there are many difficulties in devising appropriate animal models, but they provide a crucially important way of teasing apart aspects of causal mechanisms (71).

Longitudinal studies of high-risk groups are required in order to identify the mechanisms involved in transitions across developmental changes in psychopathology (33). Thus, this is needed when studying how the prodromal features of schizophrenia lead on to schizophrenic psychoses in some individuals but not in others. Similar needs apply to the transitions from the broader phenotype of autism to a severe handicapping disorder.

There is certainly a need for more, and better, studies of treatments (both psychological and pharmacological); these need to be accompanied by designs that can test the mediators of therapeutic effectiveness and the causes of individual differences in response. Pharmacogenetics provides one important focus with respect to individual differences, but a broader range of strategies need to be employed. There is an especial need to identify the mechanisms involved in age differences in response to drugs and to major hazards. It is decidedly curious that these issues have received so little systematic research attention up until now.

Past research has provided many pointers on possible modes of prevention of child and adolescent psychopathology, and there is a certain amount of evidence that well planned preventive measures can be effective. Developing further preventive strategies, it will be important to take on board the fact that most forms of mental disorders in young people (as in adults) are recurrent or chronic, as well as recognizing the need to consider the biology (72). Accordingly, evaluations must be concerned with long-term effects (both beneficial and damaging); planning also needs to be sensitive to the times when preventive interventions may be effective and when they will be received positively by those to whom they are offered.

With respect to both preventive and therapeutic interventions, we need to appreciate that causation often, and probably usually, involves multiple pathways. This is nothing special to psychopathology but is something that applies across the whole of biomedicine. It has come to be accepted, too, that most genes have multiple effects and that most environmental influences also affect a range of different outcomes (71). Currently, there is much attention paid to the issue of supposed comorbidity, but it needs to be appreciated that much of this co-occurrence is likely to be artefactual, and that the identification of co-occurrence is a starting point for research and not an end point. Insofar as the effects are real, we need to determine the mechanisms involved. There is not a single research strategy that is appropriate for this task, but what is clear is that research designed to pit alternatives one against another is likely to be the most informative.

In that connection, it is also obvious that the official classification systems contain far too many individual diagnoses. There are many of these diagnoses that are rarely, if ever, used, and it is quite impractical to suppose that even the most skilled and experienced clinicians can carry in their head the rules required to make some 400 or more diagnoses. It is very much to be hoped that revisions of the ICD and DSM classifications will simplify systems, as well as making them more scientifically validated and more clinically useful (73). In the case of child psychopathology, this will require better coverage of preschool disorders, and especially the development of diagnostic systems that are usable in primary care (both medical and non-medical) where time and constraints prevail. One specific issue that will require attention is the use of dimensions. On the one hand, there is much evidence across the whole of biomedicine that there are dimensional features to most disorders, and that most risk factors operate dimensionally, rather than categorically. On the other hand, clinical decision-making has to involve categorical decisions. It makes no sense to think that you can have a little bit of medication or a little bit of hospital admission. Accordingly, it is to be hoped that dimensions will form a part of diagnostic approaches, but that careful attention will be paid to finding workable ways of coming to categorical decisions.

Post-mortem studies have proved of value in the study of disorders in adult life and, potentially, they should be informative with respect to mental disorders in childhood (51). Practical problems stem from the fact that most young people with mental disorders do not die young and when they do die young they are often atypical in many crucial respects. There are also the practical problems associated with the fact that most deaths in early life are unexpected and have to be subject to scrutiny by coroners. Nevertheless, it is important that brain-banks be established and used in a collaborative manner.

There are several issues that are new and of high importance in the field of genetics. For example, there is now good evidence that copy number variations (CNVs; meaning submicroscopic deletions and substitutions within DNA sequences) play a causal role in relation to both autism and schizophrenia (and probably other conditions as well). Two major issues require attention. First, most CNVs are not familial and arise *de novo*. This means that although they can be demonstrated to play an aetiological role, they do not account for familiality. In addition, even when there is familiality, it is clear that the effects are probabilistic and not determinative because some family members with the CNV do not show the condition being studied. The second issue is a different one and concerns why the rates of CNVs (and also chromosome anomalies and minor physical anomalies) are much more common in individuals with autism or schizophrenia than they are in the general population. They probably arise randomly through stochastic chance variation, but the question remains as to what non-genetic factors, such as raised parental age, make variations more likely. The relative importance of rare and common variants with respect to genetic influences warrants continuing study, given that many of the rare variants are associated with atypical phenotypes which have an uncertain relevance for the broader run of conditions. In addition, we need to ask why conditions such as autism or schizophrenia, in which there is markedly reduced fecundity, do not become extinct. Different genetic mechanisms may operate than in conditions where fecundity is not affected. Expressed more generally, we need to move away from an exclusive focus on gene hunting and seek an understanding of the biological mechanisms implicated in genetic effects. This endeavour will certainly have to involve basic science strategies looking at what genes 'do' in terms of their effects on proteins and, more crucially, how the protein effects lead to the phenotype under consideration.

Problems and concerns regarding the future

As is implicit in all that has been said with respect to the past, it is essential, in the future, to avoid the ideologies that seek to escape the need for empirical evidence. That applies as much to pharmacological evangelism and biological determinism, as to psychoanalysis, family therapy, and attachment theory (65). Second, we need to work with industry because their involvement is going to be essential in drug developments but, equally, it is crucial that we guard against the biases and control (as well as the personal greed) that may come in with the tide (74). Third, we have to avoid reliance on single treatment methods. That applies even to methods, such as CBT, that have proven efficacies in certain circumstances. The point is that there is no treatment that provides the 'silver bullet' and deals with all the problems and, moreover, developments in science may bring new circumstances for which the currently favoured treatment is no longer the method of choice. Clinical training has to involve an appreciation of diverse treatment approaches and not just one.

Finally, we need to recognize that, in recent times, child and adolescent psychiatrists have played a rather limited role in the major areas of innovative research. I have indicated some important exceptions, and there are many more that I could have listed. Also, of course there are many more now doing very good research (albeit not innovative to the extent required for inclusion in this review), but there is a paucity of people doing top-level international research likely to open up new avenues and challenge the 'wisdom' of the day. It is this sort of creative iconoclastic style that I have focused on in my historical overview and it is those researchers who are in short supply. Adult psychiatrists and psychologists have increasingly taken over leadership in many of the high-priority areas. Their involvement is positively to be welcomed and it would be quite wrong to seek to marginalize them. To the contrary, their leadership has been a major positive benefit for child and adolescent psychiatry. Even so, we have to act to ensure that future generations of child and adolescent psychiatrists include really able individuals who receive systematic research training, and who are capable of moving in a creative fashion to develop new concepts and new approaches.

There is much that is good in both child and adolescent psychiatry research and clinical practice, but notable weaknesses exist that require remedial action. Steps are being taken to strengthen the discipline and all members of the profession must play their part in doing all that can be done to further strengthen research and the clinical practice so that the younger generation is in a position to move strongly ahead in the future.

Acknowledgement

This essay is based on a previously published paper in *European Child & Adolescent Psychiatry* (2010) **19**, 689–703 and is printed here with the publication's permission.

References

1 Rutter, M. (2010). Child and adolescent psychiatry: Past scientific achievements and challenges for the future. *European Child & Adolescent Psychiatry* **19**, 689–703.

2 Rutter, M. and Stevenson, J. (2008). Developments in child and adolescent psychiatry over the last 50 years. In: Rutter, M, Bishop, D., Pine, D. et al. (eds.), *Rutter's child and adolescent psychiatry* (5th edn). Oxford: Wiley-Blackwell, pp. 1–17.

3 Maddox, B. (2006). *Freud's wizard: The enigma of Ernest Jones*. London: John Murray.

4 Bowlby, J. (1951) *Maternal care and mental health*. Geneva: World Health Organization.

5 Bowlby, J. (1969/1982) *Attachment and loss, Vol. 1: Attachment*. London: Hogarth Press.

6 Rutter, M., Kreppner, J., and Sonuga-Barke, E. (2009). Emanuel Miller lecture: Attachment insecurity, disinhibited attachment, and attachment disorders: Where do research findings leave the concepts? *Journal of Child Psychology and Psychiatry* **50**, 529–43.

7 Robertson, J. and Robertson, J. (1971). Young children in brief separation: A fresh look. *Psychoanalytic Study of the Child* **26**, 264–315.

8 Levy, D. (1943). *Maternal overprotection*. New York: W. W. Norton.

9 Kanner, L. (1943). Autistic disturbances of affective contact. *Nervous Child* 2, 217–50 Reprint (1968) in *Acta Paedopsychiatrica* **35**, 100–36.

10 Kanner, L. and Eisenberg, L. (1956). Early infantile autism 1943–55. *American Journal of Orthopsychiatry* **26**, 556–66.

11 Lipman, R. S. (1974.) NIMH–PRB-support of research in minimal brain dysfunction in children. In: Conners, C. K. (ed.) *Clinical use of stimulant drugs in children*, Amsterdam: Excerpta Medica, pp. 202–13.

12 Hewitt, L. E. and Jenkins, R. L. (1946). *Fundamental patterns of maladjustment: the dynamics of their origins*. Springfield, MI: University of Michigan.

13 Robins, L. N. (1966). *Deviant children grown up: a sociological and psychiatric study of sociopathic personality*. Baltimore, MD: Williams & Wilkins.

14 Moffitt, T. E., Caspi, A., Rutter, M., and Silva, P. A. (2001). *Sex differences in antisocial behaviour: conduct disorder, delinquency, and violence in the Dunedin Longitudinal Study.* Cambridge: Cambridge University Press.

15 Ferguson, D. M. and Horwood, L. J. (2001). The Christchurch Health and Development Study: Review of findings on child and adolescent mental health. *Australia and New Zealand Journal of Psychiatry* 35, 287–96.

16 Laub, J. H. and Sampson, R. J. (2006). *Shared beginnings, divergent lives: delinquent boys to age 70.* Harvard, MA: Harvard University Press.

17 Nylander, I. (1979). A 20 year prospective follow-up study of 2 164 cases at the child guidance clinics in Stockholm. *Acta Paediatrica Scandanavia* (Suppl.) 276, 1–45.

18 Academy of Medical Sciences. (2007). *Identifying the environmental causes of disease: how should we decide what to believe and when to take action?* London: Academy of Medical Sciences.

19 Feighner, J. P., Robins, E., Guze, S. B. et al. (1972). Diagnostic criteria for use in psychiatric research. *Archives of General Psychiatry* 26, 57–63.

20 Rutter, M. and Plomin, R. (2009). Pathways from science findings to health benefits. *Psychological Medicine* 39, 529–42.

21 Rutter, M., Graham, P., and Yule, W. (1970). *A neuropsychiatric study in childhood.* London: William Heinemann Medical.

22 Rutter, M., Tizard, J., and Whitmore, K. (1970). *Education, health and behaviour.* London: Longman.

23 Rutter, M., Tizard, J., Yule, W., Graham, P., and Whitmore, K. (1976). Research report: Isle of Wight Studies, 1964–74. *Psychological Medicine* 6, 313–32.

24 Rutter, M., Maughan, B., Mortimore, P., and Ouston, J. (1979). *Fifteen thousand hours: secondary schools and their effects on children.* Cambridge, MA: Harvard University Press.

25 Rutter, M. (2008). Developing concepts in developmental psychopathology. In: Hudziak, J. J. (ed.) *Developmental psychopathology and wellness: genetic and environmental influences.* New York, NY: American Psychiatric Publications, pp. 3–22.

26 Rutter, M. (1970). Autistic children: Infancy to adulthood. *Seminal Psychiatry* 2, 435–50.

27 Weinberger, D. R. (1987). Implications of normal brain development for the pathogenesis of schizophrenia. *Archives of General Psychiatry* 44, 660–9.

28 Rapoport, J. L., Buchsbaum, M. S., and Weingartner, H. (1980). Dextroamphetamine: cognitive and behavioural effects in normal and hyperactive boys and normal adult males. *Psychopharmacology Bulletin* 16, 21–3.

29 Vargha-Khadem, F., Isaacs, E., van der Werf, S., Robb, S., and Wilson, J. (1992). Development of intelligence and memory in children with hemiplegic cerebral palsy. The deleterious consequences of early seizures. *Brain* 115, 315–29.

30 Brown, G. W. and Harris, T. O. (1978). *Social origins of depression: a study of psychiatric disorder in women.* London: Tavistock.

31 Rutter, M. (2007). Proceeding from observed correlation to causal inference: the use of natural experiments. *Perspectives of Psychological Science* 2, 377–395.

32 Kendler, K. S. and Prescott, C. A. (2006). *Genes, environment and psychopathology: understanding the causes of psychiatric and substance use disorders.* Boston, MA: Guilford Press.

33 Rutter, M., Kim-Cohen, J., and Maughan, B. (2006). Continuities and discontinuities in psychopathology between childhood and adult life. *Journal of Child Psychology and Psychiatry* 47, 276–95.

34 Thomas, A., Chess, S., Birch, H. G., Hertzig, M. E., and Korn, S. (1963). *Behavioural individuality in early childhood*. New York: New York University Press.

35 Bell, R. Q. (1968). A reinterpretation of the direction of effects in studies of socialization. *Psychological Review* **75**, 81–95.

36 Kendler, K. S., Gruenberg, A. M., and Strauss, J. S. (1981). An independent analysis of the Copenhagen sample of the Danish Adoption Study of Schizophrenia. II. The relationship between schizotypal personality disorders and schizophrenia. *Archives of General Psychiatry* **38**, 928–84.

37 Reid, W. J., and Shyne, A. W. (1969). *Brief and extended casework*. New York, NY: Columbia University Press.

38 Malan, D. (1979). *Individual psychotherapy and the science of 1300 psychodynamics*. London: Butterworth.

39 Shure, M. B. and Spivack, G. (1972). Means-ends thinking, adjustment and social class among elementary school-aged children. *Journal of Consulting and Clinical Psychology* **38**, 348–53.

40 Beck, A. T. (1963). Thinking and depression 1: Idiosyncratic content and cognitive distortions. *Archives of General Psychiatry* **9**, 324–33.

41 Meichenbaum, D. H. and Goodman, J. (1971). Training impulsive children to talk to themselves: A means of developing self-control. *Journal of Abnormal Psychology* **77**, 115–26.

42 Cassidy, J. and Shaver, P. R. (eds.) (2008). *Handbook of attachment: theory, research, and clinical applications* (2nd edn). New York, NY: Guilford Press.

43 Harrington, R., Fudge, H., Rutter, M., Pickles, A., and Hill, J. (1990). Adult outcomes of childhood and adolescent depression. I. Psychiatric status. *Archives of General Psychiatry* **47**, 465–73.

44 Roden, D. M., Altman, R. B., Benowitz, N.L, et al. (2006). Pharmacogenomics: challenges and opportunities. *Annals of Internal Medicine* **145**, 749–58.

45 Folstein, S. and Rutter, M. (1977). Infantile autism: a genetic study of 21 twin pairs. *Journal of Child Psychology and Psychiatry* **18**, 297–312.

46 Plomin, R. and Bergeman, C. S. (1991). The nature of nurture: genetic influences on 'environmental' measures. *Behavioral and Brain Sciences* **14**, 373–427.

47 Rutter, M. and Silberg, J. (2002). Gene-environment interplay in relation to emotional and behavioural disturbance. *Annual Review of Psychology* **53**, 463–90.

48 Moffitt, T. E., Caspi, A., and Rutter, M. (2005). Strategy for investigating interactions between measured genes and measured environments. *Archives of General Psychiatry* **62**, 473–81.

49 Caspi, A. and Moffitt, T. E. (2006). Gene-environment interactions in psychiatry: joining forces with neuroscience. *Nature Reviews Neuroscience* **7**, 583–90.

50 Meyer-Lindenberg, A. and Weinberger, D. R. (2006). Intermediate phenotypes and genetic mechanisms of psychiatric disorders. *Nature Reviews Neuroscience* **7**, 818–27.

51 Meaney, M. J. (2010). Epigenetics and the biological definition of gene x environment interactions. *Child Development* **81**, 47–79.

52 Hermelin, B. and O'Connor, N. (1970). *Psychological experiments with autistic children*. Oxford: Pergamon Press.

53 Baron-Cohen, S., Leslie, A. M., and Frith, U. (1985). Does the autistic child have a 'theory of mind'? *Cognition* **21**, 37–46.

54 Frith, U. (ed.) (1991). *Autism and Asperger syndrome*. Cambridge: Cambridge University Press.

55 Frith, C. (2003). What do imaging studies tell us about the neural basis of autism? In: Bock, G. and Goode, J. (eds.) *Autism: neural basis and treatment possibilities*, Chichester: John Wiley and Sons, pp. 149–76.

56 Bronfenbrenner, U. (1979). *The ecology of human development: experiments by nature and design*. Cambridge: Harvard University Press.

57 Sampson, R. J., Raudenbush, S. W., and Earls, F. W. (1997). Neighbourhoods and violent crime: a multilevel study of collective efficacy. *Science* 27, 918–24.

58 Rutter, M. and Maughan, B. (2002). School effectiveness findings 1979–2002 *Journal of Child Psychology and Psychiatry* 40, 451–75.

59 Thornberry, T.P, Krohn, M. D., Lizotte, A. J., and Chard-Wiershem, D. (1993). The role of juvenile gangs in facilitating delinquent behavior. *Journal of Research in Crime and Delinquency* 30, 55–87.

60 Caspi, A., Moffitt, T. E., Morgan, J. et al. (2004). Maternal expressed emotion predicts children's antisocial behavior problems: using monozygotic-twin differences to identify environmental effects on behavioral development. *Developmental Psychology* 40, 149–61.

61 Costello, E. J., Compton, S. N., Keeler, G., and Angold, A. (2003). Relationships between poverty and psychopathology: a natural experiment. *JAMA* 290, 2023–9.

62 Jaffee, S. R., Caspi, A., Moffitt, T. E. et al. (2004). The limits of child effects: evidence for genetically mediated child effects on corporal punishment but not on physical maltreatment. *Developmental Psychology* 40, 1047–58.

63 Rutter, M., and Sonuga-Barke, E. J. (2010). Deprivation-specific psychological patterns: effects of institutional deprivation. *Monographs of the Society for Research in Child Development* 75, 1.

64 Winnicott, D. W. (1963) Symposium: training for child psychiatry. *Journal of Child Psychology and Psychiatry* 4, 85–91.

65 Pollack, P. (1997). *The creation of Dr B: A biography of Bruno Bettelheim*. New York, NY: Simon & Schuster.

66 Eisenberg, L. (1986). Mindlessness and brainlessness in psychiatry. *British Journal of Psychiatry* 14, 497–508.

67 Weisz, J. and Kazdin, A. E. (eds.) (2010). *Evidence-based psychotherapies for children and adolescents* (2nd edn). New York: Guilford Press.

68 Bowlby, J. (1988). *A secure base: parent-child attachment and healthy human development*. New York, NY: Basic Books.

69 Rutter, M (ed.) (2008). *Genetic effects on environmental vulnerability to disease*. Chichester: John Wiley and Sons.

70 Rutter, M. (ed.) (2008). *Genetic effects on environmental vulnerability to disease*. London: Novartis Foundation/Wiley.

71 Rutter, M. (2006). *Genes and behaviour: nature-nurture interplay explained*. Chichester: Wiley-Blackwell.

72 Shonkoff, J. P., Boyce, W. T., and McEwen, B. S. (2009). Neuroscience, molecular biology, and the childhood roots of health disparities: Building a new framework for health promotion and disease prevention. *JAMA* 301, 2252–9.

73 Rutter, M. (2011). Child psychiatric diagnosis and classification: concepts, findings, challenges and potential. *Journal of Child and Adolescent Psychiatry* 52, 647–60.

74 Eisenberg, L. and Belfer, M. (2009). Prerequisites for global child and adolescent mental health. *Journal of Child Psychology and Psychiatry* 50, 26–35.

Psychiatry of old age

Catherine Oppenheimer

Introduction

I have built this essay on five interlocking themes: *developing services, mapping the diagnostic landscape, scientific background, advances in treatment,* and *the political and social context.* Inevitably my story refers mainly to the United Kingdom, often specifically to Oxford, sometimes only to personal experience. I apologize to the rest of the world, for neglecting the story of old age psychiatry there.

Textbooks are useful milestones on the journey, crystallizing the achievements and culture of their time (1, 2). I have drawn on successive editions of the textbook (1) edited by Robin Jacoby and myself to cover the period from 2008 back to 1991; and for the decade before that, Raymond Levy and Felix Post's *The Psychiatry of Late Life* (3), my bible as a newly appointed consultant in 1984. My 50-year milestone is a major British textbook (4) of that time: *Clinical Psychiatry* by Mayer-Gross, Slater, and Roth. William Mayer-Gross and Martin Roth were pioneers in the psychiatry of old age, and the text itself is full of historical perspectives. (Doubtless, filial affection (5) also influenced my choice.)

First theme: developing services

The early years

Compassion for older people in want or distress is as old as humanity; and so are efforts to construct systems for meeting their needs. But it would be fair to give to the United Kingdom the credit for inventing psychogeriatrics as a distinct medical discipline. Its roots were in Scotland at the Crichton Royal Infirmary in Dumfries in the 1940s, and it spread from there to the Maudsley Hospital in London with Felix Post, Newcastle with Martin Roth, Klaus Bergmann and David Kay, Manchester with David Jolley, and Nottingham with Tom Arie.

Many of the pioneers had stumbled on the care of older people by accident; many had unconventional backgrounds and little formal training. Poorly resourced, accepting responsibility for uncharted numbers of community-living older people and for the hidden cases of depression or dementia among them, they used their charisma and determination to create pragmatic, humane services which could do something to relieve the distresses they uncovered. Often that 'something' proved sufficient to avert an admission to hospital, throw a lifeline to a family carer, or reassure a residential home that it would not be ignored when it asked for help.

The pioneers had no grandiose plan. They expected to build up services by small steps, seizing whatever chance opportunities arose. As pragmatists they absorbed every valuable idea of their time; and having only minimal premises and staff, they understood the need to collaborate with other local powers—social services, geriatricians, fellow-psychiatrists, and general practitioners. The founding principles of the specialty came from community and social psychiatry, recognizing the power of family and neighbourhood-networks, and of teamwork between colleagues with complementary skills. The typical scientific attitude was epidemiological—taking responsibility for whole populations of older people together with the ill people embedded in them, at home, in hospital, or in residential care.

In the 1970s, I came as a junior doctor into psychiatry from general medicine, where I had worked with Leo Wollner, a geriatrician who epitomized the dauntless approach to geriatric illness pioneered in the United Kingdom in the 1940s by Marjorie Warren. Psychiatry of old age to me meant only the long-stay asylum wards I had seen as a medical student: austere rows of white-painted hospital beds with raised cot sides; the pitiful sight of patients with contractures, remotely uncommunicative or endlessly calling for help, being carefully tended by nurses in white coats and plastic aprons.

A decade later, towards the end of my psychiatric training, I saw a different side of old age psychiatry. During the 1950s and 1960s the former county asylum, Littlemore Hospital, had developed an active programme of community nursing and resettlement of patients with chronic psychotic illness, and this emphasis on psychiatry in the home was maintained into the 1970s, when Oxford's first old age psychiatrist and first community psychiatric nurse for older people were appointed. John Robinson, the psychiatrist, had come originally from a background in general practice; Steve Corea's first profession was teaching. Together they travelled around Oxfordshire in John's old green Morris Minor car, laying the foundations for older people of home assessment and community care. As a trainee in the specialty I was given responsibility for my own small patch of Oxfordshire, and from their expertise I started to appreciate the beauties of community psychiatry and the rewards of working with older people.

Second theme: mapping the diagnostic landscape

In 1969 Slater and Roth wrote (6):

> The modern era in geriatric psychiatry began with the differentiation of senile dementia, arteriosclerotic dementia and the presenile psychoses from one another and from other organic psychoses, such as neurosyphilis. . . . Affective and paranoid disorders were regarded . . . as forms of senile psychosis which led eventually to deterioration of personality and intellect. . . . When the introduction of electroconvulsive therapy (E.C.T.) for elderly patients began to make it plain that some depressive . . . syndromes responded to this treatment, the practical importance of the distinction between the clinical varieties of mental illness in the aged became clear. The view that irreversible pathological changes of senile degenerative and arteriosclerotic nature provided the whole explanation for such disorders began to be called in question.

Systematic mapping began in the 1950s with Martin Roth's careful analysis of older people admitted to mental hospitals. He classified them

'. . . on the basis of psychiatric features into five groups: affective disorder, late paraphrenia, acute or subacute delirious states, senile psychosis (i.e. senile dementia) and arteriosclerotic psychosis, and these groups were found to differ sharply in pattern of outcome at six months and two years after admission. . . . Follow-up studies 7–8 years after admission to hospital revealed the differences between the groups still to be clearly evident although mortality due to ageing had to some extent blurred them . . .'

We can trace the evolution of Roth's five diagnostic groups (in reverse order) over the following 50 years.

Arteriosclerotic psychosis

Slater and Roth distinguished this condition from senile dementia by '. . . the presence of cerebrovascular lesions, a markedly remitting or fluctuating course, the preservation of the personality, a large measure of insight until a relatively late stage, explosiveness or incontinence of emotional expression, and epileptiform attacks'. Onset was typically around the ages of 60 to 70, and men were more commonly affected than women. High blood pressure was a major cause: hypotensive medication was then risky and unpleasant to take, and was used only in severe cases.

In 1982 Levy and Post wrote 'The term multi-infarct dementia has now displaced that of arteriosclerotic dementia, as increasing evidence has accumulated to demonstrate the presence of infarcts of various sizes and situations in postmortems of patients'. They noted the 'well-known stepwise progression' and the emotional lability seen in post-infarct patients, easily mistaken for affective disorder. Multi-infarct dementia was then estimated to account for 15–20% of cases of dementia in elderly people, and infarcts co-existing with 'senile degenerative change' for a further 10–15%.

In the 1990s a new term 'vascular dementia' became current, recognizing the role that cerebrovascular pathologies such as haemorrhage and vasculitis might also play in dementia; some types of vascular dementia did not have a history of strokes or focal neurological symptoms, but rather a gradual, progressive clinical decline. The advent of brain imaging (CT, MRI, SPECT, and PET) made it possible to establish the location of cerebrovascular lesions more precisely, and clarified the clinical pictures associated with them.

In 1993, the report 'Vascular dementia: diagnostic criteria for research studies' was published by an international working group (NINDS-AIREN), a sibling to the criteria agreed for Alzheimer's disease (AD) by a similar consensus group (NINCDS-ARDRA) a decade earlier. But alongside these efforts towards diagnostic precision in research, accumulating epidemiological, clinical, and pathological evidence undermined the sharp distinction between the two types of dementia in clinical practice.

In his survey of this diagnosis in 2008 Robert Stewart (7) pointed out that secular change affects not only ideas and technology but also the *populations* of patients whom we study. Those described in the 1960s by Slater and Roth died younger and came to post-mortem with more severe pathology than do our patients now, who commonly die in their ninth and tenth decades, with mild levels of cerebrovascular disease which may make only a partial contribution to their dementia, or is merely coincidental.

Senile dementia

Slater and Roth saw the relationship between senile dementia and normal ageing as simply quantitative—senile dementia becoming manifest when the degenerative changes of old age pass a critical threshold. 'Though the possibility that senile dements are qualitatively apart in respect of some pathological change that remains to be discovered cannot be excluded'.

They considered AD separately under the heading of the presenile dementias (a category introduced in 1898 by Binswanger and applied to AD by Kraepelin in 1909), and commented that 'the clinical features of Alzheimer's disease are admittedly different from those of senile dementia, but pathologically no sharp distinction exists'.

Levy and Post, in *The Psychiatry of Late Life* (1982), while still using the term 'senile dementia', dealt crisply with these questions of definition. 'Alzheimer himself considered his eponymous disease as a variant of senile dementia but opinions have been divided ever since.... The current [majority] view is that Alzheimer's disease and senile dementia are one and the same and this is reflected by the increasing use of the term senile dementia of Alzheimer type (SDAT)'.

By the time of Wilcock's and Jacoby's account in *Psychiatry in the Elderly* (1991), the use of 'Alzheimer's disease' to refer to the condition in older people was firmly established, though the previous term SDAT was mentioned in passing. The old question of the relationship to normal ageing was left open, but a different kind of boundary was clearly enunciated: 'Strictly speaking, . . . AD is a pathological diagnosis, although a characteristic clinical syndrome corresponding to the distinct post-mortem appearances in the brain can often be distinguished. To assign a *clinical* diagnosis of AD, therefore, is to make an informed guess.'

This gradual change in nomenclature between the 1960s and the 1990s was far from trivial. To say that an older patient 'is suffering from AD' rather than 'has senile dementia' carries considerable symbolic weight. There is a dignity in being afflicted by a disease, rather than falling into predestined and ignominious decay. And where there is a disease, there may be a cure.

Other dementias

Besides these two major causes of dementia in old age, a number of specific dementia syndromes were recognized, some (e.g. Huntington's disease) with ancient pedigrees, some described only in the 20th century (such as progressive supranuclear palsy in 1964, and idiopathic normal pressure hydrocephalus in 1965). Pick's disease dates back to the early 20th century: the defining pathological changes (regional atrophy of the frontal and temporal lobes, and Pick bodies in neurons) were described by Alzheimer. Like AD, it was originally regarded as a presenile dementia, but it was recognized by neuropathologists (8) as also occurring in older people, though comparatively rarely. It was an important condition to recognize in life, not because there was any treatment available, but because of the relief that clarity could bring. Grave as the diagnosis was, it gave some meaning to the distressing and often infuriating changes endured by the afflicted family.

Meanwhile, the parallel category of 'dementia of frontal lobe type' was refined through the detailed clinico-pathological studies of the Lund group in Sweden and

Neary in Manchester, leading to an international conference and the publication of consensus criteria in 1994. So 'Pick's disease' (with a specific pathology) gave way to the clinical concept of frontotemporal dementia (FTD), and to recognition of variant forms: frontal (fv-FTD) and temporal (known also as semantic dementia and progressive non-fluent dysphasia). Though relatively rare, FTD is a fertile source of insights into regional cerebral function, but the neurobiology of the condition and its treatment are still barely understood (9).

In the 1980s, in the early years of our community team, we saw the occasional perplexing patient with striking visual hallucinations coupled with mild cognitive impairment, quite unlike the familiar AD. Some had delusional explanations for their experiences, but (unlike schizophrenic patients) they suffered severe adverse effects from antipsychotics even in low doses. Or we might be called urgently to visit a confused old person causing havoc in the home, only to find the situation calm once more, and a charmingly lucid patient quite unable to understand everyone's anxieties.

Nowadays every medical student (if we have taught them properly) would suspect that these were people who had *dementia with Lewy bodies* (DLB). Recognition of this distinct form of dementia came gradually in the 1980s. Neuropathologists showed that abnormal intracellular inclusions, first described by Lewy in 1912 in the substantia nigra in Parkinson's disease, were widely distributed in the brain, and especially in the neocortex. These cortical Lewy bodies were difficult to detect routinely and were much better revealed when immunostaining specific for ubiquitin was used. Gradually the features of the syndrome crystallized—fluctuating cognitive impairment resembling delirium, hallucinations, mild extrapyramidal signs, sensitivity to antipsychotic medication.

Diagnostic criteria defining the boundaries between AD, DLB, and Parkinson's disease (PD), were published in the 1990s and refined thereafter. The 2005 criteria recognized data from imaging of the basal ganglia, and the association of REM sleep behaviour disorder with the condition. In 2008 McShane (10) described the 'tautological' process by which clinical diagnosis in DLB was used to validate pathological criteria, and pathology in turn to validate clinical criteria—a fair comment, in fact, on the nosological progression of all the dementias.

It was rewarding to witness the emergence of a new concept in old age psychiatry, which made sense of cases that had previously bewildered us, and which became established as part of our collective knowledge. The studies of DLB made sense too of the other end of the Parkinsonian spectrum. PD was regarded originally as purely a movement disorder, but as patients have lived longer, so the cognitive, emotional, and autonomic aspects of the disease have been recognized, and the dementia of PD is seen to run a different course from that of AD.

Other rarer syndromes included Creutzfeldt–Jakob disease and the dementias associated with physical disorders (such as B_{12} deficiency, thyroid disease, and HIV-AIDS). Because of these conditions, as well as the frequent coexistence of physical and mental disorders in older people, old age psychiatrists mostly understood the need to maintain their medical skills and their knowledge of geriatrics and neurology. Whether older psychiatric patients should routinely be investigated for medical disease was a live issue in the 1970s and 1980s, and resurfaced in the 2000s when memory clinics were becoming established. Evidence of important medical conditions being missed in older psychiatric patients is scanty, but every psychogeriatrician has their cautionary tale to tell, whether of the patient in prediabetic coma referred with 'confusion' or (as happened in our team) the patient with 'hysteria' who in fact had tertiary syphilis.

Mild cognitive impairment

Often in the history of psychiatry, there is an interaction between new treatment possibilities and the delineation of disorders suitable for that treatment. In the 1980s there was no effective treatment for dementia, so efforts to distinguish in life between AD and vascular dementia seemed unnecessary. Later, the theoretical origins of cholinesterase inhibitors made them the choice for AD rather than for vascular dementia, and the distinction between the two conditions acquired practical significance. Public awareness of possible treatments for AD brought the question of early diagnosis into sharper focus, and people with mild or subjective failures in memory began to consult their GPs, worrying that they might have dementia, hoping for a treatment that might prevent it.

The study of *mild memory loss in old age* dates back to the late 1950s when Kral described 'benign senescent forgetfulness': loss of incidental details in recalling past events (details which might be remembered accurately on another occasion), without the disorientation, confabulation, or other types of cognitive difficulty which are seen in 'malignant' senescent forgetfulness (i.e. dementia). He showed that people with malignant memory loss had a mortality rate twice that of fellow-residents in the old people's home, and that during the follow-up period, the malignant memory loss progressed, while the benign loss was unchanged.

In the 1970s and 1980s, opinions differed over the legitimacy of a diagnosis for people who did not meet the criteria for dementia but had concerns about their memory. Were these just symptoms of anxiety or depression? Should people with impaired practical or social functioning (but normal memory) be included? International efforts to produce agreed criteria for 'age associated memory impairment' (1987), or 'ageing associated cognitive decline' (1994) had little impact, on either clinical practice or research.

In our day-to-day work we assumed that some kind of mild memory loss existed which was neither 'just age' nor dementia proper, and that while a proportion of these people would progress to dementia, others would remain stable. Frankly sharing this understanding was often helpful to people worried about their memory, though the possibility of dementia in future was not denied.

In the 1990s Petersen and colleagues at the Mayo Clinic began their longitudinal studies of older people with carefully defined 'mild cognitive impairment' (MCI) (11), giving the concept a stability of meaning capable of underpinning repeatable research. Can any treatment of people with MCI reduce their risk of progression to dementia? So far, trials of treatment with cholinesterase inhibitors have been disappointing, but some vitamins (the B complex) look promising (12) and, intriguingly, also lithium (13).

Acute and subacute delirious states

I cannot do justice here to this category of illness. Of course the phenomenon of altered consciousness should be profoundly interesting to psychiatrists, and it is essential for every practising doctor to have the skills to recognize it. But most of the causes of delirium, both acute and subacute, and the means for investigating and treating the patients, are the province of general physicians and geriatricians in particular. Practice has rightly changed since the time of Slater and Roth, and patients with delirium no longer form a major category in the work of psychiatric hospitals. Instead, old age psychiatry has tried to develop ways of meeting the psychiatric needs of patients in general hospitals, whether through joint units (as pioneered in Nottingham by Tom Arie), liaison teams, or individual consultation. Although these practical arrangements have been difficult to achieve and to sustain, nevertheless the understanding of delirium, its prevention and its management, has made significant progress (14).

Paranoid illness in old age

Paranoid illnesses arising in old age were included indiscriminately with 'non-organic psychoses of the senium', until Roth in the 1950s classified them in a separate category—'late paraphrenia'. He showed that these patients had a lower mortality than their coevals with dementia, but higher rates of institutionalization than those with affective disorders. Understanding of these patients was subsequently enriched by Post's detailed long-term study in the 1960s of 'Persistent persecutory states of the elderly'.

This work raised several new questions. First, was paranoid illness with onset in old age a condition distinct from schizophrenia, or the same condition but with delayed onset? Post classified his patients into groups defined by their phenomenology and their similarity to schizophrenia; but in fact these groups were not stable over time, and in a given patient the index illness and later relapses might fall under different descriptive headings. Second, was delusional disorder in old age always a consequence of degenerative brain disease, or were pathological findings at post-mortem (such as vascular damage) merely incidental? Naming was also a problem: critics argued that 'late paraphrenia' was a misleading reminder of Kraepelin's 'paraphrenia', which described a very different condition.

Arguments rumbled on through the 1980s and 1990s, not helped by international systems of classification: the third edition of the *Diagnostic and Statistical Manual* (DSM-III), for instance, restricted the diagnosis of 'schizophrenia' to cases with onset below the age of 45. The dilemmas were summarized by Naguib and Levy (15): 'For day-to-day clinical purposes, it does not matter what we call these states, provided that we make it clear what we mean. For research and statistical purposes, it is essential that we adopt a . . . classification which allows for the retrieval of cases with late-onset delusional states, whatever these are called.'

Eventually in 1998 an international consensus group considered all the available evidence and agreed that cases of schizophrenia with age of onset from 40 to 59 should be called 'late onset schizophrenia', while illnesses with onset after 60 were different in significant ways and should have their own name—'very late onset schizophrenia-like psychosis' (VLOSLP). As Robert Howard wrote (16), 'The latter term is long-winded and unmemorable but is at least unambiguous, and it received the unprecedented support of both European and North American old age psychiatrists.' And for us watching on the sidelines of this long academic wrangle, it seemed a significant moment for the international and scientific standing of our specialty.

Affective disorders

Conceptual progress has here come not through the invention of diagnostic entities but through clarification. In old age we see the affective disorders familiar to us from younger patients, but it has taken time to understand the effects of ageing on their expression.

'Involutional depression' as a diagnostic category has disappeared. 'Depressive pseudo-dementia' is no longer a live concept, and the differential diagnosis between severe forms of dementia and depression, much discussed in the literature of the 1970s and 1980s, has become less problematic—perhaps because we more often see patients close to the onset of their illness, and (as Felix Post taught) it is the early histories of the two conditions that help us to distinguish them.

A different perspective on mixed affective and cognitive symptoms is captured in the concept of 'vascular depression', proposed on clinical grounds in 1997 by Alexopoulos and colleagues, and later amplified by the demonstration on MRI scans in these patients of ischaemic lesions in subcortical areas of the brain, in both white matter and grey. Typically in vascular depression the symptoms are more apathetic than melancholic, cognitive impairment lies mainly in executive function, and the response to treatment is disappointing. The more severe the radiological findings, the worse the outcome appears to be. However, not all authorities accept the idea of a specifically vascular depressive syndrome, seeing the brain instead as subject to a variety of damaging pathological processes, interacting together to precipitate the illness.

'Manic-depressive psychosis in the senium' was well-recognized by the pioneers of old age psychiatry, although manic episodes were then thought to be rare. In *The Psychiatry of Late Life* Post, referring to the study he carried out with Shulman at the Maudsley, described 'the preponderance of surly, hostile affects in elderly manics' by contrast with the euphoria often seen in younger patients; and he called attention to the phenomenon of 'slow flight of ideas' in which the characteristic thought disorder of mania is coupled with depressive retardation. Later studies found no consistent difference in the symptoms of mania between young and old, but they confirmed Post's observations on mixed affective states, and showed that in old-age bipolar affective disorder these are at least as common as are pure manic or depressive presentations.

Patients who bear the lifelong burden of bipolar affective disorder are both a reward and a challenge for an old age psychiatrist. Those in whom the illness was recognized in youth reflect in their case-histories the whole story of 20th-century psychiatry. One of my 80-year-old patients had her first episode of manic illness in 1916, which was recorded as 'nymphomania' and treated with belladonna and tincture of opium. And those in whom bipolar disorder is finally recognized can be given some explanation for the chaotic unpredictability of their lives, and can benefit from the stability offered by treatments developed over recent decades for young and old alike.

First theme again: developing services further

During the 1960s and 1970s in Britain there was a steady growth of ideas, creative practice, concrete evidence, and national policy on the theme of community care for older people. Typically it was individual practitioners who saw the possibilities for new services, striking examples being Joshua Carse and his day hospital in Worthing, and Duncan Macmillan and his integrated assessment unit at Mapperley Hospital in Nottingham. But the support of local powers (both in the NHS and in social care) was also crucial. The final necessary ingredient was evidence. It tells us something important about the climate of those years that these innovations were properly studied and the findings fed directly into policy: a process well illustrated by a government-sponsored seminar on community old age psychiatry in 1982 (17).

At this time of optimistic growth in services at a national level, Oxfordshire also saw developments in its psychogeriatric service, precipitated by changes in the county boundary. The new segment of the county, till then minimally provided for, acquired half a consultant, a dedicated community psychiatric nurse, six beds on an old long-stay ward, and an enlightened charge nurse (with experience as a district nurse) to lead the hospital team. Full of enthusiasm for the model of early ascertainment and community provision, fortified by *The Psychiatry of Late Life*, we went out to meet the general practitioners in our new sector. They were welcoming and courteous; some were already convinced of the value of supporting older people at home instead of in hospital, others were deeply sceptical, predicting that within months our beds would be immovably filled, the waiting lists as long as before, and the new model of care an empty promise.

Our best allies at this time were the staff of the local social services department, already blazing the trail for home support for older people; and a voluntary day centre in a church hall, nurtured from birth by Steve Corea, by then a senior nurse in the Oxfordshire service.

In the 1980s, collaboration between the NHS and social care was encouraged by new legislation. 'Joint funding' grants became available for projects created in partnership by local medical and social services. Our joint invention was 'patch teams'—local outposts of the parent services—the key professionals in a patch team being a community psychiatric nurse and a social worker for older people. Each received training from the 'opposite' parent, so that, as far as possible, nurse and social worker could each offer the same range of skills, information, and networks. They sat together in an office located in the community they served, helped and taught each other, and managed a joint case-load. They shared in the time of the sector consultant, occupational therapist, and (when possible) psychologist, and everyone met weekly in their premises. The model worked well. The patients, their families, and general practitioners approved.

These patch teams, granted creative freedom, invented the 'flexible carer': carers employed simply to give time, doing whatever tasks the person concerned identified as *their* priority. (The idea was sparked when a grieving client asked for someone to help dig a grave for her beloved cat.) At first employed opportunistically, flexible carers were later adopted and managed as a service by Oxfordshire Age Concern.

In the 1990s and the new millennium, upheavals in culture and politics occurred at levels of power beyond our ability to influence. Funding was constrained in both health and social services, and their partnership was undermined. New managers dictated nationwide changes in policy and in the shape of services. A small local invention could not survive, and the patch teams were closed down. Though we still visited patients at home, and tried to work collaboratively with social service colleagues (for whom we had much respect and affection), we could no longer give our patients a service as 'close to home' as we had always intended.

National leaders at this time were celebrating 'reform' in the NHS. At the coal face we did not feel we had anything to celebrate. Rather, these centralized reforms signalled for us a doctrinaire eradication of local partnership, and the erosion of responsiveness to actual needs.

Third theme: the scientific background to clinical work

Structures in the brain

Just as technical advances (especially the use of silver stains for microscopy of brain tissue) allowed Alois Alzheimer in 1906 to describe the 'peculiar appearances' in the brain of his patient Auguste D., so further technical developments have illuminated the histopathology, chemistry, and genetics of the pathological features that he described.

The 1960s began a new era in the study of the brain. Electron microscopy helped to visualize the fine structure of neurons and the neurofibrillary tangles (NFTs) and inclusion bodies within them. Examining neural tissue stained with Congo red under polarized light identified amyloid as a component of AD pathology, especially in plaques and in the walls of blood vessels. Counting cells under the microscope by hand, and later by automated methods, brought a quantitative approach to the differentiation of dementia from normal ageing.

Corsellis (18), reviewing the pathology of dementia in 1969, predicted that 'an amyloid substance in the aged brain . . . could well repay further study, particularly by biochemists and immunologists'. Concerning the relation between cerebral degeneration and dementia, he wrote: 'it has often been contended . . . that the structural state of the brain is of relatively minor importance when compared with the influence of environmental and psychological factors'; but himself argued for the opposite view, quoting the work of Blessed and Tomlinson who had shown in 1965 that intensity of degeneration, measured by counting the plaques in brain tissue, correlated with the clinical severity of dementia.

The quantitative approach was developed further during the 1970s. Initially, laboratories each devised their own criteria for diagnosis in 'senile dementia', based on the distribution and density of plaques and tangles; in later decades shared criteria, such as the CERAD protocol (1991), were gradually accepted.

Meanwhile, neurochemical studies were establishing new ground. I remember as a medical student in the 1960s being told that the chemical study of neurotransmission in the brain (by contrast with peripheral organs) might never be possible, because of the speed with which self-digestion of brain tissue takes place after death. It was wonderful later to find that this pessimism had not prevailed—it acted only as a provocation to scientists to find ways round the problem. By studying the relevant enzymes rather than the transmitters directly, by carefully matching post-mortem tissue samples according to the physiological conditions at the time of death, and by exploiting rare opportunities to study brain biopsies taken for diagnostic purposes, abnormalities in noradrenergic and cholinergic neurotransmitter systems were identified. Through the 1970s, scientists in different centres—Bowen, Davies, the Perrys, and others—made crucial observations linking the clinical and pathological signs of dementia to the laboratory finding of impaired cholinergic neurotransmission. Thus in 1983 the 'cholinergic hypothesis' (that AD is 'a disorder of cortical cholinergic innervation') was formulated. But in time it became clear that this could not be the whole story.

Meanwhile, animal studies revealed the anatomy of the cells implicated in these chemical changes. As the Perrys explained in *The Psychiatry of Late Life*, in 1982, 'the majority of cholinergic nerve processes [in the cortex] are terminal axonal processes thought to be derived . . . from cell bodies situated in the nucleus of Meynert . . . in the substantia innominata region', and by 1997 (19) textbooks were depicting four distinct groups of neurons, each arising from its own subcortical nucleus, each releasing its particular neurotransmitter from axons projecting diffusely into the cortex.

A significant form of connectivity between different brain regions was studied by Pearson and Powell, Braak and Braak, and others in the 1980s. They found a gradient in the severity of lesions of AD, in a logical sequence along known anatomical pathways from one region to the next, suggesting a spread of the disease process from origins in the entorhinal cortex to hippocampus, to the temporal cortex, and thence to other cortical association areas. The olfactory cortex and olfactory mucosa also show pathological changes very early in AD. Clues, perhaps, to the unknown aetiology of the disease?

Also through the 1980s, the structure, chemistry, and origins of NFTs and of the amyloid in senile plaques were being clarified. Electron microscopy in the 1960s had shown NFTs to be helically paired filaments formed from abnormal protein. Now they were found to be derived from microtubules (part of the internal transport structure of neurons). In the early 1990s the microtubule-associated protein tau was extracted from NFTs, and was found to be highly phosphorylated in that situation, possibly making it functionally different from normal tau.

The amyloid protein identified as beta-A4 (or beta-amyloid) was isolated from senile plaques in 1985, and in 1987 was shown to be derived from a much larger molecule, amyloid precursor protein (APP). During the normal metabolism of APP it is divided enzymatically at specific points along its length; if cleavage occurs at a different point, an abnormal fragment of APP is produced which is then deposited as amyloid. Hardy and Higgins in 1992 proposed the 'amyloid cascade hypothesis', suggesting that 'the mismetabolism of APP and deposition of beta-A4 is the seminal pathogenic event in AD'.

In the 1990s, studies of intracortical signalling showed that glutamate, a metabolically important molecule, acts also as a cortico-cortical and hippocampal neurotransmitter. The pathways concerned degenerate quite early in AD. Glutamate can be toxic to neurons, and such excitotoxicity, probably important in cerebrovascular disease, may be relevant to AD as well.

Finally the genetic discoveries of the 1990s must be mentioned. The genetic coding for APP is found on chromosome 21 (recalling the raised incidence of AD in trisomy 21); and mutations affecting the structure of tau are associated with chromosome 17. In 1995, studies of families with early-onset AD yielded the genes presenilin-1 and presenilin-2, on chromosomes 14 and 1 respectively. The gene for a protein (Apolipoprotein E) which is secreted by astrocytes and binds to beta-amyloid was shown to influence the prevalence of late-onset AD—possibly by accelerating its onset. This gene was found on chromosome 19.

These are the bare bones of the discoveries in the last 50 years. Four areas of current ignorance call for future exploration. First, the relationship between plaques and NFTs is still obscure. Diffuse plaques precede NFTs in the course of AD, but plaques alone, unlike NFTs alone, are not always associated with dementia. Secondly, the study of glial cells (oligodendrocytes, astrocytes, microglia) has barely begun. Equally difficult is the exploration at subcellular level of whole neurons, from cell body to furthest dendrites, which means that the connection between pathological events in different parts of a cell that spans different regions of the nervous system can only be inferred. Lastly, the distinction between phenomena (chemical or histological) which signal the direct effect of disease and those which reflect adaptive responses is only gradually being unravelled.

OPTIMA: the Oxford Project to Investigate Memory and Ageing

David Smith (professor of pharmacology), Margaret Esiri (neuropathologist), Kim Jobst (clinical director of the project), and Elizabeth King (senior research nurse) were the initiators in 1988 of this meticulously planned and executed study, in volunteer patients and healthy controls, of the natural history of cognitive and non-cognitive decline in dementia. A founding principle of the study was that, since no treatment was on offer, participants must be given instead the best care then available—warm and expert support, regular contact, truthful information, and the knowledge that they and their families were contributing to research at the forefront of scientific knowledge. Participants received a complete medical and radiological examination initially and annually till death, and were visited regularly by their own Optima research nurse. At entry to the study they were invited to consider donating their brain for autopsy after their death. The success of this approach was shown by the very high rate (97%) of participants who agreed to brain donation and in whom (with their relatives' permission) autopsy was eventually carried out (20).

The studies generated by the Optima project (in neuropathology, in imaging, in clinical syndromes such as depression and DLB, in therapeutics and prevention) are too many to list here. What I most affectionately remember is the strong collaborative ethos of the research group—both internally and in its relationships with local colleagues. For the old age clinicians in the region, Optima's monthly clinico-pathological meetings were a source of knowledge and inspiration, giving a level of importance to our daily work that only participation in active research can provide.

Imaging the brain

In the early years of geriatric psychiatry, options for imaging the brain were extremely limited. Plain radiographs of the skull could show only its bones and its cavities. Occasionally a tumour might be detected, but living brain was virtually *terra incognita* for radiology. Electroencephalography (EEG) seemed to promise better, and was used by some researchers and enthusiasts, but in the United Kingdom at least (except when epilepsy was suspected) it never entered routine psychogeriatric practice.

It was different when CT emerged in the 1970s, first as a research tool, and much later for clinical use. In 1980 Jacoby and Levy employed this new technology in a study of patients with dementia and patients with affective disorder, compared to age-matched cognitively normal people. They confirmed that the cerebral atrophy of dementia would show up on CT scans; and devised a reliable method for quantifying brain volume which allowed patients and controls to be validly compared.

In routine practice the diagnosis of dementia was based on patients' histories and their clinical features. CT (then an expensive investigation) gave little additional information in straightforward cases, so its use was limited to excluding other intracranial disease. But participants in Optima did get scanned as part of the protocol, and the research staff found that showing the images to patients and their families and explaining their interpretation was therapeutic in itself. Opinions at that time were strongly divided as to whether patients with dementia should be told their diagnosis, but in this population of research volunteers, freely sharing the clinical information was undoubtedly beneficial.

Optima developed a technique for imaging the medial temporal lobe by angling the CT scan along its length, and with this method hippocampal atrophy (now an accepted diagnostic feature in AD), could be quantified. In some of the cases, serial scans showed an accelerated rate of atrophy accompanying a sharp deterioration in the patient's cognitive state.

The next advance in imaging concerned the physiology of the living brain, using radioemitting chemicals in PET and (more practically) SPECT, to provide information about metabolic function in different brain regions. The characteristic picture on SPECT scans of parietal hypometabolism, combined with atrophic changes demonstrated by CT, made the diagnosis of AD more accurately than either technique on its own.

In the 1990s as brain MRI came into use it tended to supplant the older methods (except that confused patients find CT less frightening). We take for granted the precision and beauty of its images, which would have astounded researchers just a few decades ago. They could not have conceived it possible to read the neurochemical activity of a brain while it engages in active thought—as is nowadays made possible by functional MRI.

Fourth theme: advances in treatment

Pharmacological approaches to dementia

This most stigmatizing of Roth's five diagnostic categories has become the domain of high-prestige research. Few conditions offer the same transparency of connection between disordered brain and afflicted mind. The exploration of that connection becomes ever more arcane, the world of the super-scientist not the everyday clinician, but the discoveries of impaired neurotransmission in dementia also led directly to the development of practical drug regimes, promising alleviation, if not cure, for a disease formerly thought beyond therapeutic reach (21).

Tacrine was the first compound targeted on defective cholinergic neurotransmission (22) that could be used in dementia, and clinical trials in the 1980s and 1990s showed clear, though limited, benefit to patients. The drug could cause serious side effects (especially hepatotoxicity) and never entered routine psychogeriatric practice, but it led the way for the 'second-generation' cholinesterase inhibitors, donepezil, rivastigmine, and galantamine.

Donepezil was licensed in the United Kingdom in 1997, but it was clearly not cura-tive. The evidence that it could at least help to delay the progression of AD accumulated only gradually, and the cholinesterase inhibitors were not accepted for prescription by the NHS until 2001. The body responsible for this decision, the National Institute for Health and Care Excellence (NICE), bases its reasoning less on the efficacy of a drug under research conditions than on its cost-effectiveness in practice—i.e. the health benefit attributable to the drug as opposed to an implicit alternative use of the same money. This is often a controversial position to adopt, and NICE's successive recom-mendations on the treatments for dementia provoked fierce scientific, economic, and political argument. Public opinion (led by the patients' advocacy organizations) was roused; a campaign of legal challenge funded by the drug companies began; and in 2011 NICE removed its restrictions on the prescribing of cholinesterase inhibitors in the NHS.

Other experimental approaches to treatment are being investigated. The demonstra-tion of a link between cognition and alterations in glutamate and aspartate neurotrans-mission in the cortex (the 'glutamatergic hypothesis') underpin the development of memantine, used in moderate and severe AD. Experimental attempts to reduce the deposition of amyloid beta-peptide in the brain by immunotherapy looked promising until a trial in 2001 was aborted when some subjects developed severe side effects. Gor-don Wilcock, reviewing these developments (23), concluded: 'Not only is symptomatic treatment a reality, albeit at a modest level . . . , but disease-modifying, i.e. neuroprotec-tive, treatments may be on the horizon. There is considerable hope for the future.'

By contrast, the search for drugs to modify behaviour in dementia has been less ra-tional. From the 1960s onwards, doctors have turned mainly to the antidepressants and antipsychotics to treat the agitation, aggression, confusion, paranoia, sleeplessness, and wandering of their older patients. There was little reason for preferring one drug over another, but the pressure on the doctor from struggling families or exasperated nursing staff to do something to help could be very intense. Occasionally the effects of medication were almost miraculous—for example, when a depressive illness had been unrecognized in the context of the patient's dementia. The counter-argument to using medication was concern over side effects, given added force when the exceptional vul-nerability to antipsychotics in Lewy body dementia was discovered. For patients with depressive symptoms the newer antidepressants (SSRIs and others) had been a decided improvement over the tricyclics, and for a time the atypical antipsychotics were simi-larly welcomed, until it was found, first, that they accelerate the dementing process (24) and second, that they carry an increased risk of serious cardiovascular events in people with dementia (25).

In the last few decades, there has been a second counter-force to the use of medi-cation in dementia—recognition of the power of a psychological approach. In severe dementia the necessary shift in perspective was to consider the patient's behaviour as a meaningful response to their situation (which includes the specific cognitive limi-tations imposed by their illness), rather than simply as a symptom determined by neurobiological factors. Interpretation of troublesome behaviour requires a detailed contextual analysis by the psychologist, while the help must come from people surrounding the patient (family or care staff) with their responses shaped by the understanding derived from the analysis (26).

General opinion, especially that of family carers, is usually sympathetic to psychological approaches and wary of medication—rightly so where antipsychotics are concerned. Expert advice and guidelines now set strict limits to the use of antipsychotics in dementia, but practice is slow to change, and vigilance by carers and specialists remains essential.

Pharmacological treatment in depressive disorder

Older people have shared in the advances over the last half-century in the pharmacological treatment of depression, particularly from the emergence of safer drugs with fewer side effects. In the 1990s, ahead of practice at younger ages, many old age psychiatrists kept their patients on antidepressant medication for at least 2 years after a severe depressive illness, and often for life, to prevent relapse or recurrence. A multicentre trial (in which many of us participated) of such a continuation regime (27) showed that older patients on placebo were more than twice as likely as treated patients to suffer relapse or recurrence over the 2 years of the trial.

Electroconvulsive treatment

Mayer-Gross's introduction of electroconvulsive treatment (ECT) was an important advance at the dawn of old age psychiatry, and it has continued as a safe and effective treatment for older patients, especially in severe depression and when pharmacological treatment has failed. Post in 1982 recommended unilateral (non-dominant) application to minimize post-treatment confusion and to prevent memory impairment afterwards. But in 1991 Baldwin (in *Psychiatry in the Elderly*) noted 'the negative public image suffered by ECT', the reluctance of clinicians and the practical obstacles to its use, and he feared that patients were sometimes left ineffectively treated.

In the 1970s and 1980s public suspicion and opposition to ECT were strong enough to influence policy. Fortunately these pressures during the preparation of the 1983 Mental Health Act did not succeed in outlawing ECT altogether, and the legal mechanisms enacted to constrain its use proved workable. In those years it was often hard to convince staff who had no experience of ECT and who were appalled at the thought of such 'barbaric' treatment of a gravely ill old patient, that the cruelty lay rather in withholding effective relief for their suffering. With families, likewise upset at the idea of ECT for their relative, each discussion had to begin at the beginning, and indeed one could sympathize with their disbelief that electricity would be safer than medication for a frail and unreachable 90-year old. One form of treatment which we practised without the benefit of hard evidence was maintenance ECT in patients with recurrent episodes of medication-resistant depression. (Maintenance ECT involved treatment of the patient, with perhaps one application per month, on a regular basis without waiting for any sign of relapse of the depression, in order to prevent relapse.) Such patients and their families often became the strongest supporters of the treatment plan.

In the 2000s, the Royal College of Psychiatrists, aware of failings in the quality of ECT practice across the United Kingdom, took action to improve it by creating a system of regular and rigorous audit to which hospitals could subscribe. In the Oxford ECT service this brought about striking improvements, thanks to the leadership of a committed psychiatrist invested by management with the authority to carry the audit and its recommendations through in every detail.

The College also sought out the views of patients who had undergone ECT, and their own accounts of memory loss. It is now clear that loss of autobiographical memories, invisible to routine memory tests, is a genuine effect of ECT and the one that most distresses patients. The risk of this memory loss is not increased by age; ECT can safely be given for depression in patients with dementia; and it still holds an important place in the practice of old age psychiatry (28).

Psychological treatments

Psychological and psychotherapeutic treatments were not considered in the first textbooks of old age psychiatry. It was assumed that clinicians would apply the same generic skill to older people that they had learned in the setting of general psychiatry. But from the late 1990s and early 2000s, psychological techniques devised for younger age-groups were increasingly adopted into work with older people. Most systematic studies of psychological interventions in old age date from those years, and by 2008 the subject occupied 55 pages (29) of the *Oxford Textbook of Old Age Psychiatry*. Older people are now most often offered cognitive-behaviour therapy, interpersonal psychotherapy, or problem-solving therapies. Family and systemic therapies and psychodynamic psychotherapy are less widely available. Psychological and pharmacological treatments are often used together, and it is also common to offer psychological help to a patient and to their caring relative in parallel. The greatest obstacle to the use of psychological treatments in old age is the shortage of staff with appropriate skills—not only psychologists but also members of other disciplines who elect to train in these methods.

Should services for older people be subsumed under (or integrated into) the 'mainstream' psychiatric service in each area? Or is there still a case for old age psychiatry as a specialism in its own right? An integrated service might ensure better access to psychological treatments, since a special interest in old age is relatively new among psychologists. The United Kingdom Department of Health in 2005 strongly advocated integration on this principle, declaring that separate specialist services perpetuate ageism. Against this view, clinicians in the specialty argued that psychiatric illness in old age frequently coexists with physical illness or disability, often together with cognitive impairment, so that clinical practice is genuinely different from that in 'adults of working age', and its practitioners need a different range of attitudes and skills. These clinicians also suspected that pursuit of an age-blind principle would instead separate dementia services from mainstream psychiatry, disadvantaging the many older patients who need help from both disciplines. Where psychological therapies are concerned, these arguments are fairly evenly balanced, and different providers will resolve the question in different ways.

Fifth theme: political and social context

The National Health Service and social provision in the United Kingdom

The creation of the NHS in 1948 united three different categories of health provision: general practitioners and primary care; secondary care in hospitals, including the mental hospitals; and services provided by the local authorities (which included hospitals for the chronic sick, the seed-bed for the future development of geriatric medicine). In a history of the NHS written for its 50th anniversary, Geoffrey Rivett wrote (30):

> At the outset the NHS had accepted responsibility for the long-term care of the chronic sick, although the standard of care was often unacceptably low. Over the years the NHS service improved, with an accent on rehabilitation. Categorization of people into those needing health provision (that was free) and those requiring social support (that was chargeable) was difficult. Although frail elderly people often required both social support and health care, such responsibilities increasingly passed to the social services and the private sector.

This uneasy boundary between health and social provision runs through the story of older people's care in the United Kingdom, along with the constant battle to ensure that psychiatric illness is not forgotten when strategies for older peoples' health are written.

The national strategy for psychiatry in the 1960s was to move provision out of the large old mental hospitals and into small assessment units situated in district general hospitals, backed by care 'in the community' supported by local authority services. Statistical predictions from the Department of Health of a continuing steep decrease in the number of beds required for psychiatric admissions underpinned this strategy. Clinicians doubted whether the kind of community support needed by relocated patients would materialize, and whether anyone had thought about elderly or chronically ill patients left behind in long-stay wards while resources went to the young and newly ill in the general hospital units.

Politicians did recognize that not everything ideal could be afforded. In 1976 the Department of Health and Social Security published *Priorities for Health and Personal Social Services*, in an attempt to 'move resources to the care of elderly people and those who were mentally ill'. At ground level, psychogeriatric teams struggled especially with inadequate provision for long-term care, at that time confined mainly to the back wards of hospitals under pressure to close, and to residential homes run by the local authorities.

In the late 1970s, funding of long-term care underwent a major political change. Previously, local authorities had funded *places* in residential homes which they provided and controlled. Now the funding was to come from the national social security budget, by means-tested allocation to *individuals*, regardless of the ownership of the home in which they sought a place. This move uncovered a relentlessly growing demand (partly reflecting demographic forces) for long-term care. The independent sector duly responded, so that from the 1970s to the end of the 1990s there was a fivefold increase in the number of places in independent sector homes, and correspondingly enormous pressure on the social security budget.

So in 1990 the politics changed again. Responsibility for funding people in residential and nursing homes was taken away from the Department of Social Security and given back to the local authorities. 'An open-ended and rapidly expanding budget was replaced by a limited one based on individual assessment of need . . . Local authorities became the principal budget-holders for state-financed long-term-care' (31).

No country has yet found an ideal and affordable arrangement for funding the care of its elderly. In the United Kingdom a Royal Commission proposed a solution in 1999 which was quietly shelved, and new recommendations made by the Dilnot Commission in 2011 still await a political response.

Since the reforms to the NHS in 1989–90, repeated reorganizations have largely been premised on the model of acute services and have done little to help older people with mental illness, though exceptions exist. The 1990 contract with general practitioners required annual health checks for all patients over 75, and though many GPs thought this a fruitless exercise, on balance its effects have been positive. 1999 saw a National Service Framework for Mental Health, backed by funds to ensure the implementation of its directives. Older people with mental illness were supposedly included, but the prescribed models of care were not designed for their needs. The National Service Framework for Older People in 2001 was less prescriptive, but it had no money behind it.

Only in 2009 did the psychiatric needs of (some) older people take centre stage, with the publication of the National Dementia Strategy. (Functional psychiatric illness in old age was not included.) From this strategy emerged the National Dementia Declaration, and the launch of the Dementia Action Alliance, which 'seeks radical change in the way that our society responds to dementia.'

The declaration listed the shortcomings of current social arrangements, and outlined in detail the seven desired outcomes of the strategy, couched in the imagined voice of a person with dementia. Whether these outcomes can be achieved is questionable, but the language alone is interesting for the light it throws on historical change in culture and perspective. It is hard to imagine the words 'I live in an enabling and supportive environment where I feel valued and understood' (outcome 5) being formulated in 1969.

Quality control in services for older people

'Elder abuse', the maltreatment of older people, became a serious topic of research only in the 1980s, yet neglect and cruelty have surely as long a history as do care and benevolence. In 1967 Barbara Robb wrote *Sans Everything*, documenting much neglect and mindless cruelty towards elderly people in long-stay institutions. The next year, a government enquiry into standards of care at Ely Hospital in Cardiff revealed similar abuses, and in response to its recommendations the Hospital Advisory Service was created, with responsibility for investigating hospitals for mentally ill, elderly and learning disabled patients. Revelations of the abuse of vulnerable patients in hospital continued through the 1970s, and in a book published in 1984 (32) the part repeatedly played in these scandals by incompetent management, inadequate staffing, professional isolation, and internal corruption was convincingly depicted. For a few decades there were no further horror stories on this scale, and many hoped that the closure of the old inward-looking institutions would likewise eliminate the conditions that led to abuse.

It was too much to hope. As the patients needing long-term care moved from hospitals into residential and nursing homes, or returned to their own homes to be looked after there, the potential for abuse moved with them. Once again, as risk was recognized, systems for inspection and regulation were created, initially in local social service departments and later through national regulatory bodies. Once again there were media reports of cruel or incompetent treatment of vulnerable people, where regulators had failed to intervene. In 2011 the Equality and Human Rights Commission found 'that the care of elderly people in their own homes is so poor that it breaches basic human rights'; while in the same year the Health Service Ombudsman (33) found poor communication, a dismissive response to suffering, and 'an apparent indifference ... to deplorable standards of care' among staff caring for older people. Governments would sooner respond by redesigning the systems for inspection, than by probing the factors identified in Martin's 1984 analysis. The effectiveness of this approach cannot be assumed, and the voices of relatives, of staff prepared to be whistleblowers, and of the media are still indispensable.

In the 1990s a different approach to raising standards was tried. *Clinical audit* was incorporated into 'clinical governance', a mechanism established (by analogy with corporate governance in business) in the NHS for safeguarding the quality of its services. Good audit depends crucially on choosing the right measure of the qualities that need improvement. When badly chosen, measuring instruments become parasitic and divert resources from the service into their own growth and renown. In our field the national audit of ECT overcame this danger, but many aspects of psychiatric care in old age are less clear-cut, and suitable measures are harder to find. The quality of the care given to people with dementia comes down to the details of practice, to sound training, to the moral attributes of care staff, and the nurturance and respect that the staff receive. Measurement of these intangibles, without letting measurement itself distort the care, is difficult. The best and most influential instrument so far devised is Dementia Care Mapping, the work of Tom Kitwood and the Bradford Dementia Group (34).

Mental health law

Older psychiatric patients were beneficiaries (equally with younger patients) in the replacement of the 1959 Mental Health Act by the 1983 Mental Health Act in England and Wales. It is beyond the scope of this essay to discuss those legal arrangements, though they were important in securing better treatment for older people under detention, and in protecting their rights under the law.

An important area not covered adequately by the 1983 Act was the status of people who lacked *capacity to consent*, whether to hospital admission or to treatment. The two most important groups of patients affected by this lack of legal provision were those with learning disability and people with dementia. The 1959 Act had marked a decided move away from involuntary committal, and enlarged the scope for voluntary psychiatric treatment. The 1983 Act, libertarian rather than paternalist in its philosophy, sought to constrain infringements of rights within legal boundaries. People who did not object to admission or treatment simply because they could not understand enough either to give or to withhold their consent were poorly served by that framework.

In 1989 the Law Society published a discussion document on *Decision-Making and Mental Incapacity*, calling for new legislation. After 18 years of repeated consultations, delays and redraftings—a salutary example of the obstacles which confront even widely welcomed reforms—the Mental Capacity Act 2005 was brought into force in 2007.

During this long gestation, 'non-competent non-objecting' patients were still treated as if they were voluntarily consenting. Few advocates for such patients were happy with this. When the United Kingdom's Human Rights Act 1998 was enacted, it became obvious that these rights applied fully to psychiatric patients, and a route was opened up for legal challenge by the advocates of patients who had *not* been formally detained when perhaps they should have been. The Mental Capacity Act 2005 and its 2008 Code of Practice were therefore written to ensure that proper process is followed, when patients who lack capacity are necessarily deprived of their liberty.

Though critics of the Mental Capacity Act view its procedures as legalistic and cumbersome, its system of prescribed visits may supplement with its own searchlight the roles of national inspectorates. And the status of intellectually impaired people—whether impaired from birth or in old age—has been enhanced, I believe, by the prolonged and respectful attention that was given to their rights by parliament, the relevant professions, and the public at large.

Carers and patients speak out

The word 'carer' does not appear in the index of *Clinical Psychiatry* in 1969, nor in *The Psychiatry of Late Life* in 1982. Of course this does not mean that the role of families and friends was then ignored—quite the opposite. From its beginning, geriatric psychiatry understood its dependence on collaboration with the social networks which sustained the patient at home.

Systematic epidemiological and social surveys of older people living in the community were published in the 1960s and 1970s, and the enormous role played by family members (and others) in sustaining older people in their homes began to be measured. These people were unpaid, usually unsupported, subject to desperate pressures, their work unrecognized. An influential report on carers commissioned by the National Institute for Social Work was published in 1989 (35), initiating a large and growing field of research. The term 'carer' (with its ambivalent connotations of both love and toil) was not ideal, but no better alternative was found. For the resident daughter of a parent with late dementia to be called an 'informal carer' seemed only to trivialize the weight of her emotional and practical burden; while others were offended by the implication that anyone not giving physical help to a relative did not 'care' for them, however loving their relationship.

A phenomenon of increasing importance has been the emergence of national charities to represent the interests of carers and their dependants. Carers UK was founded in 1965, and Age Concern in 1971, merging with Help the Aged in 2009 to become Age UK. The first branch of the UK Alzheimer's Disease Society (following the example of the United States) was initiated in Oxford in 1979. Originally the influence of such charities was through their local branches, bringing together groups of carers for mutual support and education. These soon engaged with the health and social providers in their area, and advocated (or themselves established) new facilities such as daycare centres. The national organizations gradually raised their public profile, providing a point of reference, a newsletter, education and advice for their members; political lobbying and media contacts; publicity for the cause and an accessible website; and fundraising for research.

Medicine has long taught us to learn from our patients, and personal accounts of illness have been a precious source of insight down the ages. In old age psychiatry we have the accounts of carers as well; they do not substitute for the voice of the person with dementia, but they are invaluable in themselves. In hearing these stories, new carers see the reflection of their own struggles and know that they are recognized. An early excellent source in 1985 was Mace and Rabins' *The 36-hour day: caring at home for confused elderly people* (36). Although compiled by professionals, it is in essence a direct and honest expression by carers of all the problems and rewards of caring. I cannot count how often I have lent my copy to families I was seeing at home, or taught my students from it.

It is rare to find personal accounts of dementia written while the disease takes hold of the writer. *My journey into Alzheimer's disease* by Robert Davis, an American pastor, was published in 1989 by his wife (37). It is a revelation to read his 'view from inside' of the signs of dementia coolly described by clinicians 50 or 100 years earlier, and since enshrined in textbooks. Especially memorable are his descriptions of the panic-stricken exhaustion that comes simply from sensory or cognitive overload, and the security that a stable routine provides.

When John Bayley, Professor of English at Oxford, wrote the memoir of his wife Iris Murdoch, the novelist (38), the depiction of dementia moved into mainstream literature (and subsequently into film). Other well-known figures such as Ronald Reagan had AD or, like the author Terry Pratchett, have been willing to say openly that they have it and to help in the fight against misunderstanding and stigma. In general, public sympathy for older people with mental illness is growing, for a combination of reasons: with greater numbers surviving into advanced old age, younger people are more likely to be acquainted with (or caring for) an old person with some form of psychological need; advances in neuroscience make good-news stories and are widely reported; and discrimination against any disadvantaged group has steadily become socially unacceptable.

Coda

I have tried to depict the evolution of old age psychiatry as both a scientific discipline and a social entity enmeshed in its specific place and time. Sustained by commitment to the welfare of mentally ill older people, it has tried to reach out further—to the earliest stages of illness or to the end of life, to independent people or to those in institutional care—and to a society which recognizes their needs, even while trying sometimes to deny them.

References and endnotes

1 Jacoby, R. and Oppenheimer, C. (1991). *Psychiatry in the elderly*. Oxford: Oxford University Press. Also (1997) second edition; and (2002) third edition.

2 Jacoby, R., Oppenheimer, C., Dening, T., and Thomas. A. (2008). *Oxford textbook of old age psychiatry*. Oxford: Oxford University Press.

3 Levy, R. and Post, F. (1982). *The psychiatry of late life*. Oxford: Blackwell Scientific Publications.

4 Slater, E. and Roth, M. (1969). *Mayer-Gross, Slater and Roth, Clinical psychiatry* (3rd edn). London: Bailliere, Tindall and Cassell.

5 Eliot Slater had four children, of whom I am the third.

6 Slater, E. and Roth, M. (1969). *Clinical psychiatry* (3rd edn), London: Bailliere, Tindall and Cassell, pp. 548–9.

7 Stewart, R. (2008). Clinical aspects of dementia: vascular and mixed dementia. In: Jacoby, R., Oppenheimer, C., Dening, T., and Thomas, A. (eds.) *Oxford textbook of old age psychiatry*, Oxford: Oxford University Press, pp. 443–52.

8 Perry, R. and Perry, E. (1982). The ageing brain and its pathology. In: Levy, R. and Post, F. (eds.) *The psychiatry of late life*, Oxford: Blackwell Scientific Publications, pp. 9–67.

9 Pasquier, F., Deramecourt, V., and Lebert, F. (2008). Frontotemporal dementia. In: Jacoby, R., Oppenheimer, C., Dening, T., and Thomas, A. (eds.) *Oxford textbook of old age psychiatry*, Oxford: Oxford University Press, pp. 461–72.

10 McShane, R. (2008). Dementia in Parkinson's disease and dementia with Lewy bodies. In: Jacoby, R., Oppenheimer, C., Dening, T., and Thomas, A. (eds.) *Oxford textbook of old age psychiatry*, Oxford: Oxford University Press, pp. 453–9.

11 Petersen, R. C., Smith, G. E., Waring, S. C. et al. (1999). Mild cognitive impairment: clinical characterization and outcome. *Archives of Neurology* 56, 303–8.

12 De Jager, C., Oulhaj, A., Jacoby, R., Refsum, H., and Smith, A. D. (2012). Cognitive and clinical outcomes of homocysteine-lowering B vitamin treatment in mild cognitive impairment: a randomized controlled trial. *International Journal of Geriatric Psychiatry* 27, 592–600.

13 Forlenza, O. F., Diniz, B. S., Radanovic, M. et al. (2011). Disease-modifying properties of long-term lithium treatment for amnestic mild cognitive impairment: randomised controlled trial. *British Journal of Psychiatry* 198, 351–6.

14 Hogg, J. (2008). Delirium. In: Jacoby, R., Oppenheimer, C., Dening, T., and Thomas, A. (eds.) *Oxford textbook of old age psychiatry*, Oxford: Oxford University Press, pp. 506–17.

15 Naguib, M. and Levy, R. (1991). Paranoid states in the elderly and late paraphrenia. In: R. Jacoby and C. Oppenheimer (eds.) (1991). *Psychiatry in the elderly*. Oxford: Oxford University Press, pp. 758–778.

16 Howard, R. (2008). Late onset schizophrenia and very late onset schizophrenia like psychosis. In: Jacoby, R., Oppenheimer, C., Dening, T., and Thomas, A. (eds.) *Oxford textbook of old age psychiatry*, Oxford: Oxford University Press, pp. 617–26.

17 Bergmann, K. and Jacoby, R. (1983). The limitation and possibilities of community care for the elderly demented. In: *Research contributions to the development of policy and practice*. Essays based on the seminar 'Support for elderly people living in the community' sponsored by DHSS and held at the University of East Anglia, September 1982. London: Her Majesty's Stationery Office, pp. 141–67.

18 Corsellis, J. A. N. (1969). The pathology of dementia. Reprinted in Silverstone, T. and Barraclough, B. (eds.) (1975). *Contemporary psychiatry: selected reviews from the British Journal of Hospital Medicine*. British Journal of Psychiatry Special Publication No. 9. Ashford, Kent: Headley Brothers, pp. 110–18.

19 Procter, A. W. (1997). Neurochemical pathology of neurodegenerative disorders in old age. In: Jacoby, R. and Oppenheimer, C. (eds.) *Psychiatry in the elderly* (2nd edn), Oxford: Oxford University Press, pp. 104–22.

20 King, E. M.-F., Smith, A. and Jobst, K. (1993). Autopsy: consent, completion and communication in Alzheimer's disease research. *Age and Ageing* **22**, 209–14.

21 Francis, P. T., Palmer, A. M., Snape, M., and Wilcock, G. K. (1999). The cholinergic hypothesis of Alzheimer's disease: a review of progress. *Journal of Neurology, Neurosurgery and Psychiatry* **66**, 137–47.

22 The 'cholinergic hypothesis' proposes that the activity of the neurotransmitter acetylcholine in the brain is reduced in AD. If the enzyme acetyl cholinesterase, which catalyses the destruction of acetylcholine, can be prevented from acting, then the level of acetylcholine at the synapse can be maintained for longer, and so achieve more effective transmission of the nervous impulse. Hence the use of *inhibitors* of acetyl cholinesterase in Alzheimer's disease.

23 Wilcock, G. K. (2008). Clinical aspects of dementia: specific pharmacological treatments for Alzheimer's disease. In: Jacoby, R., Oppenheimer, C., Dening, T., and Thomas, A. (eds.) *Oxford textbook of old age psychiatry*, Oxford: Oxford University Press, pp. 483–91.

24 McShane, R., Keene, J., Gedling, K. et al. (1997). Do neuroleptic drugs hasten cognitive decline in dementia? Prospective study with necropsy follow-up. *BMJ* **314**, 266–70.

25 Schneider, L. S., Dagerman, K. S., and Insel, P. (2005). Risk of death with atypical antipsychotic drug treatment for dementia: meta-analysis of randomised placebo-controlled trials. *JAMA* **294**, 1934–43.

26 James, I. A. and Fossey, J. (2008). Psychological treatments: non-pharmacological interventions in care homes. In: Jacoby, R., Oppenheimer, C., Dening, T., and Thomas, A. (eds.) *Oxford textbook of old age psychiatry*, Oxford: Oxford University Press, pp 285–96.

27 OADIG (Old Age Depression Interest Group) (1993). How long should the elderly take antidepressants? a double-blind placebo controlled study of continuation/prophylaxis therapy with dothiepin. *British Journal of Psychiatry* **162**, 157–82.

28 O'Connor, D. W. (2008). Electroconvulsive therapy. In: Jacoby, R., Oppenheimer, C., Dening, T., and Thomas, A. (eds.) *Oxford textbook of old age psychiatry*, Oxford: Oxford University Press, pp. 201–14.

29 Wilkinson, P. (2008). Psychological treatments. In: Jacoby, R., Oppenheimer, C., Dening, T., and Thomas, A. (eds.) *Oxford textbook of old age psychiatry*, Oxford: Oxford University Press, pp 241–96.

30 Rivett, G. (1998). *From cradle to grave, fifty years of the NHS*, London: King's Fund, p. 406.

31 Rivett, G. (1998). *From cradle to grave, fifty years of the NHS*, London: King's Fund, p. 407.

32 Martin, J. P. (1984). *Hospitals in trouble*. Oxford: Basil Blackwell.

33 The Parliamentary and Health Service Ombudsman (2011). *Care and compassion. Report of the Health Service Ombudsman on ten investigations into NHS care of older people*. London: The Stationery Office.

34 Brooker, D. (2008). Person centred care. In: Jacoby, R., Oppenheimer, C., Dening, T., and Thomas, A. (eds.) *Oxford textbook of old age psychiatry*, Oxford: Oxford University Press, 229–40.

35 Levin, E., Sinclair, J., and Gorbach, P. (1989). *Families, services and confusion in old age.* Aldershot: Avebury.

36 Mace, N. L. and Rabins, P. V. (1985). *The 36-hour day: caring at home for confused elderly people.* London: Hodder & Stoughton.

37 Davis, R. (1989). *My journey into Alzheimer's disease. Helpful insights for family and friends.* Wheaton, IL: Tyndale House.

38 Bayley, J. (1998), *Iris. A memoir of Iris Murdoch.* London: Gerald Duckworth.

The forensic psychiatric specialty: from the birth to the subliming

Paul E. Mullen and Danny H. Sullivan

Introduction

Some 30 years ago the first conference of the newly formed Forensic Section of the British and Irish College of Psychiatrists took place. 'Conference' is a grand title for a gathering comfortably accommodated in a modest-sized lounge room. Across the Atlantic the American Association of Psychiatry and the Law (AAPL) was better established, but still a small organization. Professors and departments of forensic psychiatry were few in the United Kingdom, having only John Gunn at the Institute of Psychiatry, although given the immense contribution he was to make, 'only' is not the right word. Many psychiatrists working in forensic hospitals or appearing in court would have identified themselves as general psychiatrists. No recognized training or certification existed. Forensic psychiatry had a history graced by such figures as Haslam (1817), Maudsley (1876), and Rey (1838) (1–3), but in the latter part of the 20th century, it was nascent.

Today conferences of both the UK and Australasian College Forensic Sections attract hundreds of attendees. AAPL meetings are even larger, and largest of all are conferences which embrace all the forensic mental health specialties. We have become, for better or for worse, a major psychiatric specialty claiming a significant slice of mental health funding. Forty years ago the psychiatrist portrayed in films, television, or novels was likely to have been a psychoanalyst, a madman, or both. Today our screens are full of fictional forensic psychiatrists and forensic psychologists, many with extraordinary powers to divine the motivations and identities of the obligatory serial killers. Even today's psychiatrist-lunatics, like Hannibal Lecter, are drawn from the ranks of forensic psychiatry. The extent to which the forensic psychiatrist has become established as a cultural trope is illustrated by a recent exchange with the dean of Monash University. He complained that those interviewed for places at the medical school were more likely to express the desire to grow up to be forensic psychiatrists than to become surgeons. He did not say what influence such a preference may have had on their selection.

This essay will focus on areas of forensic psychiatry concerned with the criminal justice system. Civil forensic practice concerned with issues such as compensation for psychological damage, competence to author a will, and child custody, will not be covered. This is not because they are unimportant but because they are largely outside of the authors' experience and have evolved somewhat separately.

Today we work as forensic mental health specialists alongside other professionals from psychology, nursing, social work, and occupational therapy, all of whom share training and expertise in the forensic arena. One of the stories of the last three decades is the birth of forensic psychiatry as an independent discipline. The growth of other forensic specialist disciplines has followed that of psychiatry, but this multidisciplinary endeavour could not have been foreseen 50 years ago.

Do we really care?

The ultimate purpose of a medical specialty is to provide care and treatment to patients. The most important question is therefore whether the care and treatment of mentally abnormal offenders has improved since the 1970s. The answer is neither simple nor consistent.

On the positive side, mental health services to prisoners have improved in most jurisdictions. The large secure hospitals have shared, to some extent, in the increased emphasis on treatment and rehabilitation which transformed other mental hospitals. In general adult psychiatry, recent decades have seen decreases in bed numbers with the ultimate disappearance of many large institutions (see Leff, this volume). In contrast, despite shorter stays, the population in forensic inpatient services has steadily increased, together with the number of such facilities, although today medium- and low-security hospitals tend to be far smaller than previously. The increase of forensic community-based services has been modest in comparison to the growth of their inpatient counterpart, the reverse of trends in general psychiatry.

What was once a minor part of all psychiatric inpatient services has now become a major and still growing part. General psychiatric beds are to a limited extent being replaced by forensic beds, but accessing these requires the qualification of criminality. The nature of the requisite criminality varies. In the United States, so-called sexually violent predators fill many existing and newly commissioned forensic beds. In California, some of yesterday's large psychiatric hospitals are reappearing as secure forensic hospitals (e.g. in the Napa Valley). This is in response, primarily, to the escalating numbers of those designated sexual predators who enter, but rarely leave, the forensic services.

The temptation for those sceptical about the progress of deinstitutionalization is to suggest that we are transferring patients from the care of general psychiatry to the control of prisons and forensic hospitals. There are more mentally ill people in prison, but there are also far more people in prison today than previously. What is not clear is whether the increased prison musters have been disproportionately selected from the mentally ill. There are more people in forensic hospitals, many of whom might well have occupied beds in the old asylums. But were they better off in the locked back wards of yesterday's psychiatric institutions?

Where mentally ill offenders reside defines only part of the quality of care they receive. Thirty years ago, treating mentally ill offenders often began and ended with treating the active symptoms of their psychotic disorder. One undoubted benefit from the research into the risk factors for offending in those with and without mental illness is the recognition that many of the important criminogenic factors—those associated with offending risk—are similar in both groups. Just like the general run of repeat offenders, the recidivist mentally abnormal offender is more likely to have a history of childhood disadvantage and abuse, conduct disorder progressing to juvenile offending, difficulties in interpersonal relationships, educational failure and unemployment, self-centred and callous personality traits, and disregard for social constraints. The reason why they have similar histories and current characteristics may, however, be very different. If we understood why some who will develop a form of schizophrenia show deficits which affect their social and intellectual development and function, as well as erode the integrity of their personalities, we might be able to provide different management strategies. In the continuing absence of such knowledge, management strategies developed for the criminogenic factors in other offenders remain the best guide to managing the mentally ill offender.

Offenders with psychotic disorders fall on a spectrum. At one end is the young, antisocial, often substance-abusing repeat offender. At the other is the older, often reclusive person who does not abuse substances, has no significant history of antisocial behaviour either as a child or as an adult, and who commits a single, often violent, offence. This is a skewed distribution, with most being at the young recidivist end of the spectrum. The older, one-off offender is likely to be a deluded individual whose offending is apparently out of character. These used to form the bread and butter of forensic psychiatry and once filled the secure forensic hospitals. The more disorganized young psychotic men and women who offended repeatedly used either not to be recognized as ill, or their offending was attributed to antisocial personality rather than their illness. They almost always ended up in prison, and untreated.

Epidemiological studies examining the relationship between major mental disorders, in particular schizophrenia, and offending behaviours have revealed the extent and complexity of the associations. Some continue to argue that psychosis is not causally related to offending. This fails to explain why offending is not only several times more frequent among those suffering from schizophrenia, but disturbed backgrounds, conduct disorders, substance abuse, and educational failure are also more common in the offending group of people with mental illness. Either these environmental factors generate both crime and schizophrenia, or there is something about the early development of those suffering from schizophrenia which makes them more vulnerable to developmental difficulties (see McGuffin and Murray, this volume).

For the sake of patients accumulating untreated in prisons, particularly in the United States, we can only hope that the link between the vulnerabilities which accompany certain forms of psychosis and criminal behaviour will be recognized and accepted. Without that acceptance, no progress is likely in either reducing offending, or preventing reoffending among those with serious mental illness. Forensic psychiatry now accepts the necessity of addressing criminogenic factors in parallel with 'symptom control' or suppression of features of mental illness.

In an ideal world, forensic mental health would be engaged primarily in preventive work with vulnerable patients living in the community. Early recognition and early intervention in those whose disorder increases the chances of offending or reoffending, is where forensic mental health resources should be focused. The care and containment of those mentally ill people who have committed serious crimes will hopefully take place predominantly in units integrated with community and rehabilitation services, to ensure for most a safe transition back to the community. For a small number, the nature of their crimes and the nature of their disorder will make long and perhaps permanent secure containment unavoidable. For these the challenge will continue to be maintaining hope and providing the best possible existence within the constraints of enforced incarceration.

'Praise the Lord and pass the risk' assessment forms

The rise and rise of risk assessment has wrought dramatic changes in forensic mental health practice. Assessing the risk of patients becoming violent has become central to forensic expertise. The study of potential risk factors and the creation of ever more instruments to assess the chances of each and every conceivable form of bad behaviour are now our primary research fields and most profitable occupations. Major shifts in the balance of power have resulted, both externally between forensic and general psychiatry, and internally between psychiatrists and psychologists. Some gainsayers write of the damage to patients when they are regarded first and foremost as embodiments of risk; others mutter darkly of pseudoscience and statistical infelicities (4–6). Nevertheless, the risk assessment bandwagon continues to accelerate, strewing academic and financial benefits on its followers.

The dominant figures in the new risk assessment orthodoxy tell a tale of clinical and scientific progress (7–9). Once upon a time, so the story goes, there were many psychiatrists and a few psychologists who labelled patients as 'dangerous' only on the idiosyncratic insights of personal experience. Then came the researchers and psychometricians, drawn largely from the ranks of psychologists, who replaced guesswork with systematic, usually actuarial, instruments based on empirical data. These were so transparent and simple that anyone who had paid the fees for the training could carry out reliable, reproducible, and objective risk assessments.

There may well have been psychiatrists who pronounced on dangerousness merely on the basis of personal prejudice. We never had the misfortune to meet these straw men, but that is not to say they never existed. In the 1970s the leading figures in forensic psychiatry who wrote on dangerousness (10–13) struggled with a quite different problem. It was known that the evidence pointed to a number of predictors of future offending: being male, being young, having offended previously, and having experienced disturbed and abused childhoods. Research into childhood backgrounds (14,15) set the evidence that childhood factors could exert distant effects not merely in mental disorder but also in offending outcomes.

Equally, it was well known that having regular employment and a stable emotional and sexual relationship militated against reoffending. The construct of antisocial personalities (psychopathy) was debated, though most accepted it in one form or another (16). The problem for these much maligned assessors of the past was the question of whether clinical assessment and psychiatric history added anything to the crude predictors of gender, age, past behaviour, and apparent personality.

The error to which these earlier seekers after dangerousness were prone stemmed from a number of sources. They believed that mentally abnormal offenders were qualitatively different from other criminals, in that positive symptoms in the form of delusions and hallucinations were the major drivers of their offending. This left clinicians predisposed to overestimating the capacity of clinical features to modify the crude demographic and behavioural predictors. The lack of a systematic approach to assessment, combined with an absence of follow-up studies, further stymied progress in the clinical prediction of dangerousness among the mentally ill.

In the 1980s studies began to appear which could have advanced the stalled clinical approach to the prediction of dangerousness in the mentally ill. Most notable were the pioneering studies of Häfner and Böker (17) and Taylor and Gunn (18). These demonstrated an association between the schizophrenias and a range of criminal behaviour including the violent and homicidal. Later researchers extended these pioneering studies by teasing out the features which separated those with a schizophrenia at greater risk of violence, from those who presented little or no threat.

The clinical importance of this research was however obfuscated by vigorously promoted actuarial risk assessment tools, which arose in the 1990s. Only with the gradual emergence in the last decade of the 'structured professional judgement' approach has this body of research been systematically applied to risk assessment (19).

Actuarial assessment is systematic, transparent, and based on empirical research. The usual methodology is to evaluate retrospectively the records of a specific group, such as discharged patients or released prisoners, and establish associations to subsequent offending. This data forms the basis of the risk assessment instrument. Assessments using the instruments were, in theory, reproducible and independent of examiner bias. The old clinical approach struggled to make sense of a multiplicity of variables impacting on a specific individual. The new actuarial approach assigned individuals to specific groups with known levels of risk on the basis of a remarkably small number of variables. The most widely used of all such instruments, the STATIC-99 (20), uses only 10 factors (99 refers to the year of publication, not the number of variables!).

The language of 'risk' was claimed to be preferable to that of 'dangerousness'. Dangerousness was criticized as an all-or-nothing property which could be misunderstood as an abiding quality of the individual. Risk, on the other hand, was a variable of which an individual could have more or less. On the downside, only a few patients were labelled dangerous whereas now all patients pose some level of risk; Assessment instruments do not have a 'no risk' category. In the 1970s assessments of dangerousness were usually only made in cases where there was a history of serious offending and consideration was being given to whether or not to discharge the patient. Today a violence risk assessment is part of the mandatory processing of each and every patient coming in contact with psychiatric services. In practice many such risk assessments do not employ psychometrically established instruments, but instead rely on locally generated variants of unknown probity (21).

The unmodified actuarial risk assessment instruments, despite their apparently varied content, all share a common set of core factors. These are: prior history of offending, an irresponsible lifestyle, criminal attitudes (e.g. psychopathy), and substance abuse (22,23). To these can be added age, which is increasingly recognized as a major modifier of the scores on such instruments. In short, these are essentially the same factors which the old-fashioned assessors of dangerousness employed, although with the advantage of a consistent and structured application.

The limitations of the actuarial approach have been recognized. Quite apart from judging on the basis of group membership (the very essence of prejudice), the limited number of variables can result in absurd and even perverse implications. One case we were involved with was determined to have a high risk of reoffending on the STATIC-99 (20) and the Violence Risk Appraisal Guide (VRA) (24)—two of the most widely used actuarial risk assessment tools. The fact that during the 15 years of his imprisonment he had not only entered the ranks of the elderly, but had gone blind and lost the use of his legs, found no place in the opinions expressed by the experts who relied on actuarial instruments.

Structured clinical judgement instruments (SCJI) have been developed in an attempt to combine the derided clinical approach with the use of relevant empirically established risk factors. Here the empirical variables are drawn from a broadly based review of the existing literature on risk factors for offending. SCJIs allow the assessor to take individual characteristics into consideration, including loss of use of one's eyes and legs. This approach is a major improvement over the earlier methodology of unstructured clinical assessment as it ensures the relevant variables are systematically considered and provides at least some weighting to strong influences, like age and past behaviour, as against weaker influences such as current clinical state. The problem with SCJIs as opposed to strict actuarial approaches is that they depend on the rater having experience and common sense, neither of which can be guaranteed.

In theory SCJIs are more open to influence by rater bias than strict actuarial approaches. In fact, both actuarial and clinical judgement instruments are open to biased ratings, depending on who the rater is working for, be it prosecution or defence, plaintiff or defendant (25). At least because today's risk assessors tend to use the same instruments it has been possible to demonstrate the influence of bias. Yesterday's clinicians could not be exposed to similar scrutiny, though we have encountered a case where the psychiatrist assessed the same man on two occasions, once for the prosecution and once for the defence (two different offences 2 years apart) and provided totally contradictory opinions based on essentially the same information and observations.

The greatest problem for the SCJIs is that there have been no large validation studies, which would confer the appearance of empirical solidity on the actuarial approaches. Some, like the current iteration of the HCR-20, still incorporate Hare's Psychopathy Check List (PCL-R), which in our view is a most unfortunate confection that blends social prejudice, the obvious, and the clinically insightful. The greatest strength of SCJIs is that they identify factors which can be modified by psychological, social, and psychiatric interventions to reduce the chances of future offending. Given that health professionals should be in the 'business' not just simply of labelling and stigmatizing, but of managing and assisting, this is a critical advantage.

The face of clinical psychiatry, not just the forensic specialty, has been transformed by the rise of a perceived need to assess all psychiatric patients for their risk of harming others. Given the limitations of risk assessments—practical, theoretical, and ethical—their use in general psychiatry remains questionable, particularly as the frequency of serious violence among the mentally ill, though higher than in the general population, is low. In forensic psychiatry their value is primarily in the direction of management, by identifying factors which, when modified, are likely to reduce risk (19). The success of the risk assessment 'industry' owes, in our opinion, a small debt to science, but far more to the current culture of fear and control, combined with the financial and professional rewards provided to the purveyors of such practices (26,27).

And for my next witness I call the DSM-IV-TR

Thirty years ago, the authority accorded psychiatrists in court derived largely from their professional status. Today, authority increasingly derives from texts. The expert witness has always created a problem for our adversarial court procedures. Evidence is tested by examination and cross-examination in terms of its coherence and compatibility with the totality of the evidence before the court, but the expert often appeals to matters outside that domain. Considerable latitude is usually granted to the expert in using what would in other circumstances be hearsay. Experts once used to be allowed to ground their opinion in experience and knowledge without being examined in any detail. The expert was expected to provide what was a generally accepted view—within their profession—and if they deviated from this, to inform the court they had done so, and to explain why. When courts were faced with conflicting opinions from experts, they often fell back on giving greater credence to those with the most august credentials or professional status. Occasional resort would be made by counsel to quoting textbooks as embodiments of the accepted *status quo* in an attempt to challenge the expert. Even the less adroit expert could, however, usually skip around any apparent contradiction between their own view and that in the quoted book. Perhaps more irritating to jurists were disagreements by experts over diagnosis, invariably claiming that their diagnosis was correct and would be made by any other psychiatrist—with the sole exception of the opposing expert.

The difficulty with evaluating experts reached crisis point not with mental health witnesses but with those from more clearly science-based disciplines such as engineering, pharmacology, and chemistry. The issue is usually framed in terms of how the courts could accommodate novel scientific evidence (28). 'Novel' here was used to cover recent advances in the expert's science which contradicted the generally accepted viewpoint. The senior expert, occupying a prestigious position, might indeed be less well informed about the current state of their science than a young tyro still actively engaged in research. In the legal profession, position and status are central to authority; but in science, at least in theory, status flows only from knowledge.

The other pillar of authority in law is the text—the text of legislation, the text of precedence, the text of interpretations from higher courts (29). The response of the law to novel scientific evidence was to focus on the authority of the text itself, on who authored it and where it was published. Impact factors of professional journals began to be bandied about in courts almost as frequently as in an academic promotions committee.

Lawyers, however, are used to arguing about which precedents and interpretations best fit the facts of a case. Cross-examination began to be accompanied by the exchange of downloaded publications and the drawing of attention to page and line numbers, abstracted as if they were independent units of fact. An energetic legal team linked to Google now had the ability to generate quotes capable of challenging and discomforting even the best-prepared expert.

Psychiatry might have dodged these latest legal bullets. The third revised edition of the American Psychiatric Association's *Diagnostic and Statistical Manual* (DSM-III-R) and its sibling the International Classification of Diseases (ICD-10), however, prevented any such escape from the so-called progress of the law. These texts were manna from heaven for the courts, which now had access to a 'gold standard' of psychiatric diagnosis with which to confront an expert. Notwithstanding disclaimers in the manuals, notwithstanding attempts to explain the tentative and committee-generated compromises behind the manuals, and notwithstanding the limitations of the checklist approach, the manuals have come to dominate the forensic mental health discourse.

Clinical psychologists were often the first to embrace the use of the DSM, sometimes going as far as to append to their reports copies of what they considered the relevant pages from the manual. The status of psychologists in the courts, particularly when it came to issues of diagnosis, had been uncertain; but with the manuals they acquired parity with their psychiatric colleagues, as in their own mind did many a counsel and judge. Psychiatric diagnosis, and all that flowed from it jurisprudentially, was demystified and made transparent in the manual's text.

To the cross-examination of mental health experts by 'manual', has now been added 'duelling downloads'. In a recent case, the defence counsel attempted to undermine the expert's evidence on what is known about children's responses to sexual abuse by presenting a series of recently published papers and quoting lines from them, apparently at odds with the expert's evidence. This was an able lawyer who had a remarkable, if circumscribed, grasp of the literature. It was, however, a grasp based on filtering out anything that did not fit his argument. Responding in a manner which was neither defensive, dismissive, nor difficult for a jury to understand was a considerable challenge. All too easily, the expert's evidence, which was in this case far from novel, and firmly in the area of the well established and generally accepted, could have been made to look dubious or biased. The undermining of an authority based on position and the dubious benefits of many years since qualification is to be welcomed. Replacing this with the authority of the best available research would be wonderful. A court is not, however, a place for such miracles.

Sexual offenders

The latter part of the 20th century saw a remarkable transformation in the status of sexual offending, particularly against children. What had previously been dismissed as the eroticized longings for women to possess their own penis, or unconscious love for their fathers, came to be recognized as an epidemic of sexual molestation of children.

Although there remains a lack of clarity about actual rates, it is now starkly clear that sexual abuse of children is a major social problem. However, there remain a range of unconfirmed associations and inferences which arise from a history of childhood sexual abuse. Indeed, it has been argued that the pendulum has swung too far from the denial or minimizing of the seriousness of the long-term sequelae of sexual abuse. Critics contend that these is now an 'industry' of mental health specialists providing much-needed validation of victimization, but not simply understanding and support but also compensation and status as a victim. At its peak, uncritical therapists were actively engaged in enrolling unwitting patients into a witch-hunt by manufacturing claims of sexual abuse occurring at the hand of Satanists and other ritual molesters (30).

Unfortunately, the same degree of attention paid to putative victims has not been accompanied by commensurate focus upon understanding, treatment, and eventually, moves towards prevention of sexual offending. It is not clear why this is so. It could be simply that since sexual abusers are the pariahs of convicted offenders, the stigma attached to their offences also attaches to its treatment. Another possibility is that sex offender treatment has been sequestered as an activity of correctional agencies, and is not perceived as core business for forensic mental health services. Research into sexual offenders has focused on risk assessment and prognosis and it is only in recent years that evaluation of treatment has become a focus; aetiology and epidemiological considerations have been little considered.

The consequences of this neglect of a psychiatric focus on sexual abusers is seen in the limited funding available for the treatment of sexual abusers outside the correctional system. More alarming is the resurgence internationally of legislation designed to detain indefinitely a small proportion prolific offenders. Sadly, this inordinately expensive strategy strips funding from other valuable areas and will, in all likelihood, make an unappreciable impact upon overall rates of sexual offending.

Consequently, the unusual status of paraphilia as a diagnostic category is, it appears, soon to be remedied by a politically driven diagnostic category which will enable repeat offenders to be detained indeterminately as sexually violent predators, with recurrent behaviour taken as indicative of a mental disorder which impairs their capacity to control such deviant sexual impulses. The reification of offending behaviour into a mental disorder has been accompanied by the huge growth of long-term secure units for the confinement of sexual offenders; and an industry sadly focused on assessment to assist the judicial determination of those to be confined, but not with a commensurate interest in treatment.

Increasingly those forensic psychiatrists who perceive that sexual offenders may benefit from treatments such as medications and sustained psychological therapies find themselves hamstrung by the control exerted by correctional authorities preventing early and constructive engagement. What was previously a relatively transparent ethical process in negotiating consent to treatment, has been muddied by the potential for lifelong restrictions to be imposed on sexual offenders. The capacity of a person to consent to medications, or the choice to participate in assessment and treatment, is overshadowed by the potential for clinical engagements to be discoverable by correctional agencies, or to be used as evidence to construct a legal case for indefinite detention or supervision. Many offenders faced with such decisions will opt not to engage rather than face the risk of their disclosures in therapy providing support for their confinement. Similarly, for forensic psychiatrists to participate in these legal processes requires a clear consideration of the ethics of involvement when this is geared almost exclusively to considerations of public safety, often devoid of reference to evidence about reoffending, and negating any real potential for therapeutic interventions.

Involvement of forensic psychiatrists in the treatment of sexual offending illustrates the fundamental issue facing forensic mental health as a specialty, with the challenge perhaps greater than the need to develop humane treatment options in prison hospital and community. That task is to move away from the tertiary prevention of mentally disordered offending, the provision of treatment after a person has entered the forensic mental health system by virtue of an earlier act or acts. Ideally, the challenge will be to move to secondary prevention—that is, providing targeted interventions for those considered to be at markedly escalated risk of future offending—and eventually to primary prevention through addressing the social circumstances which predispose to both the development of mental disorder and to antisocial behaviour. Such interventions have historically been seen as outside the province of forensic mental health and have remained in the province of child and adolescent psychiatry or social and family agencies.

Back to the future

Psychiatrists in the 19th and early 20th centuries were not shy in advancing theories about criminal behaviour. Atavism, degeneration, moral imbecility, and repressed guilt all had their advocates. The baleful results of such speculations had by the 1960s reduced the hubris of the profession. Few were still willing to step outside of the core tasks of assessing and treating the mentally disordered.

What makes a patient 'forensic' is first and foremost their behaviour. In the 1970s forensic psychiatry identified itself increasingly with the assessment and management of the mental abnormality in the offender. Mental abnormality was reduced to the notion of psychosis, or to use the ponderous terminology of the time 'formal mental illness'. Psychiatrists largely abandoned the study of behaviour to psychologists, retaining only the boutique area of sexual perversions. There were, in the United Kingdom and Australia, even moves to exclude personality disorders entirely from the purview of forensic psychiatry. These changes were linked to ideological shifts in the whole field of psychiatry as the pharmaceutical industry and its apostles in biological psychiatry began to redefine the nature of the psychiatric enterprise.

The brute reality of forensic practice prevented the narrowing of focus to 'formal mental illness' alone. Shoplifters, child molesters, violent and disorganized juveniles, thieves, wife batterers, and conmen continued to be referred by courts, prison authorities, and colleagues. Formal mental illness was in short supply among this population of the distressed, angry, and disturbing. The attempt to shrug off the troublesome areas of personality deviation and 'bad' behaviour had led to psychologists who took up these burdens acquiring greater and greater influence. The hegemony of psychiatry over the forensic field was weakened and in terminal decline.

It should not be said, however, that medicine abandoned its areas of influence without a fight. The counter-reformation came in the form of the DSM-III-R and onwards. Sexual perversions were miraculously rebirthed as mental disorders under the rubric of paraphilias. Impulse control disorders multiplied to incorporate thieving and assaulting, and it seems likely that raping will be added before long. Addiction extended to medicalize even the realm of the romantic afflicted by postcoital guilt, who could now protest they required treatment for sex addiction. Criminal, irresponsible, and morally dubious behaviours were converted into disorders—'formal mental disorders' no less, for what is more formal than a listing in the DSM or the ICD? As for personality disorders, these were reclaimed from the careless hands that let them drop into the laps of psychologists. They were given clear medical definitions by the manuals, combined with hints of neurobiological substrates.

In practice, medicalizing bad behaviours and promoting clear definitions of personality disorders did not clarify the field. Our patients tended, according to the manuals, each to have multiple (i.e. comorbid) overlapping personality disorders and a number of impulse control disorders and addictions. Applying the manual to the complexities of the human condition might sound good in court but was useless as a guide to understanding and managing forensic patients.

One trend that emerged from this muddle was an attempt to redefine the primary object of forensic psychiatry as the offending behaviour itself. This 'problem behaviours model' is of use primarily in the context of community assessment and management of those who have repeatedly committed the same offences, examples being fire setting, stalking, or threatening to kill (31). It is not applicable to those with a wide spectrum of offending, or those who have committed one serious crime of violence, for whom motivations may be singular or complex, but are not so readily understood as repetitive and maladaptive patterns of managing conflicts and provocative situations.

The focus is on the nature of the problem behaviour, its motivation, its triggers and the patient's resistance to, or embracing of, the behaviour; this does not exclude standard psychiatric and psychological assessments. Again, when it comes to management, the offending behaviour and the elements contributing to that behaviour have primacy, although the treatment of co-occurring mental disorders is, however, also included. In our experience, the co-occurring mental disorders, particularly if in the affective range, are as likely to be the result of the behaviour and its consequences for the offender, as part of the genesis of the problem.

In many ways the problem behaviours approach is turning the clock back to the days of Maudsley, Freud, and Lombroso. There are risks in medicalizing deviance and dissident behaviour (32). The problem behaviours approach does not treat behaviour as if it was mental disorder but rather as a range of activities open to modification by psychological, social, and psychiatric means. This involves a sustained and continuous exploration of the behaviour, its motivations and manifestations, in order to target individualized interventions. These, when effective, can assist the hapless to refrain from actions which are harmful to others, and may consume them in ultimately futile pursuits.

What are libertarians doing in a place like this?

The doctor–patient relationship in inpatient psychiatry, unlike almost every other medical specialty, commonly occurs against a background of compulsion. We can force ourselves on our patients. Our advice can become instructions, our understanding a denial of legitimacy to the patient's beliefs, and our care can become control. The hopes some entertained in the 1960s that compulsion would disappear from psychiatry came to nothing. In the state of Victoria in Australia, where we work, some 70% of admissions to public hospital psychiatric units occur as a result of the psychiatrist invoking the compulsory powers of mental health legislation. As in much of Australia, these compulsory powers follow the patient into the community when they are discharged. In the United Kingdom significantly more admissions are ostensibly voluntary, but the threat of compulsion still hangs over the head of any psychiatric patient with the temerity to go against medical advice. In forensic psychiatry in the criminal jurisdiction, coercion governs most of our interactions with patients except, interestingly, in prison. Here the writ of the Mental Health Act does not run, though many other sources of discipline and control do operate. The prison psychiatrist is one of the few members of the prison staff whom an inmate can defy with impunity.

Given the close relationship of forensic psychiatry to social systems that discipline and punish, it is a strange place to find a libertarian. Working in forensic psychiatry has persuaded us that mental disorders do not of themselves justify control or constraint, irrespective of whether the justification is in terms of competence or capacity. Paradoxically, however, a forensic psychiatrist can work in a world where the power to compel is in the hands of those—i.e. judges—to whom society delegates the power to punish and control. With a little care, and more than a few weasel words, a forensic psychiatrist can avoid operating as an advocate for control. Our patients have had their civil rights curtailed, not because of their mental disorders, but because of their criminal acts. These criminal acts would have attracted prison sentences or other restrictions had not a mental health disposal been considered by the courts as more appropriate. The discharge of patients, and whether they will remain under any restrictions once back in the community, at least in our system, remains the responsibility of the court which imposed the initial order for detention.

Some of our psychiatric colleagues are of the view that forensic patients should be detained and discharged solely on the basis of their psychiatric status. This is theoretically and practically problematic. In the Australian state of Queensland their unique laws once made this a possibility. The result was that offenders, including homicide offenders, were discharged back into the community as cured, or at least stable, sometimes only a matter of months after their trials were completed. Reoffending, including in some cases repeat homicides, created the predictable public scandals. Had this occurred in the United Kingdom or North America the careers of those psychiatrists responsible for the discharge decisions would have been over. Fortunately, Australia retains an essential respect for doctors, and for those who act as the law allows. As a result the obloquy fell largely on politicians and the laws which permitted such practices. Though it may offend medical sensibilities, the nature and length of the restrictions placed on mentally abnormal offenders are largely determined by the nature of their offending and the chances of further serious violence. The patient's mental state and the likely stability of any remission are relevant primarily to the issue of the chances of future offending.

Some would argue that this reduces forensic mental health services to being extensions of the prison and community correctional services. In the 1970s, when the Maudsley and Bethlem Hospitals agreed to build a medium-secure forensic unit, Professor Michael Shepherd, a true doyen of psychiatry, referred, at every opportunity, to the hospital's 'little prison with walls of only medium height'. There are, or there should be, dramatic differences between being detained as a patient in a forensic service or being subjected to imprisonment.

Prisons are about confinement and incapacitation, that is, removing criminals from the community to prevent, at least for a while, further offending. For a forensic mental health service, on the other hand, therapy and rehabilitation is the purpose. The culture of correctional services is that of control and discipline. The culture of forensic mental health should be that of care in the context of maximizing patients' control over their own lives. Of course, secure hospitals restrict the ability of patients to leave without consent, but this should be, if not the only, by far the most obvious restriction. Therapy needs to be directed not just at managing the patient's mental disorder but actively addressing criminogenic factors, those elements which sustain the risk of reoffending. In most modern services patients return to the community earlier than they would have from prison. The reoffence rate is usually negligible compared to the tragically high rates among ex-prisoners.

Those who appear before our courts charged with criminal offences are drawn disproportionately from the dispossessed and disadvantaged of society. Those with mental disorders have often never been adequately assessed, let alone treated. Of all those who come into the mental health services in the advanced world, the mentally abnormal offender is the most gratifying to treat. Even the basics of attention, concern, and simple remedies, pharmacological, psychological, and social, often produce life-changing responses.

Early in the 20th century, William Osler is said to have obtained a massive grant from the US Federal Government for Baltimore's Johns Hopkins Hospital on the basis of a promise to cure cancer in 10 years. Much good came from the money, if not the cure for cancer. Perhaps the trick could be repeated if forensic psychiatrists promised to cure crime.

Afterword

This essay had a difficult gestation, as the editors will attest. Among the reasons for the procrastination is a belief that those who try to recall the past almost always end up constructing an imaginary history tied to legitimizing today's claims to authority. History is a bad teacher because its recounting, and textural exegesis, are often in thrall to the authority of the present. Science is an anarchistic enterprise, constantly seeking to subvert received truths and yesterday's authority (33). The measure of a scientific paper is that it will be superseded and usually forgotten. As scientists, we do not stand on the shoulders of giants but ascend stairways of methodology and mathematics built by the labour of thousands. Only fictions and their authors persist over time. Perhaps that is why psychiatry is so tied to yesterday's heroes and their semi-fictional productions.

References

1 Haslam, J. (1817). *Medical jurisprudence*. London: Callow;.
2 Maudsley, H. (1876). *Responsibility in health and disease*. London: H. S. King & Co.
3 Rey, I. (1838). *A Treatise on the medical jurisprudence of insanity*. Boston, MA: Little, Brown.
4 Szmukler, G. (2001). Violence risk prediction in practice. *British Journal of Psychiatry* **178**, 84–5.

5 Large, M. M., Ryan, C. J., Singh, S. P. et al. (2011). The predictive value of risk categorisation in schizophrenia. *Harvard Review of Psychiatry* **19**, 25–33.

6 Mossman, D. (2009). The imperfection of protection through detection and intervention. lessons from three decades of research on the psychiatric assessment of violence risk. *Journal of Legal Medicine* **30**, 109–40.

7 Quinsey, V. L., Rice, M. E., Harris, G. T. et al. (2004). *Violent offenders; appraising and managing risk.* Washington, DC: American Psychological Association.

8 Monahan, J. and Steadman, H. (2001). *Rethinking risk assessment; the macarthur study of mental disorder and violence.* New York: Oxford University Press.

9 Steadman, H. J., Silver, E., and Monahan, J. et al. (2000). A clarification tree approach to the development of actuarial violence; risk assessment tools. *Law and Human Behaviour* **24**, 83–100.

10 Scott, P. D. (1977). Assessing dangerousness in criminals. *British Journal of Psychiatry* **131**, 127–42.

11 Walker, N. (1978). Dangerous people. *International Journal of Law and Psychiatry* **11**, 37–50.

12 West, D. J. (1969). *Present conduct and future delinquency.* London: Heinemann Educational Books.

13 Hamilton, J. R. and Freeman, H. (1982). *Dangerousness; psychiatric assessment and management.* London: Gaskell Press.

14 Rutter, M., Tizard, J., and Whitmore, K. (1970). *education, health and behaviour.* London: Longmans.

15 Farrington, D. P. and Coid, J. (2003). *Early prevention of adult antisocial behaviour.* Cambridge: Cambridge University Press.

16 Lewis, A. (1974). Psychopathic personalities: a most elusive category. *Psychological Medicine* **4**, 133–40.

17 Hafner, H. and Böker, W. (1982). *Crimes of violence by mentally abnormal offenders,* translated by H. Marshall. Cambridge: Cambridge University Press.

18 Taylor, P. J. and Gunn, J. (1984). Risk of violence among psychotic men. *BMJ* **288**, 1945–9.

19 Mullen, P. E. and Ogloff, J. R. P. (2009). Assessing and managing the risk of violence towards others. In: Gelder, M., Andreasen, N., López-Ibor Jr, J., and Geddes, J. (eds.). *New Oxford textbook of psychiatry* (2nd edn). Oxford: Oxford University Press.

20 Hanson, R. K. and Thornton, D. (1999). STATIC-99: improving actuarial risk assessments for sex offenders. <http://courtdiagnostic.com/Static%2099-02.pdf> [accessed 6 June 2012].

21 Carroll, A. (2007). Are violence risk assessment tools clinically useful?*Australian and New Zealand Journal of Psychiatry* **41**, 301–7.

22 Kroner, D., Mill, J., and Reddon, J. (2005). The coffee can, factor analysis, and the prediction of antisocial behaviour: the structure of criminal risk. *International Journal of Law and Psychiatry* **28**, 360–74.

23 Skeem, J. and Monahan, J. (2011). Current direction in violence risk assessment. *Current Directions in Psychological Science* **20**, 38–42.

24 Quinsey, V. L., Harris, G. T., Rice, M. E., and Cormier, L. A. (1998). *Violent offenders: appraising and managing risk.* Washington, DC: American Psychological Press.

25 Otto, R. K. (1989). Bias and expert testimony. *Behaviour Science and Law* **7**, 267–73.

26 Simon, J. (2007). *Governing through crime.* Oxford: Oxford University Press.

27 Garland, D. (2001). *The culture of control: crime and social order in contemporary Society.* Oxford: Oxford University Press.

28 Monahan, J. and Walker, L. (2010). *Social science in law; cases and materials* (7th edn). New York: Foundation Press.

29 Mullen, P. E. (2010). The psychiatric expert witness in the criminal justice system. *Criminal Behavior and Mental Health* **20**, 165–76.

30 McHugh, P. R. (2006). *Try to remember: psychiatry's clash over meaning, memory, and mind*. New York: Dana Press.

31 Warren, L. J., MacKenzie, R., Mullen, P. E., and Ogloff, J. R. P. (2005). The problem behavior model: the development of a stalkers clinic and a threateners clinic. *Behavioural Science and Law* **23**, 387–97.

32 Bloch, S. and Reddaway, P. (1977). *Psychiatric terror: how Soviet psychiatry is used to suppress dissent*. New York: Basic Books.

33 Feyerabend, P. (2010). *Against method*. London: Verso.

Trauma and psychiatry

Arieh Y. Shalev

Introduction

My personal experience with trauma started at the age of three when our home was ruined by an explosion during Israel's war of independence. I still have remote but clear recollections of that experience, of my injured brother, and of myself, wondering about the sound of sewing machines outside (they were actually machine guns, but I hadn't heard those before).

My father's death, when I was five, was a founding trauma—though not a traumatic event as would be currently defined. His legacy combined strict science and a humble, humane approach. Not having him alive, to revolt against, I may have attempted to prolong his existence by following that path.

At the time of writing this text, governments are involved in the killing and torture of their own citizens. To draw attention to their agenda, belligerent organizations indiscriminately assassinate civilians in open markets. Natural disasters have created unimaginable devastations. Rape and other forms of interpersonal violence and traumatic accidents occur daily. The inescapable consequences of these events—death, injury, loss, misery, degradation, relocation, or starvation—shatter survivors' lives.

Life-shattering events have been documented since the beginning of history. The biblical narration of Job's predicament includes many of their pertinent protagonists: innocent victim ['*There was a man in the land of Oz . . . perfect and upright, and one that feared God, and eschewed evil*']; utter surprise ['*There came a great wind from the wilderness, and smote the four corners of the house, and it fell upon the young men, and they are dead*']; evil forces [*And Satan went forth from the presence of the LORD, and smote Job with sore boils from the sole of his foot unto his crown*'], a breach of duty by an ever-observing Providence ['*And the LORD said unto Satan, Behold, he is in thine hand*'], the breaking of a man's spirit [*'After this, opened Job his mouth, and cursed his day.*'] and the bewilderment of sympathetic observers, such as Job's three friends who ['*lifted up their eyes afar off, and knew him not*'].

Job's story is wrapped in the then-prevalent moral and theological discourse. Later, the consequences of human trauma become parts of tragic tales, involving courage, defeat, and remorse (Lady Percy's monologue in Shakespeare's *Henry IV*):

> *In thy faint slumbers I by thee have watch'd,*
> *And heard thee murmur tales of iron wars;*
> *Speak terms of manage to thy bounding steed;*
> *Cry 'Courage! To the field!' And thou hast talk'd*

Of sallies and retires, of trenches, tents,
Of palisadoes, frontiers, parapets,
Of basilisks, of cannon, culverin,
Of prisoners' ransom and of soldiers slain,
And all the currents of a heady fight.
Thy spirit within thee hath been so at war
And thus hath so bestirr'd thee in thy sleep,
That beads of sweat have stood upon thy brow
Like bubbles in a late-disturbed stream.

Along with other forms of human suffering, psychiatry embraced the maladaptive consequences of life-shattering events, construing them as mental disorders and subjecting them to clinical recognition, pathogenic reasoning, and prescribed therapies. Related emotions and behaviours came to be seen as 'symptoms'—this is, salient identifiers of underlying illness.

As medical objects, the maladaptive consequences of life-shattering events are construed as affecting individuals (rather than groups, families, or communities), stripped of moral significance, and resulting from strict (though admittedly complex) natural causes. Limitations to their understanding, diagnosis, and treatment are seen as transient, surmountable in principle, and requiring further inquiry and better discovery tools.

This view does not negate the moral, humanitarian, and historical aspects of extreme events. However, as a medical discipline psychiatry claims to identify, among other consequences, severe, disabling, prolonged, or otherwise inappropriate disease-like entities that require special care. Following transient romances with the terms 'shock', 'fatigue', 'situational reaction', or 'neurosis', psychiatry eagerly borrowed the surgical term 'trauma' to designate the injurious mental health effect of extreme events. By an additional twist of language, the latter became known as 'traumatic events'. The analogy between physical and psychological injury became a powerful, captivating metaphor.

Psychiatric consequences of extreme events were repeatedly described during the 20th century. Survivors of ship explosions in Toulon in 1907 and 1911 exhibited 'recapitulation of the scene, terrifying dreams, diffuse anxiety, fatigue, and various minor phobias' (1, p. 147). Symptoms of World War II 'operational fatigue' (2, p. 210) comprised irritability, fatigue, difficulties falling asleep, startle reaction, depression, tremor, evidences of sympathetic overreactivity, difficulties in concentration, mental confusion, preoccupation with combat experiences, nightmares and battle dreams, phobias, and personality changes. Symptoms of 'traumatic neurosis' (3, p. 86) comprised fixation on the trauma, typical dream life, contraction of general level of functioning, irritability and proclivity to explosive aggressive reactions.

Post-traumatic stress disorder and other developments

The definition of post-traumatic stress disorder (PTSD) in the third *Diagnostic and Statistical Manual* of the American Psychiatric Association (DSM-III, 1980) produced a unifying and prescriptive description of the psychiatric consequences of extreme events. As with other disorders in DSM-III, the diagnosis of PTSD relied on explicit identifiers (diagnostic criteria) and decision rules. Subsequent editions of DSM modified some features of PTSD but kept the guiding principles: a symptom template with explicit decision rules descending from experts' deliberations and shaping practice and research.

The extent to which PTSD is the proper descriptor of the consequences of traumatic events has been fiercely debated. Nevertheless, the inclusion of PTSD in DSM-III was *the* formative step in the recent history of mental trauma in psychiatry. It structured clinical observations, created much-needed consistency in diagnostic routines, and provided a necessary precondition for empirical research.

Other developments that have significantly affected our understanding of traumatic disorders include the universal availability of computational power, the exponential growth of neuroscience, model-based animal research, and molecular genetics. Together with advances in research methodology and higher standards of medical evidence, these developments have truly revolutionized the field.

There is nothing surprising, therefore, in saying that current knowledge about mental trauma and its consequences is both extensive and very different from what it was 40 years ago: the brain has opened itself to functional observations; there is better agreement about measurements, data analytic approach and reporting; novel evidence quickly becomes an object data-informed corroboration—or criticism; research production increased by an order of magnitude (as discussed later in this essay).

The need for theory

Given such productive power, the quality of underlying theories and the accuracy of research hypotheses are critical. Non-theoretical by intent, the robustness of DSM specified disorders depends on uncovering their underlying biomedical structures, and this, in turn, must be guided by generic principles and ultimately by theory. The success of theory-based cognitive behaviour therapy (CBT) for PTSD, and the relative stagnation of trial-and-error-based pharmacotherapies, are salient examples of the added value of having a theory.

As expanded below, the translational gap between biological hypothesis, animal models, and clinical interventions in trauma research has been particularly narrow. Several animal models have directly informed human treatment trials with varying degrees of success, but with consistent record of teaching lessons. Without guiding theory, however, the crucial question is whether the field of traumatic stress has truly advanced or just expanded. Or could it have been blown off course by side winds?

Side winds and other hurdles

PTSD was born to an age of increased sensitivity to social justice, human rights, protective networks, and duties of care. From its inception, therefore, the disorder was associated with *advocacy* and a sense of mission among many of its proponents. PTSD has also been used extensively to identify and infer psychological damage and claim *compensation*. Surpassing its intended role as a descriptor of a mental disorder, PTSD has become a social, cultural, and economic object.

Additionally, because of its captivating simplicity, PTSD was quickly reified. Rather than descriptor of an underlying condition PTSD became the condition itself, the sought-after outcome of traumatic events. Referring to PTSD as a real and distinct entity, while useful for 'diagnostic and statistical' reporting, might have made it too easy to forget the underlying heterogeneity. In other words, the disorder's forced phonotypical coherence can easily camouflage an underlying ontological confusion.

By another DSM rule, complex clinical presentations that follow trauma are subsumed as comorbidities—that is, coexisting but distinct disorders. PTSD and major depression, for example, overlap in over 40% of the cases at any given time, and co-occur in 95% of the cases in a lifetime perspective. PTSD and major depression are nonetheless seen as distinct entities—particularly when it comes to defining research groups and subsequently recommending or licensing therapies. The amount of information lost by anchoring research and practices to categorical entities is hard to estimate.

Similarly, in a typical post-hoc attribution error ('after this, therefore because of this') the association between PTSD and the antecedent event was quickly perceived as causal. Part of the popularity of PTSD is due to its symbolizing such highly desirable, simplified, intuitive causal attribution. As we shall see, this is also one of the most contentious areas in the PTSD literature.

A ceiling to progress

Finally, advances in the clinical management of PTSD have not followed the accelerated path of neurobiological discovery. PTSD remains chronic, disabling, and frequent. The prevalence of PTSD among US veterans of recent conflicts, for example, matches that seen after the Vietnam war. Not unrelated to the latter, the US Institute of Medicine's (IOM) 2008 report used uncompromising language to describe this state of affairs: 'The studies conducted over the nearly three decades since *Diagnostic and Statistical Manual of Mental Disorders* (DSM) adoption of the PTSD definition do not form a cohesive body of evidence about what works and what does not.'

There is therefore room for both pride and critical reflection. This essay explores both. It outlines progress, delineates boundaries, and offers reflections about ways to go forward. The essay is also a personal account, reflecting my own professional and personal encounters with trauma, addressed in the last section.

The rise of PTSD

PTSD migrated to Israel with slight delay, the country's official classification during the 1980s being the ninth edition of the International Classification of Diseases (ICD-9). In January 1983, along with another psychiatrist of the Israel Defense Forces Medical Corps, I interviewed and carefully documented symptom progression in 120 combat stress casualties of the 1982 Lebanon War. Choosing to ignore DSM's 'Americanism', we used ICD-9 and 'war neurosis' descriptions to collect data. However, at the time of preparing this work for publication, the prominence and the desirability of PTSD symptom criteria were such that our work was seen as reflecting an obsolete construct.

How PTSD gained such prominent status is unclear. Illustrating a quantifiable dimension of that success, the number of yearly publications on trauma and PTSD increased from fewer than 100 before 1984 to over 1000 from 2004 on, thereby reaching the order of magnitude of publications on schizophrenia or major depression. Studies concerning PTSD were published in *Nature, Science,* and the *New England Journal of Medicine.* PTSD has also been a prominent subject of lay publications, as attested by 20 dedicated articles in the *New York Times,* 12 in *The Times* and over 100,000 YouTube entries on PTSD in 2011 alone.

Trauma before PTSD

To fully appraise the progress in this field one must go back to the ways in which trauma was perceived and managed before DSM-III. As illustrated above, World Wars I and II generated eloquent descriptions of combat stress reactions and their management. However, knowledge gained during armed conflicts was not readily translated into civil trauma and, in the absence of notable wars between 1945 and 1968, the topic lost its prominence. Consequences of different events were described under different headings (e.g. 'concentration camp (KZ) syndrome', 'war neuroses' or 'rape survivor's syndrome'). Kardiner (4) described the situation as follows: 'it is hard to find a province of psychiatry in which there is less discipline that in this one. . . . Every author has his own frame of reference—lengthy bibliographies not withstanding.'

Distressed survivors of traumatic events were nonetheless seen and treated, often under the heading 'traumatic neurosis'. The construct of traumatic neurosis combines a reactivation of pretrauma vulnerabilities and trauma-induced dysfunction of intrapsychic regulatory processes (e.g. 'ego functions'). Healthy subjects, accordingly, should show only transient responses to traumatic events. Developing a chronic condition implied an underlying weakness. Therapies were supposed to explore and correct trauma-induced symptoms in the context of the person's entire life experience. McHugh and Treisman (5) refer to this approach as 'bottom-up' assessment:

> By this method, a psychiatrist drew diagnostic formulations from a 'bottom-up' assessment that evaluated a subject's full biography and took into account his previous psychological problems, temperament, and mental state in explaining presenting complaints. When thinking 'bottom up', a diagnostician naturally considered all the various forms of psychological maladjustments that people, soldiers or not, experience and express with mental symptoms.

Within such an assessment, specific symptoms were somewhat less important than the particularities of the patient's history as related to his or her current response. Treatment could proceed without much emphasis on diagnosis and categorization. Theory had an important role, and therapies often followed 'schools of thought' and local traditions. Therapists learned their art from paradigmatic case reports and oral tradition. Neuroses were generally considered 'non-biological' and their pharmacological management seen as mainly calming and sedating. This view was held despite the availability of antidepressants and major tranquilizers, the first reports of using antidepressants taking place shortly after the delineation of PTSD (reviewed in 6).

The belief that neuroses should be treated 'from the root', i.e. by exploring the underlying conflicts, did not encourage either symptom-oriented therapies or symptom-based outcome measurement. Nonetheless, symptom-focused interventions, often consisting of punishment-based behavioural retraining, were attempted during World War I (e.g. 7), but rarely followed afterwards. World War I also generated a debate between symptom-based and meaning-based (e.g. 8) treatment for psychological casualties, a debate that resonates in a current discussion between exposure-based and cognition-based therapies for PTSD (e.g. 9,10).

Another important construct was that of 'abreaction'—that is, the therapeutic discharge of trauma-induced repressed recollections and related suppressed emotion. Abreaction-based therapies were used for treating combatants during World War II, and, at times, with traumatized civilians. What remains of this view is the vague belief that 'one must fully remember in order to be cured'. One can find an echo of the latter in the more recent exposure-based therapies and debriefing.

Finally, the understanding that messages provided by survivors' immediate environment can shape the way in which they make sense of their experiences, and ultimately express or attend to their symptoms, was expressed in frontline treatment of combat casualties that used the proximity, immediacy, and expectancy (PIE) principles. The PIE interventions consisted of providing rest, restoration, brief evaluation, and re-insertion in military routine with clear message that the trouble was transient and full recovery expected. PIE-based interventions continue to be practised in modern wars and still have their partisans (11,12). They failed miserably in the Vietnam war, but the voices that had claimed that 'the problem of war trauma has been solved' (13) are now heard again in today's top science magazines (14).

To summarize, before DSM-III, psychiatrists knew that severe traumatic circumstances could lead to protracted and disabling psychiatric conditions. Psychiatrists were also aware that such conditions occurred in only a minority of those exposed. They were fully aware of the difference between transient and permanent responses, perceiving the aetiology of the latter as encompassing vulnerability, exposure, and recovery factors. They could even tell that the response to trauma included both intolerable mental content and a breakdown of psychic regulatory processes. Psychiatrists were acutely aware of the limitations of therapies and had hopes invested in early, acute care.

Psychiatrists were, however, unable to decide if different traumatic events (e.g. rape, railway accident) generated distinct conditions, and were unable to convincingly formulate the communalities between responses. Further, they did not know if traumatic life events mainly exacerbated previously existing disorders. Without reliably defined object of study they were unable to empirically explore these and other questions and assemble pieces of knowledge into one picture, however patchy. Finally, as is the case today, there were serious doubts about the credibility of post-traumatic disorders and those who suffer from them.

Descriptive psychopathology

DSM-III

Delineated 7 years after the end of the Vietnam war, PTSD was originally construed as *prolonged disturbance* due to *previous* and *currently terminated* events that were *out of the realm of normal human experience*. PTSD symptoms were derived from previous descriptions (e.g. 4) and from data collected in Vietnam war veterans and rape victims. PTSD symptom criteria of 're-experiencing' and 'numbing' were additionally influenced by psychoanalytic views and descriptions of grief and traumatic loss.

As had been hoped, PTSD was found among survivors of different events and thus gained the status of a generic description. The disorder's diagnostic criteria were slightly modified in DSM-III-R and DSM-IV, but its tripartite structure (re-experiencing, avoidance/numbing, hyper-arousal) remained. More recent factor-analytic studies suggest that the avoidance criterion could be split into avoidance and numbing. With slight modifications, therefore, the construct of PTSD remains robust, replicable, and universally reported.

The definition of traumatic events, however, has radically changed. Once defined as being uniquely terrifying or 'out of this world', the traumatic event now includes virtually every negative occurrence, provided that it evokes immediate fear, horror, or helplessness. Direct exposure to the event has been replaced with 'witnessing' or 'being confronted' with it. PTSD was subsequently described after childbirth, upon receiving a diagnosis of cancer, among body handlers and, following the 9/11 terrorist attacks, among US citizens living in remote areas of the country. Because many PTSD patients had not reported fear and horror during the traumatic event (e.g. soldiers at war may, instead, 'kick their training in' and suppress their emotions) the use of this component of PTSD criterion A has been criticized.

Natural course and prediction

Longitudinal studies found that trauma survivors frequently express early PTSD symptoms, from which most of them recover with or without treatment. This has lead to seeing chronic PTSD as a disorder of recovery. Higher levels of initial symptoms, early depression, and dissociation symptoms predict non-remitting PTSD. However, these predictors have limited specificity (most individuals who have them will still recover). To improve the prediction of PTSD, DSM-IV defined acute stress disorder (ASD), a diagnostic category that includes, in addition to the PTSD symptoms, symptoms of dissociation. ASD is associated with higher prevalence of chronic PTSD. However, most chronic PTSD patients never had expressed ASD. Predicting from early symptoms, therefore, remains a challenge, and facing symptomatic trauma survivors one is still left to guess who will remain with PTSD and who might recover.

Intriguingly, recent studies of US war veterans do not show the 'progressive recovery' trajectory, making it even harder to identify risk and initiate early prevention. Within the traumatic event itself, atrocities, exposure to the grotesque, and human cruelty may be more important than life threat or participation in combat. Indeed, the relative contribution of the triggering event to the likelihood of chronic PTSD may be less important than that of enduring subsequent stressors and having inadequate interpersonal support.

Limitations

PTSD diagnostic criteria capture salient and reliably communicable behaviours. They do not, however, include elaborate states of mind, attitudes, or emotional experiences (e.g. being humiliated, defeated, shocked, or changed by trauma), although these may have significant prognostic and therapeutic value. Similarly, the psychological components of traumatic events (e.g. unexpectedness, controllability, escape) are not specified, hence a rather shallow discussion of their parameters and their effects.

Many humans are exposed to repeated, prolonged, and unending trauma (e.g. soldiers in protracted wars, civilians under siege or shelling, victims of partner violence, refugees in crowded and lawless environments). Many such victims express PTSD symptoms, but their mental health problems are not limited to PTSD. An attempt to include a diagnostic category of 'complex traumata' in DSM-IV has failed, however. The proposed 'disorders of stress not otherwise specified (DESNOS)' and the more recent 'complex PTSD' include PTSD symptoms, personality traits, and attitudes of mistrust and disbelief. In the absence of accepted diagnostic criteria, however, complex PTSD had not been properly researched and validated (e.g. 15; but see 16).

In my own clinical experience, there is more heterogeneity in the clinical presentations of people who eventually meet PTSD diagnostic criteria than those criteria would ever suggest. Many of them do not suffer from the symptoms that we use to diagnose them as much as from experiencing a profound emotional disturbance touching on their being in the world and living with others, destroying their ability to collude with our shared, tolerable, and probably factitious reality. One of my first patients recalled the worst instance in her childhood rape experience as the moment in which she suddenly realized that she was 'trapped in what is a definite evil' (17). In a world in which the internet daily throws in our faces the images of men thrown from tall buildings or broken and bruised children's bodies, I often wonder who has the right version of reality. If I were to describe what separates my PTSD patients from all others, my choice would be their terrible and endless subjugation to repeatedly re-living fear, horror, and defeat, their extreme reactivity to the environment, and their essential inability to relax or to allocate attention and emotional resources to anything but their traumatic misery.

Historical perspective

Cohabitation

The short history of PTSD can be described as tense cohabitation of strict empiricist, spirited advocates, sceptics and believers, biologists, and humanists, each group making its own impact and introducing its own bias. The leading institution in the field, the International Society for Traumatic Stress, similarly includes (and sometimes confronts) scientists, clinicians, first responders, and disaster managers. Members of the society have been involved in each step of the recent history of PTSD, from drafting its initial diagnostic criteria to exploring underlying genetics. What binds this heterogeneous group together is, I believe, the galvanizing effect of dealing with a profound source of human misery.

The formative years

Because PTSD was a new disorder, the first years after its inclusion in DSM-III were dedicated to defending its credibility and increasing its acceptance. This included assessments of the disorder's prevalence and natural course, preliminary pathogenic hypotheses, description of risk and protective factors, and preliminary testing of treatments. Journals and reviewers often rejected PTSD papers as addressing a non-valid subject, but a few editors, such as John C. Nemiah of the *American Journal of Psychiatry* and Eugene Brody of the *Journal of Nervous and Mental Disorders*, opened their doors and enabled many of the early publications.

Pertinent data became available towards the end of the 1980s. Among other founding studies, the National Vietnam Veterans Readjustment Study was published in 1988; Pitman and colleagues' studies of physiological responses to mental imagery in 1987 (18); Blake and his group's psychometric tools from 1988 on (19); studies of behavioural 'flooding' for PTSD in 1989 (20); and McFarlane's description of the compounded aetiology of PTSD in 491 Australian firefighters in 1989 (21).

Following the revision of DSM-III (DSM-III-R, 1987) the field had, at about 1990, a reliable phenotype, validated measurement tools, preliminary biological correlates (e.g. elevated urinary catecholamines) and scattered treatment studies, requiring extension and replication. Thus the years 1980–1990 can be seen as the 'phenotype validation' and 'hypothesis generating' period.

Buttressing the construct

By extension, the years 1990–2000 may be seen as the 'hypothesis testing' period. Previous reporting of therapies in small, non-representative samples was followed by major and methodologically superior studies of specific serotonin reuptake inhibitors (SSRIs) and CBT. The results of these studies have not been surpassed and still inform current treatment guidelines.

Studies of war veterans were extended to civilians, and large epidemiological surveys appeared in 1995 (US National Comorbidity Study, 22) and 1988 (the Detroit area survey, 23). These studies established the prevalence of PTSD, evaluated the conditional probability of its occurrence after different events, and buttressed previous reports of overlap between PTSD, depression, and other anxiety disorders.

The established consistency of provoking physiological responses resembling PTSD symptoms by using mental imagery of traumatic events was implemented in 'symptom provocation,' functional brain imaging studies of PTSD. Starting with Bremner's report (24), structural brain imaging studies showed reduced hippocampal volume in PTSD. Static neuroendocrine studies were supplemented by challenge tests, many of which showed an increased responsivity of the hypothalamic–pituitary–adrenal (HPA) axis. Longitudinal studies documented typical symptom trajectories and buttressed the idea that PTSD is a 'disorder of recovery' from early symptoms.

When submitted to empirical validation, early interventions, such as debriefing or minor tranquilizers, were shown to have no preventive effect, or even to harm survivors. Basic scientists (e.g. 25) formulated hypothetical analogies between animal models (e.g. fear conditioning) and human PTSD, marking the beginning of significant translational work. Towards the year 2000, the field seemed to have a rather consistent narrative supported by clusters of findings at all levels, and a preliminary grasp of the underlying biology.

Introducing complexity and uncertainty

The early years of the 21st century have been characterized by explosion of knowledge and growing realization of complexity. Few original findings survived replication, and many original successes were eroded.

Replication of the studies of SSRIs in PTSD yielded more tentative results. No other compounds were found to be similarly effective. More recent work, however, challenges the use of central tendency statistics in intervention research, and emphasized the importance of exploring response heterogeneities and their sources.

Studies of stress hormones, although still viewed as sustaining the assumption of the hypersensitive HPA axis, show heterogeneity, inconsistencies, and conditional responses (e.g. appearing among subsets of patients with PTSD). Other neurohormonal systems and peptides have been implicated in PTSD (e.g. DEHA, pregnanolol, substance P), but there is a general realization that their measurements can only explain a limited amount of the variance (for review see 26). Early interventions by adrenergic blocking agents have generally failed. Genetic association studies failed to uncover candidate polymorphic genes for PTSD. More recent studies found a conditional association between PTSD, some gene variants (e.g. the FK506-binding protein 5 or *FKBP5* gene), and a history of child abuse, thereby introducing a gene–environment model.

Animal studies supporting the fear conditioning hypothesis of PTSD moved from their original emphasis on initial acquisition to considering deficiencies in the extinction of fear response, and thence exploring the problem of extinction recall and reconsolidation. To exemplify this rapidly changing area, the initial findings of successful interference with reconsolidation of fear memories (i.e. erasure of memories during recall) have nonetheless shown time-dependent renewal of fear, as if persistent cortical- and hippocampal-mediated episodic memories that remained untouched by fear-related interventions were able to reinstate the 'erased' emotional and hypothetically amygdala-dependent fear responses.

Functional brain imaging studies similarly show a more complex picture, in which PTSD encompasses excessive fear activation, lagging cortical control, relative blindness to contextual information, and deficient emotional regulation.

Finally, barriers to the effectiveness of CBT have been shown and studies currently explore enhanced forms of CBT (e.g. by adding medication, using virtual reality, or added transcranial magnetic stimulation), as well as shorter and better-delivered protocols.

Most importantly, while comorbidity is still formally supported by the classification of mental disorders, the fact of sharing common dimensions offers a new way to 'cut across' disorders and better access their underlying biology. It is unclear, in other words, whether PTSD is the proper 'unit of analysis' for understanding traumatic stress disorders. Pessimists may say that the PTSD agenda has failed whereas optimists can hold that the PTSD template was a necessary step and is currently transcended.

Challenges to the validity of PTSD

Attacks on the diagnosis and the underlying construct

Despite growing acceptance in the professional community, and cumulative evidence, several scholars have challenged both the foundation and the validity of PTSD. Allan

Young's book *The Harmony of Illusion: Inventing Post-traumatic Stress Disorder* (27) is one of the better-developed arguments against PTSD. Young challenges the presumed aetiological role of traumatic memory in PTSD, arguing that one can only show a concurrent association between symptoms and memories. He also criticized the political nature of the introduction of PTSD into DSM-III and illustrates how belief in the aetiological role of memories can lead to biased interpretation of patients' communication and to false inference of causality. Young extends his criticism to the related stress-hormone theory of memory imprinting and conservation. He is disturbed by the moral value of a disorder that can be diagnosed in both victims and perpetrators.

Having held two public debates with Mr Young, I believe that his criticism essentially targets a reified PTSD, that is, PTSD turned into solid object. Because I believe that PTSD is a 'distal approximation', or an observable identifier of an underlying central nervous system (CNS) disturbance, I can live with Mr Young's criticism: both of us believe that PTSD is sort of illusion, a virtual object, but I submit that in the current stage of knowledge PTSD is as good an approximation how this disturbance—or disturbances—looks as one can get. After years of conducting prospective studies of the recently traumatized, I am convinced that, following trauma exposure, my patients became severely distressed and disabled in relation to that trauma.

McHugh (28) uses PTSD to illustrate 'how psychiatry lost its way', and to buttress an attack on DSM-III. According to him, psychiatry lost its way because it narrowed psychiatrists' field of observation by enforcing top-down diagnostic templates on their clinical enquiry and practice. The specific field of trauma in psychiatry, however, had used bottom-up, narrative-based case identification before DSM-III with similar, and perhaps greater, error. As for McHugh's wider criticism about imposing a less than optimal template on research and practices, this is a generic DSM problem, indeed a generic research problem: research necessarily employs generalizations, whereas clinical practice is case-by-case. Generalizations, including the DSM PTSD template, should not prevent clinicians from seeing the particularities of each patient. The problem behind neglecting patients' particularities is not in the templates which clinicians across medical disciplines are trained to translate, but rather in the current industrialization of medicine which does not leave practitioners with enough time and intellectual space to exercise their art. The collusion of industrialized medicine and captivating, time-and-effort saving diagnostic templates (and, additionally, aggregate-based, algorithmic treatment guidelines) is where the problem lies. Against the pervasive effect of that collusion I have no problem joining McHugh.

Ben Shephard's *A War of Nerves* (29) traces the history of combat-related PTSD. He fairly describes a permanent tension between neurological or biological explanations (e.g. shell shock) and psychological or humanistic understanding. Arguably we are still working within that tension, struggling to align neurobiological research with interpersonal, social, and cultural moderators of post-traumatic illness.

What might perpetuate that tension is our trying to decide between the two, or our using simplistic correlational matrices to account for their interaction. A solution to the problem that Ben Shephard appropriately raises will involve stepping back from the current reductionist and mechanistic approach, and attempting to construe some of the subjective, interpersonal, and social aspects of traumatic stress responses as emergent properties of an underlying psychobiological complexity, unaccounted for by any computed combination of its elements. This view has been developed for understanding consciousness as an emergent property of the brain's activity (e.g. 30,31). It more directly addresses the dichotomy that Shephard alludes to. The extent to which the heuristics of emergence can help understanding psychological trauma is still an open question.

Finally, in an article in the *BMJ*, Summerfield (32) attacks the 'invention of PTSD' as being culturally biased, detracting resources from urgent needs in poorer, war-prone countries, and resulting 'as much from sociopolitical ideas as from psychiatric ones'. Summerfield's ideas do not come from nowhere. Doubts about the validity of PTSD, schizophrenia, psychotherapy, pharmacotherapy, and the rest are part of what one meets along the way. I am grateful for having had real patients, PTSD and others, whose unmistaken need for help forced me to work within doubts and operate despite uncertainties. They could not wait for conceptual clarity to illuminate the field.

Overstretching PTSD and trauma

Excesses by proponents of traumatic stress are also on record, including the predictable claims of miracle cure (e.g. the early eye movement desensitization and reprocessing publications) or miracle prevention of PTSD by a single session of critical incident stress debriefing.

The 'false memory' debate, however, was arguably the most destructive mishap in the history of PTSD. In this debate, the uncontested fact that some trauma survivors do not remember parts of their traumatic experiences was expanded to suggest that memories of childhood trauma, retrieved during psychotherapy, constitute factual and legally acceptable evidence of past abuse. Fiercely defended by some experts, therapy-reconstructed memories have been shown to be factually false in several instances, and the entire issue has been largely dropped, not without creating significant embarrassment.

Considered as challenging the accuracy of traumatic recall, studies also showed that developing PTSD could be associated with progressively endorsing more negative accounts of the traumatic event. Again, this is not surprising: memory is often affected by post-hoc attributions that modify the weights and saliencies of past events (e.g. 33). Recollections are also part of interpersonal communication and thus affected by assumptions about the listener, desirability of communicating, and subtle interpersonal perception. Recall is also influenced by affective states. Ultimately, traumatic recollections should be taken for what they are: context-, affect- and intent-dependent mental productions.

On the positive side, the false memory debate illustrates an interesting boundary in listening to trauma survivors. Even when true, trauma stories often evoke scepticism: they are told in the first person, most often without corroboration; they are emotional; and they challenge the listener's reasonable expectation and assumptive world as much as they had challenged those of the victim when the trauma unfolded. Trusting a traumatized survivor is often a matter of choice. Mothers may not believe their sexually abused daughters, commanders mistrust soldiers who break down. One of the features of trauma is that it 'cannot happen', or could not have happened.

The false memory episode shows how easy it is to be biased in the opposite direction—that is, in assuming trauma behind current symptoms. It should have served as a warning to practitioners and scientists ever since.

Recognizing the need to corroborate the occurrence of traumatic events, a secondary data analysis of the seminal National Vietnam Veterans Readjustment Study used military records to corroborate combat exposure (34). The results replicated the previous finding of significant (though somewhat smaller) prevalence of PTSD among combat veterans, found little bias in former self-reporting or exposure, and described a dose–response relationship between combat exposure and PTSD.

Biological underpinning

Uncovering the biological underpinning of mental disorders has been the dream of psychiatric researchers for generations. Compared with other mental disorders, PTSD was somewhat better positioned: the disorder has a salient onset and its symptoms can be traced to specific neurobiological systems such as stress response, memory, and learning. Previously referred to as 'physioneurosis' (4), PTSD it is associated with typical bodily responses (e.g. to trauma reminder, to sudden noise).

Reviewing the biological findings in PTSD is beyond the scope of this essay. This section briefly outlines core developments, focusing on the growing complexity of findings and their interpretation and on the rapid translation of biological hypotheses to interventions typical for this field.

Early biological studies of PTSD explored two biological components of stress response: (1) the HPA axis; and (2) adrenergic transmission.

HPA axis

In an initial success, neuroendocrine studies have shown lower levels of cortisol in PTSD and heightened sensitivity of the HPA axis. They also showed higher diurnal excretion of catecholamines in PTSD. However, the resulting aetiological explanation (e.g. too much adrenaline, not enough cortisol to control the initial stress response) was not corroborated by longitudinal studies, including from our laboratory. Notwithstanding, the cortisol hypothesis has led to clinical interventions designed to prevent PTSD by using cortisol shortly after a traumatic event. The results of these studies are too weak to allow conclusions. These are daring experiments based on the somewhat naive assumption that manipulating one of many response modulators may have enough power to affect the compounded outcome of several system's responses within powerful environmental response modulators.

Adrenergic response

Another biological candidate was the body's sympathetic or adrenergic response to trauma. Again the hypothesis was based on extensive, rather convincing animal studies: higher adrenergic drive was believed to enhance the acquisition of conditioned fear response that might explain the occurrence of PTSD. Our own finding of elevated heart rate response shortly after a trauma, and subsequent replications, supported the association between PTSD and strong initial response to traumatic events (although we could not find higher levels of norepinephrine shortly after trauma). As with the HPA axis hypothesis, this was quickly translated to human intervention, with four published studies attempting to prevent PTSD by the adrenergic inhibitor propranolol. These studies have failed.

For both cortisol and propranolol, the exact timing of prescribing might be critical. Administering propranolol more than 6 hours after the traumatic event (i.e. after the first memory consolidation) might be too late. The same may be true for cortisol—and for any early intervention. As in studies of stroke, the occurrence of PTSD may involve specific, time-dependent processes about which we must know in order to better tailor our interventions.

The fear conditioning theory of PTSD

The fear conditioning theory of PTSD received significant support from animal studies that have shown that conditioned fear-driven associations are indelibly stored in the amygdala; that their extinction involved a superimposition of cortical inhibition, that such extinction required new learning and can be blocked by interfering with that learning; and (lately) by interfering with the rewriting of memories after recall ('reconsolidation').

Each step in this discovery path led to human interventions. Strengthening cortical neuronal transmission during therapy of PTSD (by the use of D-cycloserine) was supposed to improve extinction learning by enhancing NMDA-based prefrontal processing. Propranolol was used in conjunction with trauma recall and tried as an anti-reconsolidation agent. Transcranial magnetic stimulation of the prefrontal area was evaluated as a means of strengthening extinction learning. Although it is much too early to decide if these studies can yield substantial results, they already constitute a salient example of hypothesis-driven translational interventions in psychiatry.

Brain imaging studies

Structural brain imaging studies of PTSD initially revealed an association between the disorder and a modest reduction in the volume of the hippocampus—a brain structure involved in the storage and maintenance of episodic (biographical) memories and indirectly in modulating emotional memories. Animal studies of hippocampal atrophy under stress provided a convenient explanatory model. Finding a smaller hippocampus in PTSD has been rather consistently replicated, but is also found in depression, schizophrenia, and other chronic mental disorders. Our own prospective study of hippocampal volume in PTSD (35) did not show a time-dependent reduction of the hippocampus. A corroborating twin study (36) has shown that smaller hippocampi characterize both PTSD patients and their identical twins and thus should be considered a risk factor for PTSD. With the advent of high-powered MRI we now recognize that changes to the hippocampus may involve specific subsets of that brain structure and thus our original approach was rather crude. Current studies can track white matter pathways and better explore PTSD-related networks. They also go beyond the diagnostic category of PTSD and explore neurocognitive dimensions that are shared by several disorders.

The sophistication of functional brain imaging studies of PTSD has grown with time. Early studies involved provocation tests. Subsequent studies used overt or subliminal stressful stimuli (e.g. fearful faces) to explore the fear system in PTSD. Current studies challenge networks, use neurocognitive tasks, and explore resting states and spontaneous brain activities. Current evidence points to excessive responses of the amygdala, abnormally weak engagement of regulatory prefrontal brain areas, and impaired context recognition and emotional regulation in PTSD.

Based on functional brain imaging studies, our view of PTSD has evolved from seeing it as fear imprinting and fear response disorder to conceiving it as related to deficient fear inhibition, emotional deregulation, or deficient contextual appraisal or brain connectivity. This is a remarkable and very dynamic development.

Treatment and management

As with other areas in psychiatry, therapies for PTSD seem to have reached a ceiling of efficacy, and failed to reduce the prevalence of mental disorders and associated morbidity. Not that nothing has changed. In 1996 we concluded a review of the treatment of PTSD (6) by stating that although several treatment protocols may reduce PTSD symptoms, their results are very limited indeed. Between 1996 and today several CBT protocols have been consistently shown to have significant beneficial effect on both chronic and acute PTSD. SSRIs have been approved for the treatment of PTSD. The effectiveness of eye movement desensitization and reprocessing (EMDR), the protocol of which currently includes many components of CBT, was similarly validated, and other psychotherapies (e.g. brief eclectic psychotherapy) were equally supported by evidence.

Limitations to implementing trauma-focused CBT and other forms of individual therapies include their relative high cost, limited effectiveness, high dropout rate, and the requirements for the patient's commitment. These therapies are virtually absent in war- and disaster-prone areas, and the cost of their systematic implementation, even in modern facilities, is prohibitive (37). Current efforts mainly involve dissemination (e.g. CBT in the armed forces and health care systems for veterans), simplification (shorter protocols), and translation to web-based therapies. Less demanding interventions, such as stress management or need-based supportive interventions, have limited effect on PTSD, though they might mitigate its occurrence. Thus, we know much more about therapies now, but we mainly know how limited is our capacity to provide effective and efficient treatment for PTSD.

The next steps?

Prediction is a deeply embedded neurocognitive function. Proper prophecy, however, is a risky endeavour. The field of traumatic stress will probably evolve with the rest of psychiatry, trying to position itself within the uncompromising paradox of, on the one hand, having to be practical and provide for patients, while beset by serious doubts about its own taxonomy, diagnostic entities, and its failure to properly articulate social and interpersonal dimensions of mental illnesses and their expressions.

On the horizon are attempts to replace the current disorder-based classification by a dimensional grid, cutting across disorders. PTSD is perhaps best placed to incorporate the proposed research domain criteria (RDoC), or any other dimensionality, into its research and practice. In fact, there are already several attempts to treat PTSD by addressing the underlying neurocognitive dimension (e.g. the Tel-Aviv University/NIMH 'attention bias modification treatment' or Amit Etkin's training of emotion regulatory circuits).

Similarly, a growing sophistication of computational models should uncover functional networks (e.g. in genetics, CNS activity) and within such networks critical nodes that govern disease process and persistence. The rapidly improving understanding of gene-expression modulators may similarly improve our understanding of top-down, environment-to-neuron pathogenesis of PTSD. Some of that sophistication should also be used in descriptive studies of responses to trauma, to get us away from narrowly using the PTSD template as the sole or the most salient outcome of trauma.

One should also hope that treatment studies, and particularly those involving pharmacological agents, will successfully implement truly novel compounds. However, for that to happen we must, among other changes, cease using sample averages as the sole criterion for licensing new compounds, and have more respect for response heterogeneity.

A point of particular interest is the ongoing move from studying immutable risk factors (such as polymorphic DNA loci) to better understanding of genetic modulatory processes (such as DNA or RNA expression modulators), some of which are clearly affected by early life events, and possibly during traumatic events and their aftermath. Current biology seems to be getting the outside world back into the game of creating vulnerability for, defining, and modulating disease trajectories in trauma and other mental disorders. The few existing publications about gene–environment effects in the aetiology of PTSD may open the gate to better articulating the host–environment interaction that is at the core of developing and maintaining traumatic stress responses.

All this is not far from where psychiatry is now. One can predict, therefore, that mental trauma will remain within psychiatry, having a diagnostic category for itself or otherwise. Because psychic trauma is still the core category with mandatory linkage to life events, one can hope that studies of traumatic stress disorders will help to reintroduce real life into psychiatry.

A personal note

As young psychiatrist, upon examining combat veterans after the 1982 Lebanon war, the first combat stress casualty to enter my office was my best mate from high school. Here, but for the Grace of the Lord, went I: I had served in that and other wars as field surgeon, had first-person experience of fear and of what still makes me sick—distorted human bodies. I was there in the critical role of saving others' lives and, luckily, was as skilful as the situation required and was never altogether defeated. I remained irritable after wars but never had PTSD. I joined the group of PTSD researchers as soon as I was discharged from the Israel Defense Force's Mental Health division, in 1998.

Getting back to 'what it was like' to be in the thick of the action while the PTSD agenda was unfolding is a somewhat unusual exercise. Initially, this was an open field and few professionals were in it. I was curious, the questions were fundamental, and I was well placed to address some of them, having left military psychiatry to work in an academic hospital. Repeated terrorist attacks in Jerusalem provided, over the years, more freshly traumatized survivors than we could handle. Indeed, my first stab at publishing on trauma was a description of survivors of a terrorist attack on a bus between Tel-Aviv to Jerusalem. I soon realized that trauma more frequently occurs in mundane daily incidents, such as road traffic accidents, family violence, or rape. Injuring your child in a road traffic accident in which you were the driver is nothing less than total personal disaster. I opted to focus on the very early stages of trauma response—those instances that can, in one blow, change people's lives forever. What convinced me that PTSD actually existed were those survivors who came to our Emergency Department from sites of traumatic incidents, dressed and mannered as they were before the event, whom I saw transformed into fearful, irritable, besieged, and defeated men and women.

Sceptical by constitution, I felt that I had to generate my own evidence about the veracity of PTSD. Thus in our first early trauma studies my group and I simply documented symptoms and symptom progression and attempted to provide therapy. The failure to even scratch the disorder's trajectory with love and care, meaning-driven, open-ended, dynamic, and interpersonal therapies, in which I was versed, meant that the problem was serious indeed, and not amenable to intuitive improvisations. We tried benzodiazepines that had been recommended for their capacity to tame stress response, and our patients got worse. Then, guided by our friends and colleagues, we successively evaluated physiological, neuroendocrine, brain imaging, and ultimately gene expression predictors of PTSD and trajectory modulators. We discovered, and carefully introduced, novelty to the field of traumatic stress—and that was fun. The other fun part was the privilege of fully expressing polite intolerance to nonsense and false pretence—such as the debriefing agenda, the false memory shambles, blinded belief in medication, and some pretentious biological claims. I empirically tested common beliefs and had a record of publishing negative studies: no shrinkage of the hippocampus in PTSD; neither higher nor lower cortisol or norepinephrine before PTSD; negative effect of benzodiazepines; null preventive effect of SSRIs; non-specificity of early PTSD symptoms (though high sensitivity), etc. I encountered many distinguished colleagues and made lifelong friends.

More recently I was privileged to be involved in treatment research and early prevention of PTSD. With my group we could show a significant and lasting effect of CBT on early symptom trajectories and rule out a potential effect of SSRIs. Because we lived, at the time, in a terror-prone country, our contribution to prevention was particularly gratifying: at last we were directly providing, and tasting the essential challenge of touching and eventually reducing the suffering of fellow men and women.

So how was it to be a trauma researcher all those years? I don't know. I am still in that milieu. I think that humble honesty is a way to do sound research. Too much money is poured on loosely defined, over-pretentious studies. The core questions are simple and need to be squarely asked. Survivors agree to participate in studies when they perceive honest intent. We need (i.e. our patients need) more research: current therapies have reached a low ceiling of efficacy. Our object-like diagnoses—including PTSD—are a burden now. Maybe that should change. Maybe we should generate and use data to redraw the map of mental disorders.

Yet, the greatest pleasure was to see a growing stream of young, brilliant neuroscientists and geneticists fascinated by the agenda of traumatic stress responses. Having created such interest, perhaps my generation of researchers has done its bit. Now we must take care to see that the magnificent next generation of researchers gets from us, who were privileged and who carried the responsibility of having defined and promoted PTSD and trauma in psychiatry, a better phenotype and better questions commensurate with their readiness and potential. I would encourage them to produce the necessary evidence to productively dismantle the construct of PTSD and offer alternatives. For one: we use rating scales in a simple additive way (i.e. by summing up individual items' score), whereas under varying circumstances, symptom items have different weights. The same goes for evaluating neural activity, or, for that matter, gene expression. Contextual weighting of what, for lack of better computational tools, we were constrained to measure linearly, could become what Jacques Barzun has called the 'glorious entertainment' of the new generation of scientists.

Unfortunately for my PTSD patients, much of the above is quite theoretical indeed. I find it harder not to share their impatience to see a change. Many have been through several treatment attempts and endlessly receive polydrug therapy. Presumably one way to go is to, transiently, leave aside curative pretence and focus on rehabilitation. Ultimately one has to admit that PTSD is currently a disorder that, in its chronic phase, can sometimes be stabilized but rarely cured. All this calls for more emphasis on secondary prevention and early interventions. This is my personal agenda for the future.

Acknowledgement

Work supported by successive US Public Health Service/NIMH grants during the years 1997–2012.

References

1 Trimble, M. R. (1981). *Post-traumatic neurosis. From railway spine to the whiplash.* Chichester: John Wiley and Sons.

2 Grinker, R. R. and Spiegel, J. P. (1945). *Men under stress.* Philadelphia: Backiston.

3 Kardiner, A. (1941). *The traumatic neuroses of war.* New York: Hoeber.

4 Kardiner, A. (1959). Traumatic neuroses of war. In: Arieti, S. (ed.) *American handbook of psychiatry.* New York: Basic Books, pp. 245–57.

5 McHugh, P. R. and Treisman, G. (2007). PTSD: A problematic diagnostic category. *Journal of Anxiety Disorders* 21, 211–22.

6 Shalev, A. Y., Bonne, O., and Eth, S. (1996). Treatment of the post-traumatic stress disorder. *Psychosomatic Medicine* 58, 165–82.

7 Mott, F. W. (1917). Mental hygiene in shell-shock, during and after the war. *British Journal of Psychiatry* 63, 467–88.

8 Rivers, W. H. R. (1918). The repression of war experiences. *Proceedings of the Royal Society of Medicine (Section of Psychiatry)* 11, 1–20.

9 Bryant, R. A., Mastrodomenico, J., Felmingham K. L. et al. (2008). Treatment of acute stress disorder: a randomized controlled trial. *Archives of General Psychiatry* **65**, 659–67.

10 Shalev, A. Y., Ankri, Y., Israeli-Shalev, Y. et al. (2012). Prevention of PTSD by early treatment: results from the Jerusalem Trauma Outreach and Prevention Study. *Archives of General Psychiatry* **69**, 166–72.

11 Solomon, Z, Shklar, R, and Mikulincer, M. (2005). Frontline treatment of combat stress reaction: a 20-year longitudinal evaluation study. *American Journal of Psychiatry* **162**, 2309–14.

12 Jones, E. and Wessely, S. (2003) 'Forward psychiatry' in the military: its origins and effectiveness. *Journal of Traumatic Stress* **16**, 411–19.

13 Bourne, P. G. (1978). Military psychiatry and the Viet Nam war in perspective. In: Bourne P.G. (ed.) *The psychology and physiology of stress*, New York: Academic Press, pp. 219–36.

14 McNally, R. (2012). Are we winning the war against posttraumatic stress disorder? *Science* **336**, 872–3.

15 Resick, P. A., Bovin, M. J., Calloway, A. L. et al. (2012). A critical evaluation of the complex PTSD literature: implications for DSM-5. *Journal of Traumatic Stress* **25**, 241–51.

16 Bryant, R. A. (2012). Simplifying complex PTSD: comment on Resick. *Journal of Traumatic Stress* **25**, 252–3.

17 Shalev, A. Y., Galai, T., and Eth, S. (1993). 'Levels of trauma': multidimensional approach to the psychotherapy of PTSD. *Psychiatry* **56**, 166–77.

18 Pitman, R. K., Orr, S. P., Forgue, D. F., de Jong, J. B., and Claiborn, J. M. (1987). Psychophysiology of PTSD imagery in Vietnam combat veterans. *Archives of General Psychiatry* **44**, 970–5.

19 Blake, D. D., Weathers, F. W., Nagy, L. M., et al. (1995). The development of a clinician-administered PTSD scale. *Journal of Traumatic Stress* **8**, 75–90.

20 Keane, M. T. Fairbank, A. J. Caddell, M. J., and Zimmering, T. R. (1989) Implosive (flooding) therapy reduces symptoms of PTSD in Vietnam combat veterans. *Behavior Therapy* **20**, 245–60.

21 McFarlane, A. (1988) The longitudinal course of posttraumatic morbidity: the range of outcomes and their predictors. *Journal of Nervous and Mental Disease* **176**, 30–9.

22 Kessler, R. C., Sonnega, A., Bromet, E. J., Hughes, M., and Nelson, C. B. (1995) Posttraumatic stress disorder in the National Comorbidity Survey. *Archives of General Psychiatry* **52**, 1048–60.

23 Breslau, N., Kessler, R. C., Chilcoat, H. D. et al. (1998) Trauma and posttraumatic stress disorder in the community: the 1996 Detroit Area Survey of Trauma. *Archives of General Psychiatry* **55**, 626–32.

24 Bremner, J. D., Randall, P., Scott, T. M., et al., (1995), MRI-based measurement of hippocampal volume in patients with combat-related posttraumatic stress disorder. *American Journal of Psychiatry* **152**, 973–81.

25 LeDoux, J. E., Romanski, L., and Xagoraris, A. (1989). Indelibility of subcortical emotional networks. *Journal of Cognitive Neuroscience* **1**, 238–43.

26 Shalev, A. Y., Gilboa, A, and Rassmusson, A. (2011) Neurobiology of PTSD. In: Stein, D. J., Friedman, M., Blanco, C. (eds.) *Post-traumatic stress disorder*. Hoboken, NJ: John Wiley and Sons.

27 Young, A. (1997). *The harmony of illusion: inventing post-traumatic stress disorder.* Princeton, NJ: Princeton University Press.

28 McHugh, P. R. (1999). How psychiatry lost its way. *Commentary* **108**, 32–8.

29 Shephard, B. (2001). *A war of nerves: soldiers and psychiatrists in the twentieth century.* Cambridge, MA: Harvard University Press.

30 Sperry, R. W. (1969). A modified concept of consciousness. *Psychological Review* **76**, 532–6.

31 Feinberg, T. E. (2012). Neuroontology, neurobiological naturalism, and consciousness: a challenge to scientific reduction and a solution. *Physics of Life Reviews* **9**, 13–34.

32 Summerfield, D. (2001). The invention of post-traumatic stress disorder and the social usefulness of a psychiatric category. *BMJ* **322**, 95–8.

33 Slovic, P., Finucane, M., Peters, E., and MacGregor, D. G. (2002). The affect heuristic. In: Gilovich, T., Griffin, D., and Kahneman, D. (eds) *Heuristics and biases: the psychology of intuitive judgment.* Cambridge: Cambridge University Press, pp. 397–420.

34 Dohrenwend, B. P., Turner, J. B., Turse, N. A. et al. (2006). The psychological risks of Vietnam for U.S. veterans: a revisit with new data and methods. *Science* **313**, 979–82.

35 Bonne, O., Brandes, D., and Gilboa, A. (2001). Longitudinal MRI study of hippocampal volume in trauma survivors with PTSD. *American Journal of Psychiatry* **158**, 1248–51.

36 Gilbertson, M. W., Shenton, M. E., Ciszewski A. et al. (2002). Smaller hippocampal volume predicts pathologic vulnerability to psychological trauma. Nature Neuroscience **5**, 1242–730.

37 Shalev, A. Y., Ankri, Y., Peleg, T., Israeli-Shalev, Y., and Freedman, S. (2011). Barriers to receiving early care for post-traumatic stress disorder (PTSD): Results from the Jerusalem Trauma Outreach and Prevention Study (J-TOPS). *Psychiatric Services* **62**, 765–73.

Psychiatry and the addictions

Jerome H. Jaffe

Introduction

The relationship of psychiatry to the addictions has been intertwined over the years with society's changing attitudes and responses towards psychoactive substances and the people who use them. These responses affect their availability, cost, and the consequences of their use, the likelihood of becoming dependent (addicted), the treatments and research permitted or supported, and the role of the health professions. How they deal with the problem is also determined by how they are paid, how much autonomy they have in deciding which patients to accept and which methods to use, and how generously the country supports research. This essay focuses mainly on the United States and on the role of psychiatrists in relation to alcohol and drug problems. However, the field of addictions is a broad and interdisciplinary enterprise not limited to psychiatrists, but including a wide range of professionals whose research and clinical activities shape the way the problems are understood and treated. I shall consider three broad categories of drugs whose different patterns of use have led to very different levels of social concern, investment in research, and regulatory control: alcohol; the 'illicit' drugs—opiates, cocaine, and cannabis; and tobacco/nicotine. It covers selectively major developments in the second half of the 20th century and their influence on psychiatry. Furthermore, it needs to be emphasized that psychiatrists typically function within an interdisciplinary context involving psychologists, social workers, sociologists, epidemiologists, and pharmacologists. Thus, while the essay is nominally aimed at the history of psychiatry and the addictions, it is of necessity the story of an interdisciplinary endeavour.

In the mid-20th century, American psychiatry had a simple view of the multifaceted problems associated with the misuse of alcohol, illicit drugs, and tobacco. Addiction to alcohol was seen as a manifestation of underlying psychic conflict; addiction to drugs in the second category (opiates, cocaine, etc.) as part of a character disorder best left to the law; and use of tobacco as not at all relevant to psychiatry. In keeping with their placement in the first and second editions of the American Psychiatric Association's (APA) *Diagnostic and Statistical Manual* (DSM), discussion about alcohol and 'illicit' drugs in major American textbooks was found in sections with titles such as 'Psychopathic conditions, deviations, addictions.' Discussion of tobacco did not appear at all. Over the second half of the 20th century, the problematic use of the three categories became important concerns for psychiatry at different times. It was not until the 1980s, however, that all three came to be regarded as appropriate subject matter for the profession.

The mid-20th century

Drugs in the spotlight

Perhaps the most significant events leading to when and why addictions eventually became more important to psychiatry were the epidemics of drug use that emerged following World War II. Starting in the late 1940s, cannabis and heroin use began to rise among young people. It seems probable that increased availability was seen first in the United States because of its relative affluence, and the persistence of organized crime that had developed earlier during the prohibition years. Consistent with its punitive approach to illicit drug use, the United States passed laws in 1951 and 1956 that mandated progressively more severe criminal penalties for the sale or possession of opiates (especially heroin), cocaine, and cannabis. Nevertheless, their use continued to increase.

At the same time, cannabis use mounted in the United Kingdom, but the response to it was less punitive than in the United States. In Japan, an epidemic of methamphetamine use occurred following the release of military stores of the drug for general sale; this led to a sharp tightening of anti-drug laws coupled with compulsory treatment in psychiatric hospitals of methamphetamine users. Sweden also experienced an epidemic of amphetamine use, fuelled largely by some physicians who prescribed liberally. But generally, in Europe, Scandinavia, and Australia, alcohol was the dominant substance of abuse.

Whether the recognition that a predominantly criminal justice response to illicit drug use was not sufficient to stem the tide or reluctance to see penalties applied to non-minority users from 'good' families, reliance on a punitive approach had begun to decline by the late 1950s (1). An alternative to a criminal justice response was to view opiate addiction as an illness that needed a medical or public health approach. But the medical profession, and psychiatry in particular, was not well placed to take on the role. There was little interest in addictions within mainstream psychiatry, which was dominated by psychoanalysis. Psychiatrists interested in addictions were often viewed as 'odd' and risked sharing the stigma attached to patients they were trying to help. At most medical schools and hospitals, psychiatrists had minimal or no contact with addicted patients and a scanty interest in people dependent on alcohol. The typical American medical school curriculum allowed for only an hour of teaching on substance abuse, usually as part of pharmacology. The situation in the United Kingdom and Australia was not dissimilar.

In the United States, patients seeking treatment for addiction to opiates, cocaine or cannabis could find it only at a few state psychiatric hospitals or Public Health Service (PHS) hospitals. While nominally under the direction of psychiatrists, the PHS hospitals at two major centres in Kentucky and Texas were also prisons housing federal offenders convicted for drug-related crimes. Both the prisoners and the voluntarily admitted patients received the same kinds of milieu and group therapy conducted by psychiatrists and psychologists. The approach used was based on a psychodynamic understanding of underlying motives. Treatment after withdrawal was expected to last for about 6 months. Despite the belief based on patient histories and re-admissions that relapse was far more common than lasting remission, the approach to treatment persisted well into the 1960s (2).

Several physicians who made notable contributions to the understanding and treatment of the addictions (for example, Marie Lysander, Jerome Jaffe, George Vaillant, Herbert Kleberg, and Frederick Glaser) received part of their psychiatry training at the Lexington PHS hospital in the 1950s and 1960s. Clinicians and policymakers in the United States and elsewhere who would influence the development of addiction psychiatry including scientific research (among them Vincent Dole and Griffith Edwards), began their work with a visit to Lexington and its addiction research centre (ARC).

Located on the same campus as the hospital and prison, but administratively distinct, the ARC was at that time one of only three interdisciplinary research facilities worldwide dedicated to the study of addiction disorders. The Alcohol Research Foundation of Ontario and the Yale Center for Alcohol Studies were the other two. The contributions of ARC researchers in the 1950s were monumental, including the demonstration of the utility of methadone in managing opiate withdrawal; that abrupt withdrawal of barbiturates resulted in convulsions and a syndrome resembling delirium tremens (DTs); and that DTs and 'rum fits' were manifestations of alcohol withdrawal and not a form of alcohol toxicity or due to malnutrition. The finding that allophone, an opiate antagonist, could precipitate signs of withdrawal after only a few days' exposure to opiate use implied that the biological process then called physical dependence was probably ushered in with first few doses.

The work of Abraham Winkler, chief psychiatrist at the ARC, was of considerable significance for addiction psychiatry. Starting in 1955, he elaborated an alternative to the psychoanalytic view that addiction was a feature of an underlying personality problem. His model emphasized the consequences of drug-using behaviour (operant reinforcement) and the role of classical conditioning in relapse (3). These ideas evolved into a behaviourist view of the genesis and course of the addictions, and laid the foundation for an emphasis on relapse prevention, and to a reworking of the previously held psychodynamic model.

Any history of the interface of addiction and psychiatry must take note of the burgeoning studies of psychopharmacology in the 1950s. The impact of new drug treatment of the seriously mentally ill stirred the US Congress, in 1956, to fund a centre within the National Institute of Mental Health (NIMH) to stimulate research. Jonathan Cole, a psychiatrist recruited to head the new centre, interpreted his mission broadly and allocated research funds on addiction as well. This was the chief source of the modest support for research carried on outside of the ARC until the mid-1960s. By 1960, there were enough clinicians and researchers to form a new interdisciplinary society, the American College of Neuropsychopharmacology (ACNP). Psychiatrists with an interest in addiction who had been outside mainstream psychiatry were then welcomed by the new organization. Among its founding members were Jonathan Cole, Henry Brill, Alfred Freedman, Daniel X. Freedman, and Louis Jolyon West. The latter three became chairmen of university departments of psychiatry where addiction research and treatment would be a major focus. ACNP founders also included internal medicine specialists like Harris Isbell and Leo Hollister, and behavioural psychologist Joseph Brady, all major figures in shaping both research and treatment. Isbell served as director of the ARC while Hollister carried out pioneering clinical work on sedative dependence. Brady, and his students Charles R. Schuster and Travis Thompson, were among the first to use animal models of drug self-administration. Brill and Cole were also members of the National Academy of Science's research group on addiction which organized the first interdisciplinary meetings dealing with the full range of addictions. The group later was converted into a freestanding membership organization, the College on Problems of Drug Dependence (CPDD), for addiction researchers.

Drugs, crime and treatment: new trends

In the early 1960s it was left to individual states in the United States to decide how addicted people wanting treatment could obtain it; there was no national policy. As public concern began to focus on the growing numbers of heroin users and to perceive that this was directly linked to an increase of crime, states (and some cities) devised various ways to deal with the problem. For example, California instituted as part of the Department of Corrections civil commitment (compulsory treatment) of narcotic addicts; this mandated incarceration for a year in a secure facility. Several state mental hospitals began to admit opiate addicts to specialized wards but most of them had little interest in participating in psychotherapy and left soon after being detoxified. By 1965, New York also had instituted a period of compulsory treatment under the aegis of a special commission. The federal government followed suit a year later with legislation establishing a nationwide civil commitment programme—the Narcotic Addict Rehabilitation Act (NARA). Addicts deemed suitable for treatment were sent to the PHS hospitals at Lexington, Kentucky and Fort Worth, Texas for 6 months followed by counselling based in the community. An ironic aspect of the hospital-based programmes is that they were undertaken at the same time that follow-up studies of patients treated at Lexington showed a 90% rate of relapse to opiates within a year of discharge. The legislation that created NARA also contained funding to establish treatment programmes in the community; several were awarded to psychiatrists based at state departments of mental health (e.g. Connecticut and Missouri) or at medical schools. The principal investigators of two projects (Kleber at Yale and Jaffe at the University of Chicago) had trained at Lexington (4).

Three other kinds of treatment emerged during this period: therapeutic communities, methadone maintenance, and the use of narcotic antagonists. The therapeutic community movement, which expanded in the 1960s, was modelled on Synanon, an organization created and directed by Charles Dederich, a former alcoholic himself. Synanon demonstrated that under certain conditions people who had been addicted to heroin could become, and remain, drug free, crime free, and self-supporting. The organization was pointedly anti-professional and particularly disdainful of psychiatrists. Its confrontational methods were unlike anything then used by mainstream psychiatry. Yet, several of the 'second-generation' therapeutic communities, part of an expansion of this approach to treatment, were started by psychiatrists (e.g. Mitchell Rosenthal at Phoenix House and Julianne Densen-Gerber at Odyssey House). Interestingly, most clinical activities in the initial phase were carried out by abstinent former heroin users who had acquired their experience in Synanon or a similar centre.

Perhaps more significant for psychiatry and addiction in the 1960s was the launch of methadone maintenance treatment by Vincent Dole and Marie Lysander. Dole was an expert in metabolism at the Rockefeller University, Lysander a psychiatrist who had trained at Lexington and then treated heroin-addicted patients in New York. They reported in 1965 that heroin addicts who had been refractory to previous attempts at treatment could be stabilized on single daily doses of oral methadone and pursue law-abiding and productive lives. The dramatic changes in these patients led Dole and Lysander to postulate that addicts suffered from an inherent or acquired metabolic disorder, and that behaviours previously regarded as personality problems were engendered by the need to get the upload (heroin) (5). Nonetheless, their use of an opiate drug (methadone) to treat heroin addiction was sharply criticized by many professionals, including psychiatrists, who had pursued other approaches to treatment.

Methadone maintenance did not require the participation of psychiatrists, and was soon adopted by physicians in other specialties. Within a decade the widespread establishment of methadone programmes greatly affected the attitudes of those in medicine and psychiatry to the treatment of heroin addiction and they promoted the interests of the latter in the addictions.

At about the same time, a few researchers, including psychiatrists, were exploring the use of opiate antagonists and testing the ideas of Abraham Wikler and William Martin, the latter a pharmacologist who succeeded Isbell as director of the ARC, concerning extinction of reinforced behaviours and conditioned withdrawal. The antagonists then available (e.g. cyclosporine) were never widely adopted, but a less problematic antagonist (naltrexone) was under development at the ARC that later had a crucial place in treating both alcoholism and opioid addiction.

The role of psychiatry in the delivery of these treatments varied widely. Some required the participation of a physician, but not necessarily a psychiatrist. However, linking addiction treatment clinics to academic departments of psychiatry was important in bringing the addictions into the medical school curriculum and thus exposing medical students and trainees to emerging ideas in addiction science, and encouraging more psychiatrists to become addiction specialists. Two such programmes, at the University of Chicago and Yale University, compared different ways of treating opiate addiction and demonstrated that they were complementary and could be combined as part of a multimodal approach (4).

Youth, drugs, policy, progress

As the 'baby boomers', the large generation born in the immediate post-war years, reached their teens in the 1960s, there was a general rise in the incidence of non-medical drug use. Cannabis use became progressively more common. Many young people experimented with the hallucinogen lysergic acid diethyalamide (LSD), others with amphetamines, and a minority with heroin. Many adopted non-traditional, 'anti-establishment' lifestyles. Drug use was also linked with political protest about the Vietnam war. An upsurge in amphetamine use, much of it by injection, was, in part, a result of overprescribing by medical practitioners of the injectable form.

The rise of cannabis use in the United States was also paralleled in the United Kingdom, Sweden, and several other western European countries, Canada, Australia,

India, and Hong Kong (1). Increased heroin use in the United Kingdom was fuelled by physicians who prescribed it liberally for addicts. Until the late 1960s, they were legally permitted to prescribe any opiate (as well as cocaine) to any patient, including those addicted to opiates (known as the British system). Although the number of new heroin addicts was still small, there was a sharp rise in heroin use and associated deaths through overdose. This led Lord Brain (a distinguished neurologist) and his colleagues, members of a specially appointed government committee, to recommend, in 1965, the licensing of doctors to prescribe heroin or cocaine, specialized clinics for heroin addicts, reporting of addicts to the Home Office (the ministry responsible for internal affairs), more research into addiction, and setting up an advisory body to oversee and coordinate the government response to addiction (6).

The epidemics of amphetamine use enabled Western countries to learn what the Japanese had earlier so clearly observed: amphetamine and similar drugs could induce a psychosis resembling acute schizophrenia. Some observers believe that the general increase in illicit drug use in so many countries in the 1960s was linked to young drug-using Americans, whose relative affluence allowed them to travel widely, bringing their drug use and lifestyle with them (1).

By the late 1960s, addiction research was deemed to be worthy of funding. In the United Kingdom, Griffith Edwards established the Addiction Research Unit at the Institute of Psychiatry in London, the fourth interdisciplinary group dedicated to such research. In Canada, the Alcohol Research Foundation of Ontario changed its name to the Alcohol and Drug Research Foundation to reflect an expanded focus (still later becoming the Addiction Research Foundation).

Alcohol's parallel story

In the 1950s, the disease model of alcoholism in the United States had not yet completely replaced the moral model. Consequently, the treatment of alcoholic patients varied widely, depending on their socioeconomic status and circle of contacts. A few consulted psychiatrists; some received treatment in private hospitals, while others went to state mental hospitals that contained specialized units; some were admitted to general hospital psychiatry units. The few outpatient psychiatric clinics utilized a psychodynamic model. By contrast, others were arrested for public drunkenness and taken by the local police to dry out in 'drunk tanks'. A major force in promoting the disease concept of alcoholism and in changing the treatment of alcoholics was the growth of Alcoholics Anonymous (AA), formally founded in the United States in 1939. Proponents of AA viewed alcoholism as a distinct disorder, rather than as a manifestation of an unconscious conflict, and believed that recovery could be best achieved by following the '12 steps'. This perspective differed radically from the dominant psychodynamic model practiced by most psychiatrists. By the 1950s, AA members had persuaded a number of local hospitals to admit alcoholic patients for detoxification, established several rehabilitation houses operated along 12-step principles, and convinced programmes operating in some state hospitals to adopt the 12-step model using multidisciplinary teams (the Minnesota Model, named after the state where the approach was first used—at Willmar State Hospital) (7).

Psychiatrists played a central role in the 1950s and 1960s in the research leading to more effective medications for managing withdrawal; their adoption reduced the frequency of DTs and mortality associated with it. In practice, most patients admitted to publicly supported local hospitals were only treated for withdrawal and then discharged. However, the 1950s can be said to mark the beginning of a new area of specialization—addiction medicine—when physicians interested in treating alcoholism, many of whom were themselves 'in recovery', formed an organization that later evolved into the American Society on Alcoholism, and still later into the American Society of Addiction Medicine (ASAM) (7).

At the Yale Center for Alcohol Studies, E. M. Jellinek, who was not a physician, conducted his work with the help of AA members. During the 1950s, Jellinek had exerted considerable influence on the World Health Organization (WHO) Expert Committee on Mental Health, advocating for treatment for alcoholism. In keeping with his views on phases of alcoholism, he argued that most cases could be treated as outpatients. Viewing alcoholism as a disease would increase the access of those who needed help to established medical facilities. In his classic study, *The Disease Concept of Alcoholism*, published in 1960, he concluded that there were five 'species' of alcoholism; two of them, *delta* and *gamma*, involved increased tissue tolerance and withdrawal symptoms and could be regarded as addictive diseases. From a current perspective, Jellinek was prescient when he observed, 'By adhering strictly to our American ideas about 'alcoholism' (created by AA in their own image) and restricting the term to these ideas, we have been continuing to overlook many other problems of alcohol which need urgent attention' (8).

American psychiatry was not quick to respond to the need for alcoholism treatment or to the growth of AA and its view of alcoholism as a distinct disorder. In DSM-II (1968), the continued placement of alcoholism and drug addiction within 'psychopathic conditions' implied that they both were aspects of a character defect. Well into the early 1960s the dominant perspective of mainstream psychiatry was to see alcoholism and drug use as symptoms of an underlying unconscious conflict to be treated with traditional psychodynamic, uncovering-type therapies, or with periods of prolonged institutional treatment. George Vaillant wrote of his own psychiatric training at a leading American teaching hospital that there might as well have been a sign over the door reading 'Alcoholic patients need not apply' (9).

In Britain, in the 1950s and early 1960s, the National Health Service (NHS) had shown relatively little interest in alcoholism and related problems. Much of the care for persons with alcoholism was provided by churches, AA, and other non-psychiatric services. Psychiatry had neglected the problem. However, two NHS centres, one at the Maudsley Hospital and the other at Warlingham Park, did take a keen interest. Under the leadership of Max Glatt, the latter group reported good results from group therapy carried out over 12 weeks in a specialized psychiatric inpatient unit. This report influenced a 1962 NHS recommendation for setting up additional specialized inpatient units and utilizing group therapy, with a minor mention of the need for outpatient clinics and for cooperation with AA (which had established itself in the United Kingdom soon after the war.) By 1968 there were 13 such inpatient units, and these continued to increase (21 by 1975). Influenced by a 1966 study by Edwards and Guthrie, a 1968

Ministry of Health memorandum gave more recognition to outpatient care, noting that experts had found that it could be as helpful as inpatient treatment (10).

The 1970s

Drugs and alcohol a little closer together

In the United States in the 1970s, drug addiction and alcoholism were growing areas of interest within psychiatry, paralleling their increased visibility in society and political importance, and the availability of federal funding for treatment and research. It was a decade of explosive growth of treatment programmes and addiction-related science, following the establishment of the National Institute of Alcohol Abuse and Alcoholism (NIAAA) in 1970. Its creation was largely the work of Senator Harold Hughes who, as a recovered alcoholic, had championed the need to understand the causes of alcoholism and to provide necessary treatment. According to William White, NIAAA was evidence of the power of 'alcoholism constituencies' who wished to see alcoholism separated from mental health and recognized as 'a disease and public health problem in its own right. . . .' The NIAAA's mission was to expand both research and treatment and this it did successfully. Alcoholism treatment programmes expanded from about 500 in 1973 to 2400 by 1977 and 4219 by 1980 (7).

The following year, in response to continuing escalation of heroin use and crime and reports of heroin use among servicemen in Vietnam, President Richard Nixon established a Special Action Office for Drug Abuse Prevention (SAODAP) within the Executive Office of the President and gave it authority to coordinate activities in all federal agencies dealing with the 'demand side' of the drug problem—research, prevention, training, and treatment. He appointed a psychiatrist (this writer), to head the office (7). Among the staff and consultants to SAODAP were John Kramer, Peter Bourne, Benny Primm, John Ball, Vincent Nowlis, Jack Mendelson (a Harvard professor of psychiatry who had served as the first director of the NIMH Center for Alcohol Studies), Nancy Mello, and Roger Meyer. Resources for the relevant federal agencies were increased to historically unprecedented levels, two-thirds going to research, treatment and related activities, and the rest to law enforcement (11). SAODAP legislation included a provision for the later creation of a National Institute on Drug Abuse (NIDA) to give 'block grants' to each of the states for treatment and prevention activities.

Over the next 2 years SAODAP established a framework for regulation and support of methadone treatment programmes and increased grants for a wide range of treatments including therapeutic communities and outpatient clinics. From 1971 to 1973, federally funded drug abuse treatment programmes went from 54 to 214; by 1975 there were more than 1800 (7). The emphasis was on heroin addiction, but programmes for youthful poly-drug users were not ignored. There was also generous support for epidemiology, treatment evaluation, and basic science research related to addiction. The 'Career Teachers' programme provided grants to medical schools to integrate teaching about addiction into the curriculum. Any physician could be a teacher eligible for support and the programme did as much to foster the field of addiction medicine as addiction psychiatry.

Over the period from 1970 to 1980, key advisors on drug problems to Presidents Nixon, Ford, and Carter, (Jerome Jaffe, Robert DuPont, and Peter Bourne), as well as the first directors of NIAAA (Morris Chafetz, Robert Morse, and Ernest Noble) and NIDA (Robert DuPont and William Pollin) were psychiatrists. Although sound arguments were made for a single institute to deal with alcohol and other drugs, there was little possibility for this given the political forces at play.

The continuing increase in cannabis use among adolescents and young adults in the early 1970s was such a concern that governmental commissions in the United States (two members, Henry Brill and Thomas Ungerleider, were psychiatrists), the United Kingdom, and Canada (Heinz Lehman was the single psychiatrist), reviewed the appropriateness of the then prevailing criminal statutes in term of its use and possession. While these efforts were not formally coordinated, all three commissions advised some form of decriminalization; the recommendations in each case were rejected by political decision-makers. By contrast, a 1979 Australian commission, composed of a single judge, called for retention of criminal penalties. At the time, scientific evidence for cannabis dependence was sparse and very few users sought treatment.

At this time in the United States treatment programmes for drug addiction were for the most part separate from those for alcoholism. 'Alcoholics' did not want to be grouped with 'drug addicts'. AA groups wished to focus exclusively on alcoholism, but they offered help to drug users in setting up 12-step programmes for addiction to drugs (Narcotics Anonymous, NA). Although it became apparent that many alcoholics also used other drugs and that drug addicts were often dependent on alcohol, it was not until the end of the decade that a few 'chemical dependency' programmes emerged to offer treatment to those whose problem was mostly alcohol and also those whose problem was mostly drugs. These programmes, in the late 1970s and 1980s, typically entailed an inpatient or residential phase lasting 28 days based on the Minnesota Model mentioned earlier. Many private insurance plans provided payment for such care even though an evolving literature comparing longer and shorter inpatient stays found that longer residential care did not produce better outcomes than briefer periods or even day hospital or outpatient care (12).

As happened in the United States, the rise in heroin use in the United Kingdom that began in the 1960s continued through the 1970s. Most of the drug users who sought treatment from specialized clinics were polydrug-dependent, with much consumption, often intravenously, of barbiturates and amphetamines. Some private physicians, banned by new regulations from prescribing cocaine, began prescribing injectable methamphetamine and thereby fuelled an epidemic of amphetamine use. Physicians who worked at the specialized clinics associated with teaching hospitals (15 such clinics in London alone) walked a fine line between supplying addicts with drugs in order to prevent the emergence of a black market (the system failed in this respect) and the conviction that their mission was also to persuade the user to give up drugs. In practice, heroin prescribing declined sharply and that of oral methadone escalated. The clinics varied considerably in terms of what and how much was prescribed. Addiction specialists recognized the need for greater participation of physicians in the wider community but, as in other countries, prescribing to addicts was controversial and medical colleagues were reluctant to become involved (6). The first 'concept house' therapeutic community in Britain, modelled more on Phoenix House in the United States than on Maxwell Jones's innovation at the Henderson Hospital, was started in the 1960s. NA groups were launched in Britain in the early 1980s. The response to illicit drug use was destined to change again later in the decade with the development of community-based drug teams and the emergence of HIV.

In the 1970s, most people with alcohol problems in the United Kingdom did not receive treatment from the few hospital-based psychiatric units then in existence. The units selected their clientele carefully, largely ignoring vagrants, skid row alcoholics, and drunkenness offenders. Health planners advocated a shift from special treatment units to primary care teams, given research findings of the comparable efficacy of out-patient care, recognition that there would not be enough psychiatrists to handle the work and, no doubt, by the lower costs of non-specialist services. Notwithstanding, hospital admissions for alcoholism increased sharply during this period, mainly as a result of the growing acceptance of alcoholism as a disease. Thus, the rise in admissions to hospital care came even as the evidence grew that outpatient care was as effective as hospital care; minimal intervention as effective as more intensive programmes; and significant improvement could occur even without formal treatment (10). In the late 1970s, spurred by both research and economic necessity, alcoholism services were re-organized to give more responsibility to a community-based team of professionals and voluntary helpers and to link patients to primary health care providers. It was hoped that a psychiatrist in each health district would take a special interest in alcoholism and support the community team with only more complex cases referred to special treat-ment units.

Defining a disorder

Among the major developments of the 1970s in terms of psychiatry and its relationship to addiction were changes in how psychiatric disorders were classified (see Berrios, this volume, pp. 180–95). The first two editions of the APA's *Diagnostic and Statistical Manual* (DSM-I and II), and the eighth edition of the WHO International Classifica-tion of Diseases (ICD-8) had provided only brief definitions of the psychiatric disor-ders listed. Although this left clinicians uncertain about diagnostic boundaries, this was not considered a serious problem since most psychiatrists were more interested in understanding underlying dynamics.

With the advent of the psychotropics, reliability and validity of diagnosis assumed greater relevance. In 1972, Eli Robins, Samuel Guze, and colleagues at Washington Uni-versity in St. Louis published specific criteria on the basis of their research for what they regarded as formal psychiatric disorders (13). Included in their 15 categories were antisocial personality, alcoholism, and drug dependence. A diagnosis of alcoholism required the presence of symptoms from at least three of four sets whereas that of opiate addiction required depended only on evidence of withdrawal symptoms or hospitaliza-tion for drug abuse or its complications. This essentially descriptive and atheoretical approach figured prominently in the development of DSM-III.

In preparing DSM-III, Robert Spitzer and his committee developed a new set of cri-teria applicable to alcoholism and other forms of substance abuse. Meanwhile, Griffith

Edwards and Milton Gross set forth a provisional description of an alcohol dependence syndrome, focusing on seven clinical features that clustered together (elements were adopted by WHO for ICD-9). The two experts asserted further that a continuum of severity applied which could be distinguished from alcohol-derived disabilities (14). Edwards later stated that he had been influenced by Wikler (see above) and behavioural psychologists at the Maudsley Hospital (15). Gross also consulted with Spitzer's group. As a member of the Substance Abuse Advisory Committee, I felt confident that the concept of a severity continuum and the need to meet several characteristics of a cluster would be adopted by the APA and applied to all forms of drug dependence. However, DSM-III hewed more closely to the Washington University criteria, with separate sets of criteria for each drug category, its pathological use, and the occurrence of tolerance or withdrawal symptoms as essential pathognomonic features of opioid and sedative dependence. At a meeting co-sponsored by WHO and the US Alcohol, Drug Abuse and Mental Health Administration in 1980, a work group recommended that the Edwards and Gross alcohol dependence syndrome should be used for other types of drug dependence (16). In 1987, when DSM-III was revised (DSM-III-R), the alcohol dependence syndrome did in fact serve as a foundation for a general model. Diagnosis of dependence required any three of nine criteria to be met; the definition was made such that no single criterion was pre-eminent. Ultimately, the criteria used in DSM-III-R and DSM-IV became progressively closer to those deployed in ICD-9 and ICD-10.

The science behind it all

While the scope of this essay precludes chronicling the full story of addiction science, it would distort the history not to mention landmark findings. One was the discovery in 1973 of specific opioid receptors and shortly thereafter of endogenous ligands for these receptors (17). These findings not only powerfully affected neuroscience, but also facilitated new hypotheses about susceptibility to dependence and factors contributing to relapse. Other key results stemmed from adoption and twin studies (American and Scandinavian researchers collaborated in this work) that firmly established a genetic contribution in alcohol dependence and the probability of several distinct types of alcoholism (18). These studies paved the way for later investigations of the role of genetic factors in other drug categories, the search for specific genes and trait markers of vulnerability, and the matching of different types of alcoholism to a range of distinct treatment options (19). A fuller description of the remarkable advances in neuroscience underlying addictive disorders and motivational systems in the brain is dealt with in this volume by Hyman (pp. 1–21); and progress in the genetics of the addictions by McGuffin (pp. 22–44).

The 1980s and 1990s

Policy, politics, professionalization

By the 1980s there was little question that addiction was no longer confined to the backwaters of psychiatry, but no specific date can be identified for the birth of addiction psychiatry as a distinct discipline. In the United States, psychiatry training programmes were required to include the addictions. A few academic departments established divisions for the study and treatment of alcohol and drug problems comparable in status to subspecialities like child psychiatry and consultation-liaison psychiatry. Most of the psychiatrists who headed these divisions had acquired their expertise through research and clinical work.

Ironically, despite these academic developments, the US government's drug policy once again acquired a militant tone manifest as reduced support for treatment and research, and as urine testing for drugs in the workplace. Parent groups pressed government agencies to emphasize the dangers of cannabis (11). There was relatively little change in attitudes to alcohol, although concerns about drunk-driving and alcohol-related accidents led to raising the legal drinking age from 18 to 21. At about this time, changes in patterns and consequences of drug use occurred that had a marked impact on systems of treatment, addiction science, addiction psychiatry, and on social policy in many countries. Cocaine use rose sharply, as well as that of 'crack', an inexpensively produced free-base form of cocaine, especially among poorer urban African Americans.

The 1980s also saw the beginning of the AIDS saga and its causal relationship to a blood-borne virus, HIV, which could be spread through sharing of injection equipment. In response, research resources were increased. Although these funds were technically designated for research related to HIV, the net effect was an expansion of diverse research studies. The recognition of HIV transmission among drug users had a major impact on addiction programmes in Europe, and Australia; a 'harm reduction' movement gained considerable momentum. Harm reduction is a perspective about drug use that considers it more important to reduce its harms, such as spread of HIV and overdose deaths, than to reduce the drug use itself. Among the initiatives that were promoted were providing clean needles and syringes, 'safe places' to inject, and legitimate access to treatments such as methadone (20). Harm reduction did not become American national policy but was supported by many local governments.

In the United States, it became more common for private health insurance to cover the treatment of alcoholism. Many hospital-based programmes (similar to the Minnesota Model and lasting 28 days) expanded or were newly developed. In contrast to heroin addicts, those dependent on cocaine included many affluent individuals who usually were privately insured. The hospital-based treatments that had been developed for alcoholic patients were modified for cocaine addicts, also lasting 28 days. In effect, a two-tiered system evolved with much more spent on the well-to-do than on those with alcohol and drug problems who could not afford insurance (21).

With the expansion of the treatment enterprise, NIDA and NIAAA funded studies to assess the effectiveness and to understand which elements of treatment were crucial to outcome. Research aimed at identifying suitable psychological and pharmacological treatments for alcohol, opioid, and cocaine dependence resulted in notable achievements. Oral naltrexone was approved for opioid dependence (although poor compliance limited its utility) and was later found to be useful for alcoholism (22). Depot preparations became available subsequently that were approved for alcoholism and opioid dependence. Buprenorphine, originally studied at the Lexington ARC by Jasinski and colleagues in the 1970s, was granted approval for opioid dependence three decades later. A large project to determine whether various types of alcoholism responded differentially to recognized psychotherapies like motivational enhancement and cognitive behaviour treatment, or AA, found equivalent outcomes (23).

DSM-III brought new attention to diagnosis and assessment. Much of the expansion of treatments for addiction in the 1970s had occurred outside established psychiatric institutions, threatening to make psychiatry a bystander, but more careful assessment of patients in the 1980s revealed that most suffered from concurrent psychiatric disorders. Two extensive epidemiological studies showed that such comorbidity was not limited to those seeking treatment but was also found among alcohol- and drug-dependent people in the community (24,25).

Comorbidity and dual diagnosis

There are several reasons for the meagre attention given to comorbidity during the early expansion of addiction services. Firstly, psychiatrists tended to focus on psychiatric symptoms rather than dealing directly with the drug and alcohol problems. Secondly, a number of these symptoms, especially of depression and anxiety, diminished rapidly when drug or alcohol abuse was discontinued. Thirdly, the unavailability of explicit criteria prior to DSM-III meant that psychiatric diagnoses were unreliable.

The advent of DSM-III and structured interviewing led to a greater facility to identify psychiatric disorders associated with substance abuse. In one study 70% of opiate addicts had a concurrent mental illness while almost 90% met criteria for at least one psychiatric diagnosis at some time in their lives (26). Other investigations found that affected heroin users on methadone with the most severe psychiatric symptoms did not benefit as much as those with less severe states. A subsequent comprehensive literature dealing with treatment for comorbid patients showed that better outcomes are achieved when more severely affected patients receive psychotherapy from trained professionals (27).

Of equal significance for psychiatry is the high prevalence of substance abuse, mostly involving alcohol, cannabis, cocaine and amphetamines, in patients with severe mental illness (e.g. schizophrenia and affective disorders). Among these patients, the substance abuse is associated with greater morbidity and a poorer response to treatment (28).

Is addiction a brain disease?

In the mid-1990s, some government officials and a few researchers began to refer to addiction to several drug categories as a 'brain disease' or a 'chronic relapsing brain disease'. While these terms were probably intended to reduce the stigma associated with substance abuse and to reflect the consistent findings from technologically sophisticated studies of changes in the brains of people severely dependent on drugs or alcohol (e.g. PET scans, MRI), they have the disadvantage of obscuring the epidemiological data indicating that a significant proportion of people who at one time meet criteria for dependence recover without any formal treatment (29,30). Additional problems arising from the use of brain disease terminology have been considered in several critiques (31,32).

Professional societies

The 1980s and 1990s were notable for how many psychiatrists and other medical professionals formed or joined organizations to advance the status of addiction psychiatry, addiction medicine, and addiction science. A few addiction-related societies had existed for many years but many of them emerged from the 1960s onwards. Most are interdisciplinary; only a few restrict membership to psychiatrists. Edwards and Babor identified 38 national and international organizations. They all hold periodic scientific meetings and most publish journals and other material.(33) One of the first, the British Society for the Study of Addiction (SSA), was organized by physicians in 1884. SSA was relatively dormant from the 1930s to 1960s but under the leadership of Malcolm Lader evolved again into an active multidisciplinary society that publishes two scientific journals, *Addiction* (formerly the *British Journal of Addiction*) and *Addiction Biology*. The oldest of the organizations in the United States is the CPDD. As mentioned earlier, CPDD evolved from a National Academy of Science/National Research Council committee established in the 1920s; its goal for many years was the search for a non-addicting analgesic. By the 1960s, it broadened to encompass a diverse group of researchers and clinicians and to deal with a range of addiction-related problems. Its journal, *Drug and Alcohol Abuse*, founded by Hans Halbach, was first published in 1976.

Addiction medicine is often said to have its origins in meetings arranged by Ruth Fox, a psychiatrist, for physicians interested in treating alcoholism. The meetings led to the formation, in 1954, of an organization that evolved into the American Society on Alcoholism and, still later, into the American Society of Addiction Medicine (ASAM) (7). By 1990, ASAM had over 3000 members of whom an estimated 40% were psychiatrists and the rest physicians from a wide range of medical specialities. In addition to holding annual scientific meetings and publishing the *Journal of Addiction Medicine*, ASAM has offered a credential signifying the completion of an examination and published an excellent textbook, *Principles of Addiction Medicine*. Similar societies exist in other countries. For example, the Australian Professional Society in Alcohol and Other Drugs, founded in 1981, publishes the *Drug and Alcohol Review* and certifies expertise in addiction medicine through its relationship with the chapter of addiction medicine, a part of the Royal Australasian College of Physicians. The International Society of Addiction Medicine, formed in 1999, also offers certification of expertise in addiction medicine.

The Association for Medical Education and Research in Substance Abuse (AMERSA), founded in 1976 in the United States with Mark Galanter as its first president, evolved from the federally funded Career Teachers programmes (mentioned earlier in this essay). AMERSA's mission is to educate health professionals about the treatment of people addicted to alcohol and other drugs. It produces the journal *Substance Abuse*.

In 1985, a group of American psychiatrists who had devoted the bulk of their clinical and academic work to alcoholism or drug-related problems formed the American Academy of Psychiatrists in Alcoholism and Addiction, now the American Academy of Addiction Psychiatry (AAAP). Within a few years, AAAP began publishing a journal, the *American Journal on Addictions,* and offering a credential of expertise by examination to eligible psychiatrists. Successful candidates are awarded an Added Qualification in Addiction Psychiatry.

Just as relevant for professional communication and development are the sections on addiction within broader psychiatric bodies. These include, for example, the World Psychiatric Association, APA, Royal College of Psychiatrists, and Royal Australian and New Zealand College of Psychiatrists. Some convene specialized meetings during the annual congresses of the parent organizations; others schedule independent meetings. A number of them offer advanced training and credentialing.

Tobacco: is it or isn't it?

No area within the framework of the addictions underwent so radical a reassessment as that of tobacco use in the second half of the 20th century. In 1950, in most parts of the world, tobacco use, particularly cigarette smoking, was normative. Indeed, most physicians, including psychiatrists, were regular smokers. It was accepted that smoking could be a hard habit to break but the few voices that grouped smoking with addictions such as alcoholism and opiate dependence were largely ignored. Even into the mid-1970s, there was barely a mention of tobacco or nicotine using behaviours in psychiatry texts. However, studies by M. A. H. Russell and colleagues at the Addiction Research Unit of the Institute of Psychiatry in London, and by Murray Jarvik and his associates in the United States, helped to initiate a sea change of opinion. The two groups viewed cigarettes as nicotine delivery devices and argued that smoking constituted a true dependence on the drug nicotine; their position was given attention in the popular media (34). DSM-III included 'tobacco dependence' as a disorder for the first time. In 1976, William Pollin, a psychiatrist who then headed NIDA, took the critical step of increasing government funding for research in this area; many studies were carried out as a result. In particular, research by Hatsukami and his colleagues on tobacco withdrawal, and by Henningfield, Jasinski, and Goldberg on nicotine self-administration by humans and animals in tandem with a comprehensive review of the literature, facilitated a report by the US Surgeon-General in 1988 entitled *Nicotine Addiction* (35). The conclusion reached was that nicotine is a drug found in tobacco that causes addiction similar to that to drugs such as heroin and cocaine.

ICD-10 (1992) is largely compatible with DSM-IV (1994) in including tobacco in the section entitled 'Mental and behavioural disorders due to psychoactive substance use'.

Most textbooks of psychiatry, addiction psychiatry, substance abuse, and addiction medicine contain an account of nicotine dependence. Academic departments of psychiatry have generally included this topic in their curricula. In the United States, psychiatrists in training and postgraduate fellows in addiction psychiatry also cover this area. However, unlike their clinical roles in dealing with other addictive disorders, psychiatrists have not been at the forefront of providing treatment for addicted smokers. The effort in both the United States and the United Kingdom is left largely to primary care physicians and non-medical counsellors.

Funding for research on nicotine dependence, its treatment and prevention continued to grow substantially in the United States and led to new understanding of how nicotine interacts with nicotine receptors in the brain, its actions on cognitive and reward pathways, the contribution of genetics to the vulnerability to becoming dependent, and the relationship of smoking to comorbid psychiatric disorders that are sometimes observed in dependent smokers. Research on smoking has produced a number of pharmaceutical products that can help smokers quit successfully. The first of these was nicotine gum (approved for use in the United States in 1984). Since then, new forms of nicotine have become available (lozenges, nasal sprays, skin patches). In addition, buproprion, a drug once used for anxiety, and varenicline, an entirely new product, have shown efficacy.

Present and future

How one assesses the current relationship of psychiatry and addiction depends very much on the vantage point from which one surveys the field. In the more developed countries there has probably never been a time when there has been a greater interest in addiction among psychiatrists and mental health professionals. During the late part of the 20th century, in most countries, drug and alcohol disorders came to be seen more as medical and public health problems than as moral problems properly the concern only of the criminal justice system. That is not to say that most countries have abolished penalties for possession and use of drugs like opiates, cannabis, and cocaine, although a few have done so for varying periods of time. But it is now generally accepted that there must also be public health efforts as well as what is most aptly described as 'treatment'. The range and form of these efforts are often determined by other cultural values that vary from country to country. Some countries exclude any form of opioid maintenance and several still include compulsory treatment in secure facilities within the available options. Klingeman and Hunt have edited a book that provides a consideration of drug treatment from an international perspective and describes the roles of the medical, social welfare, and corrections systems at the end of the 20th century in 20 countries (36). However, very few of the chapters differentiate the role played by psychiatry from that of the medical professions in general. Whether provided on a voluntary or compulsory basis, whether on an inpatient, residential, or ambulatory basis, whether aimed at abstinence or harm reduction, societies in the 21st century must figure out how best to deliver prevention services and individual interventions. In the most developed countries the cost of health care, no matter which system is used to deliver it, appears to be outstripping resources. The pursuit of ways to reduce costs of health care is likely to impact various facets of addiction psychiatry in different ways.

As an academic discipline, addiction psychiatry is now firmly in place. There is virtually no likelihood that knowledge about the disorders related to alcohol and drug use will again be moved to the margins of psychiatry. Medical personnel and psychiatrists in training will continue to be taught about the substance use problems, the available treatment approaches, and the prevalence of comorbidity. The established academic chairs of addiction psychiatry at universities throughout the world are not likely to be eliminated any time soon.

It is in the delivery of the available treatments to those seeking help for drug use problems where the role of psychiatrists and especially those with additional training in addiction psychiatry may have already reached asymptotic levels. In many countries, such as the United Kingdom, France, Canada, the United States, and Australia, the prescribing of opioid agonist therapies (such as methadone and buprenorphine) has already been shifted largely to primary care physicians. To a lesser extent this is also the case for the prescription of naltrexone and of acamprosate for alcoholism. In many other countries the emphasis is on self-help groups (AA, NA, GA, etc.) and psychosocial treatments such as therapeutic communities (Italy, Poland) or counselling and cognitive therapy that is provided by non-professionals and professionals without medical or psychiatric training (36). In the United States, most outpatient alcohol and drug clinics are staffed by drug counsellors and social workers. Few even use psychiatrists as consultants.

Even when residential treatment is used, it is usually the case that the medical staff is drawn from addiction medicine, with the addiction psychiatrist playing only an occasional consultative role. Thus, while the healthcare system may continue to pay lip service to the importance of comorbidity of addictions with other significant psychiatric disorders, this may not translate into greater demand for psychiatrists with additional training in addiction psychiatry. In most situations there are simply not enough psychiatrists to meet treatment needs. In addition, there is quite commonly reluctance to pay salaries that sufficiently compensate for the long and costly training of a psychiatrist, especially one with additional qualifications in addiction psychiatry. It is also the case that evaluation studies of treatment have not yet shown that outcomes are better when services are delivered by addiction psychiatrists than by others with less or different training.

Not all this shift of services away from specialized psychiatric care is based on economic considerations. It is increasingly recognized that the most seriously addicted individuals who seek treatment are on the extreme of a continuum of drug/alcohol-related problems. Studies have demonstrated that much can be done to help those with less severe problems by screening, earlier identification, and brief intervention (37). Thus, only the more serious problems would be referred to specialized care. Furthermore, developments in pharmacotherapy have offered more tools for treatment to primary care physicians. These are arguments for moving initial treatment to primary healthcare delivery practitioners, as was done earlier in the United Kingdom.

In the area of addiction science, addiction psychiatry is likely to continue to flourish. The discoveries since the 1980s have had an impact that goes well beyond the area of addiction. By the early years of the 21st century the combined research budgets of NIDA and NIAAA in the United States exceeded a billion dollars. NIDA has often made the point that it funds a substantial proportion of drug-abuse-related research throughout the world, and despite the outcries for reduction in spending, the budgets of the NIAAA and NIDA have not been significantly reduced. For the present there remains a robust infrastructure that supports addiction science. In the United States there is now serious discussion of merging these two institutes, 40 years after their creation.

Psychiatrists and other researchers involved with the classification of mental health disorders are now considering what revisions will go into the DSM-V, scheduled for publication in 2013.[1] Based on the current draft, the section now called 'Substance-related disorders' will be renamed 'Substance use and addictive disorders' and will

---

[1] The DSM-V was published in May 2013.

include the addictions with the behavioural syndromes that appear to be closely re-lated, such as compulsive gambling, which will be renamed 'gambling disorder'. There continues to be discussion on the specific criteria to be included and whether what is now called substance abuse will be retained. Suggestions about the inclusion of similar compulsive-like behaviours, internet addiction and sexual addiction, have been put forward. Scholarly articles on compulsive gambling, internet and sexual addictions, their characteristics and comorbidities, have appeared in addiction specialty journals and substance abuse textbooks for a number of years, and some work on gambling has received support from NIDA.

Another sign of the stability of the infrastructure of addiction science has been the growth of institutes and special centres devoted to addiction-related issues. In 1993, Babor described the chronology of the development of these centres. Almost all were interdisciplinary, some were national, but many were associated with universities and had diverse means of support. In 1950 there were 3; by 1991, there were 84 located in 16 countries throughout the world; by 2008 there were 200. Before 1954 there were only three journals devoted to drug and alcohol studies. By 1991, this number had grown to 29; 14 were started in the 1960s and 1970s; more than 70% were published in English. Since then, the number of specialty print journals has continued to grow. There were 85 in 2008 (38,39). These have been augmented by publications that are exclusively internet based. Paralleling the growth of specialized journals has been the increase in the propor-tion of articles on addiction-related matters appearing in more general journals of psy-chiatry, psychology, psychopharmacology, and neuroscience. Scientific meetings dealing with addiction, national and international, are now almost as numerous as the learned journals where research is published. While there can be no assurance that the addiction research enterprise will continue to be as richly supported as it has been over the past decades, when a scientific infrastructure of institutes, organizations, journals, and col-legial relationships reaches a certain level it is likely to survive fluctuations in support.

It is not possible in this brief history to mention by name even a small proportion of the hundreds of individuals who have contributed significantly to the current size and shape of the field of addictions. Fortunately for historians of the field, in 1990, the journal *Addiction,* under the leadership of Griffith Edwards, began to publish a series of interviews with such individuals. That series, still ongoing, now numbers almost 100 interviews and represents 40 different countries. These have been gathered together and republished in a book series, the most recent collection in 2011 (40). Included in the series are scientists, clinicians, politicians, innovators of treatment, and directors of international agencies and national research centres, many of whom are psychiatrists. These interviews taken together constitute a remarkable oral history of the evolution of the field of addiction over the last half-century, and in the process, the place of addic-tion within the field of psychiatry.

References

1 **Courtwright, D. T.** (2001). *Forces of habit.* Cambridge, MA: Harvard University Press.
2 **Maddux, J. F.** (1978). History of the hospital treatment programs, 1935–74. In: Martin, W. R. and Isbell, H. (eds.) *Drug addiction and the U.S. Public Health Service.* DHEW Publi-cation No. (ADM) 77–434. Washington, DC: US Government Printing Office.

3 **Wikler, A.** (1973). Dynamics of drug dependence. Implications of a conditioning theory for research and treatment. *Archives of General Psychiatry* **28**, 611–16.

4 **Glasscote, R., Sussex, J. N., Jaffe, J. H., Ball, J., and Brill, L.** (eds.) (1972). *The treatment of drug abuse—programs, problems, prospects*. Washington, DC: American Psychiatric Association.

5 **Dole, V. P. and Nyswander, M. E.** (1968). Methadone maintenance and its implication for theories of narcotic addiction. In: Wikler, A. (ed.) *The addictive states*, Baltimore, MD: Williams & Wilkins, pp. 395–66.

6 **Connell, P. and Strang, J.** (1994). The creation of the clinics: clinical demand and the formation of policy. In: Strang, J. and Gossop, M. (eds.) *Heroin addiction and drug policy: the British system*, Oxford: Oxford University Press, pp. 167–77.

7 **White, W. L.** (1998). *Slaying the dragon: the history of addiction treatment and recovery in America*. Bloomington, IN: Chestnut Health Systems/Lighthouse Institute.

8 **Jellinek, E. M.** (1960). *The disease concept of alcoholism*. Highland Park, NJ: Hillhouse Press.

9 **Vaillant, G. E.** (1980). The doctor's dilemma. In: Edwards, G. and Grant, M. (eds.) *Alcoholism treatment in transition*, London: Croom Helm, pp. 31–31.

10 **Orford, J. and Edwards, G.** (1977). *Alcoholism. A comparison of treatment and advice with a study of the influence of marriage*. Institute of Psychiatry Maudsley Monographs, 26. Oxford: Oxford University Press.

11 **Massing, M.** (1998). *The fix*. New York: Simon & Schuster.

12 **Institute of Medicine Division of Mental Health and Behavioral Medicine** (1990). *Broadening the base of treatment for alcohol problems*. Washington, DC: National Academy Press.

13 **Feighner, J. P., Robins, E., Guze, S. B. et al.** (1972). Diagnostic criteria for use in psychiatric research. *Archives of General Psychiatry* **26**, 57–63.

14 **Edwards, G. and Gross, M. S.** (1976). Alcohol dependence: provisional description of a clinical syndrome. *British Medical Journal* **1**, 1058–61.

15 **Meyer, R. E.** (1988). Overview of the concept of alcoholism. In: Rose, R. M. and Barrett, J. E. (eds.) *Alcoholism: origins and outcome*, New York: Raven Press, pp. 1–14.

16 **Edwards, G., Arif, A., and Hodgson, R.** (1981). Nomenclature and classification of drug and alcohol related problems. *Bulletin of the World Health Organization* **59**, 225–42.

17 **Snyder, S. H.** (1989). *Brainstorming. The science and politics of opiate research*. Cambridge, MA: Harvard University Press.

18 **Schuckit, M. A.** (1992). Advances in understanding the vulnerability to alcoholism. In: O'Brien, C. P. and Jaffe, J. H. (eds.) *Addictive states*, New York: Raven Press, pp. 93–108.

19 **Babor, T. F., Hesselbrock, V., Meyer, R. E., and Shoemaker, W.** (eds.) (1994). *Types of alcoholics: evidence from clinical, experimental and genetic research*. Proceedings of a conference. Farmington, Connecticut, October 22–23, 1992. New York: New York Academy of Sciences.

20 **Stimson, G. V.** (1994). Minimizing harm from drug use. In: Strang, J. and Gossop, M. (eds.) *Heroin addiction and drug policy. The British system*, Oxford: Oxford University Press, pp. 248–56.

21 **Gerstein, D. R. and Harwood, H. J.** (eds.) (1990). *Treating drug problems*. Vol. 1. Washington, DC: National Academy Press.

22 **Volpicelli, J. R., Rhines K. C., Rhines, J. S. et al.** (1997). Naltrexone and alcohol dependence. Role of subject compliance. *Archives of General Psychiatry* **54**, 737–42.

23 **Project MATCH Research Group** (1997). Project MATCH secondary a priori hypothesis. *Addiction* **92**, 1671–98.

24 Kessler, R. C., McGonagle, K. A., Zhao, S. et al. (1994). Lifetime and 12-month prevalence of DSM-III-R psychiatric disorders in the United States. *Archives of General Psychiatry* **51**, 8–19.

25 Regier, D. A., Farmer, M. E., Rae, D. S. et al. (1990). Comorbidity of mental disorders with alcohol and other drug abuse: results from the Epidemiologic Catchment Area (ECA) Study. *JAMA* **264**, 2511–18.

26 Rounsaville, B. J. and Kleber, H. D. (1986). Psychiatric disorders in opiate addicts: preliminary findings on the course and interaction with program type. In: Meyer, R. E. (ed.) *Psychopathology and addictive disorders*, New York: Guilford Press, pp. 140–68.

27 Woody, G. E., Luborsky, L., McLellan, A. T., and O'Brien, C. P. (1986). Psychotherapy as an adjunct to methadone treatment. In: Meyer, R. E. (ed.) *Psychopathology and addictive disorders*, New York: Guilford Press, pp. 169–96.

28 Brady, K. T. and Malcolm, R. J. (2004). Substance use disorders and co-occurring Axis I psychiatric disorders. In: Galanter, M. and Kleber, H. D. (eds.) *Textbook of substance abuse treatment*, Washington, DC: American Psychiatric Press, pp. 529–38.

29 Robins, L. N. (1993). Vietnam veterans' rapid recovery from heroin addiction: fluke or normal expectation? *Addiction* **188**, 1041–54.

30 Robins, L. N., Helzer, J. E., Przybeck, T. R., and Regier, D. A. (1988). Alcohol disorders in the community. In: Rose, R. M. and Barrett, J. E. (eds.) *Alcoholism: origins and outcome*, New York: Raven Press, pp. 15–30.

31 Heyman, G. M. (2009) *Addiction: a disorder of choice*. Cambridge, MA: Harvard University Press.

32 Satel, S. L. (2001) Is drug addiction a brain disease? In: Heymann, P. B. and Brownsberger, W. N. (eds.) *Drug addiction and drug policy: the struggle to control dependence*, Cambridge, MA: Harvard University Press, pp. 118–43.

33 Edwards, G. and Babor, T. (2008). Closing remarks: addiction societies as valuable assets. *Addiction* **103**, 9–12.

34 Brecher, E. M. and the Editors of Consumer Reports (1972). *Licit and illicit drugs.* Boston: Little, Brown.

35 US Surgeon General (1988). *Health consequence of smoking: nicotine addiction. a report of the Surgeon General.* Rockville, MD: US Dept. of Health & Human Services, Office of Smoking and Health.

36 Klingeman, H. and Hunt, G. (1998). *Drug treatment systems in an international perspective.* London: Sage.

37 Babor, T. F., McRee, B. G., Kassebaum, P. A. et al. (2007). Screening, brief intervention, and referral to treatment (SBIRT): toward a public health approach to the management of substance abuse. *Substance Abuse* **28**, 7–30.

38 Babor, T. (1993). Beyond the invisible college: A science policy analysis of alcohol and drug research. In: Edwards, G., Strang, J. and Jaffe, J. H. (eds.) *Drugs, alcohol and tobacco: making the science and policy connections.* Oxford: Oxford University Press, pp. 48–69.

39 Morisano, D. and Babor, T. F. (2011). The global infrastructure for addiction science. Poster presentation at College on Problems of Drug Dependence meeting, Scottsdale, AZ, June 2010.

40 Edwards, G. and Babor, T. (eds.) (2012). *Addiction and the making of professional careers.* New Brunswick, NJ: Transaction Publishers.

Essay 17

Personality disorders

Edwin Harari

Introduction

As a naive medical student in a busy hospital emergency department, I once expressed scepticism about the clinical effectiveness of psychiatry to a consultant psychiatrist. I was feeling frustrated by and annoyed with a young woman, whose repeated nocturnal presentations to the emergency department over several weeks with self-inflicted lacerations to her wrists and forearms, all the while screaming drunken locker-room epithets at the harried nurses and doctors, had provided me and a couple of my friends with our basic training in surgical suturing techniques, and our first clinical experience of the borderline personality disorder.

The psychiatrist, a softly-spoken, kindly man, sighed, and uttered one of those memorable clinical aphorisms, part wisdom, part oversimplification, which abound in medicine: 'Patients with mental illness suffer, those with personality disorders tend to make others suffer; we can treat the former, the latter we try to manage'. That was in 1969. Today, over four decades later, seven treatment models of proven effectiveness are available to treat that woman's personality disorder. This represents one of psychiatry's most remarkable and least publicized achievements.

In this essay I summarize how the concept of personality disorder developed in psychiatry, mentioning some contributors of key ideas about causation, classification and treatments. Contrary to the aphorism, patients diagnosed with personality disorders *do* suffer, as do their intimates, colleagues, and clinicians. Whatever their ontological status, personality factors influence a psychiatric patient's cooperation with treatment, relationships with clinicians, 'treatment-resistance', and propensity to suicide.

Mainly history

Pre-20th century

Contemporary texts of the history of personality disorders locate the origins of the concept with Hippocrates (or the authorities subsumed under his name), who, in the 4th century BC explained disease to be caused by an imbalance in the four 'humours': choleric (yellow bile), melancholic (black bile), sanguine (blood), and phlegmatic (phlegm). Galen described personality types that corresponded to these putative humoral perturbations. This model dominated European medicine till the late 17th century, its demise hastened by William Harvey's demonstration in 1628 of the circulation of the blood and the structural and functional constitution of the human body.

A science of personality, its disorders, and its relationship to psychiatric illnesses is yet to be articulated, though recognition of such 'comorbidity' is hardly new. In 1621, the reclusive Oxford clergyman, Richard Burton, subscribed to the Hippocratic model that considered an excess of black bile to be the cause of his melancholia, but he also clearly regarded the entire human personality to be implicated: 'And who is not a Fool, who is free from Melancholy? Who is not touched more or less in habit or disposition? . . . And who is not sick, or ill-disposed, in whom doth not passion, anger, envy, discontent, fear and sorrow reign?' (1). Nor is the debate over the status of personality disorder as genuine pathology a recent phenomenon. On the eve of the Revolution, in a France awash with ideas of rationality, free will, and scepticism about divine authority, the medical superintendent of the Chartenton mental asylum declared of its most infamous inmate: 'the Marquis de Sade is not mad; his only sickness is vice'.

Soon after, Pinel famously removed the shackles of patients in the Saltpetrière Hospital. Faithful to his stance of objective observation, rational explanation, and humane care, Pinel also described a condition of 'manie sans delire' in people who harmed themselves and displayed impulsive, often antisocial acts while fully aware of the irrationality of their actions. He described: '. . . maniacs who gave no evidence of lesion of understanding, but who were under the dominion of instinctive and abstract fury, as if the faculties of affect alone had sustained injury' (2). The similarities with contemporary description of borderline personality disorder (BPD) are striking.

The historian of psychiatry Gregory Zilboorg described Pinel's views as the first victory in the history of psychiatry of the alliance between rationality and humanism. By contrast, Michel Foucault saw Pinel's therapy not as an expression of innate humanism, but as the dawn of disciplinary practices spearheaded by the emerging professions of medicine, psychiatry, education, and criminology, which deploy their expert knowledge to facilitate the surveillance and control of citizens in order to create 'normal' (i.e. compliant, productive) subjects of the state. Such historically contingent forms of knowledge (epistemes) define health and sickness, normality and disorder, the methods of inquiry, and how such knowledge is deployed. For Foucault, the domains of the epistemic/clinical are totally imbricated with the judicial/political. As examples, one might point to the psychiatric diagnosis and 'treatment' of political and religious dissidents in the 1960s and 1970s in the then Soviet Union, and recent publicity that some American soldiers charged with killing innocent civilians either while in a war zone, or upon their return home, were suffering from BPD, whose effects had been amplified by their combat experiences.

While Pinel claimed his observations to be objective, a moral dimension to this description was added in England in the early 19th century, when personality disorder was subsumed under the category of 'moral insanity', which predominated among men. By contrast, women were prone to hysteria: 'an immoderate sensitiveness, a tendency to refer everything to themselves, great irritability, senseless caprices, inclination to deception, jealousy and prevarication' (3).

The 20th century

During the 20th century, personality disorders emerged in the psychiatric nomenclature as a diagnostic category distinct from both the neuroses and the psychoses. An exception was the view of Adolf Meyer, who argued that a person was a psychiatric unity, in whom forms of psychopathology represented a spectrum of reactions to adverse environmental experiences. Meyer's views dovetailed with psychoanalytic ideas and were very influential in the United States in the middle third of the century.

Two broad streams of thought predominated: descriptive psychopathology and psychoanalysis. Both of them encompassed the notion that particular personality types predispose to the development of particular neuroses or psychoses. This is reflected in the terminology. After a period of eclipse, this view has regained credibility.

Descriptive psychopathology

Emil Kraepelin did not identify personality disorders as a separate diagnostic group until the 8th edition of his *Handbook* (1913). There he described the personality predispositions to the two major psychoses: the cyclothymic type, prone to mania, and the autistic (shy, seclusive, passive) type prone to dementia praecox (later renamed schizophrenia). Eugene Bleuler referred to the latter kind of personality as 'schizoidal'. Kraepelin described subtypes for each major personality disturbance, including the affective—people with an 'irritable' or 'excitable' temperament, who resemble contemporary descriptions of BPD.

Kraepelin relied on longitudinal observations of behaviour, and patients' reports of subjective experience, to argue that mental disorders were discrete, categorical entities. This view strongly influenced DSM approaches in the latter third of the 20th century.

Schneider's influential *Psychopathic Personalities* (1923) led to the eclipse of the terms 'character' and 'temperament', which previously had often been used as synonymous with personality, while he also restricted the term 'psychopathic' to refer to a subclass of abnormal personalities rather than an umbrella term for all forms of mental illness. Schneider did not consider personality disorders to be diagnostic categories; rather they were 'forms of being' which deviated from the social mean in either a statistical or ideal sense, wherein personality reflected 'a stable composite of feelings, values, tendencies and volitions' (4).

Psychoanalysis

The second major stream of thought concerning personality was psychoanalytic. While he saw himself as upholding the Enlightenment ideal of Reason, Freud was also influenced by romanticism. Its exemplar was the ill-fated, fictional character, Werther, in Goethe's *The Sorrows of Young Werther* (1774), who commits suicide in despair at the selfish, shallow, and callous qualities that modern life demands of people. The book triggered a wave of 'copycat' suicides among young people.

In the first half of the 20th century, modernism celebrated Freud's idea that the psychological foundations of a person's character lay veiled behind the apparent rationality and morally sanctioned practices of everyday life. In the late 20th century postmodernism claimed an affinity with yet another interpretation of psychoanalysis when arguing that personality has no foundation or 'essence'. Instead, time-honoured notions of identity and the self were comforting illusions, the products of the unconscious, contingent relational and linguistic worlds into which individuals are born and which they internalize.

Freud himself initially wrote little about personality and its disorders. The main exceptions are his description of the anal character, with its traits of orderliness, parsimony, and obstinacy, and its characteristic ego defences, and his biographical study of Leonardo da Vinci where he speculated on the relationship between personality, neurosis, and creativity.

In his charming 1916 paper 'Some character types met in psychoanalytic work', Freud sketched three character types: the 'Don Juan' character (a form of male hysteria), 'those wrecked by success' (a form of self-defeating tendencies), and 'criminal from sense of guilt' (a form of antisocial behaviour).

Building on his ideas of mourning, Freud's structural model described the unconscious process of 'identification' which influences the child's ego development. Identification involves unconsciously taking on characteristics of a loved person as a defence against the pain of losing or being punished by them. Freud also described a product of identification, the ego-ideal, derived from the child's recognition of the expectations and aspirations his parents may have of him. The ego-ideal is relevant to psychoanalytic formulations of the narcissistic personality disorder.

Freud also introduced the phenomenon of 'repetition compulsion', the recurrent attempts to master unconscious conflicts that underpin personality. These three concepts—defences, identification, and repetition compulsion—are clinically relevant and enduring ideas Freud contributed to our understanding and treatment of personality disorders. Anna Freud subsequently introduced the idea of developmental lines: that is, how each ego function evolved throughout life through the interaction of drives, maturation of ego defences, and life's challenges. Wilhelm Reich focused on how defences and the developmental conflicts they were deployed to solve constituted an individual's 'character armor'. His ideas marked an important transition in psychoanalysis from the treatment of the symptomatic neuroses (e.g. hysteria, obsessions, phobias) to that of personality (character) pathology, which became the principal domain of psychoanalytically informed therapy in the latter part of the 20th century.

This, in turn, prompted a continuing debate as to how the interpretation of conflict and defences, the hallmark of 'classical' psychoanalysis for symptomatic neuroses should be modified to treat character neuroses (i.e. personality disorders). Symptomatic neuroses reflect conflicts over unconscious sexual and aggressive drives for which therapy offers the means to recognize and 'own' them, while personality disorders refers to the patient's lack of stable identity and self-coherence, for which therapy offers a reparative experience so as to feel oneself more integrated.

Erik Erikson constructed a life-cycle model of personality based on 'developmental tasks'. Acquiring a sense of stable identity is a developmental task of adolescence, one of whose pathologies is 'identity diffusion' (5). This concept became a feature of Otto Kernberg's formulation of BPD, particularly relevant to the vexed question of making this diagnosis in adolescents. Adolescents are often moody and transiently emotionally unstable; this must be differentiated from emerging personality pathology, psychosis, or major mood disorder.

George Vaillant usefully arranged the defences in a hierarchy of developmental maturity, ranging from primitive and immature (e.g. projection, psychotic denial) seen in psychoses and severe personality disorders, to mature such as humour and altruism. Vaillant's long-term study of a cohort of American male medical students, and his biographical essays about famous individuals (6), show that while the lives of some people with personality pathology follow a seemingly inexorably doomed trajectory, significant personality change for the better may occur throughout life, facilitated by such relationships as marriage and grandparenthood, and psychotherapy.

An partial integration of aspects of Kraeplin's descriptive psychopathology and psychoanalytic conceptualizations of mental illness formed the basis of the first and second editions of the American Psychiatric Association (APA) *Diagnostic and Statistical Manual* (DSM). The World Health Organization (WHO) developed its own taxonomy, the International Classification of Diseases (ICD), which is similar in many respects to the DSM.

DSM

The first edition of the DSM (DSM-I) was developed in the United States after World War II by hospital doctors and military psychiatrists seeking a reliable nomenclature to differentiate people who were 'genuinely' mentally ill from those whose 'bad' behaviour was not a sign of an underlying mental illness. DSM-I reflected an American style of clinical practice influenced by the ideas of Adolf Meyer and psychoanalysis, buttressed by projective tests (the Rorschach and Thematic Apperception Test), and psychological questionnaires that did not differentiate clearly between personality disorders and other psychiatric syndromes.

Typified by Freud's case of the 'Wolf Man', psychiatrists had described patients who, while not displaying sustained, clear-cut anxiety, depression, or psychosis, nevertheless suffered vaguely defined, partial manifestations of such disorders, considerable emotional distress, unstable or impoverished social relationships, and recurrent work difficulties. In the 1930s psychoanalysts suggested that such patients were 'on the border' between psychoses and neuroses, and they became known as having 'borderline personality disorder'.

During their treatment three phenomena became apparent. First, the developmental issues they described were concerned with issues from the earliest phases of psychosocial development, where the patient's fundamental sense of self often appeared to be at stake, rather than the developmentally more advanced conflicts about self-assertion and sexuality Freud had described. Secondly, when treated in psychoanalysis some patients deteriorated or became caught in repetitive cycles of desperate, sometimes suicidal neediness, alternating with angry accusations of betrayal or rejection by their long-suffering psychotherapists and hospital staff. Thirdly, though often profoundly distressed and possibly suicidal, they generally did not develop a psychosis, or if they did, it was short-lived, without deteriorating into schizophrenia.

For such patients, the multiaxial DSM-III (published in 1980) introduced the personality diagnoses of BPD and narcissistic personality disorder. It provided a special designation, Axis II, for the classification of personality disorders. DSM-III claimed adherence to Kraeplin's method of objective, 'theory-free' observation. So while the terminology of borderline and narcissistic personality in psychoanalysis and DSM-III were and still are similar, they are the product of two different methods of enquiry, resulting in some confusion.

Another group of patients, who displayed subtle difficulties in cognitive processing and eccentric ways of assessing their environment, were diagnosed in DSM-III as schizotypal which, together with the schizoid personality (the loner), were formulated as lying on a biological continuum with schizophrenia.

In 1941 Hervey Cleckley (7) published his famous monograph *The Mask of Sanity*, in which he carefully described the psychopathic personality. Its core features of callousness, unemotionality, lack of remorse or guilt, lack of empathy, and an inability to accept responsibility for one's actions were incorporated by Hare (8) into an assessment scale for this disorder. In clinical practice, the manipulative, exploitative, and sometimes violent nature of the psychopath, especially one whose personality includes powerful narcissistic and sadistic traits, may confound or disturb clinicians, particularly those who have either denied the severity of the psychopathology or believed that they could save the patient from himself. The anxiety and uncertainty such patients arouse may be a factor in the ill-fated Dangerous and Severe Personality Disorder Programme (DSPD) in the United Kingdom, which has raised concerns that some psychiatrists misrepresented or misjudged the clinical and ethical difficulties involved in its implementation.

Controversy still attends the failure of DSM-III to differentiate clearly between psychopathy and antisocial personality disorder (ASPD). The pathology of the former is probably genetically, neurobiologically, developmentally, and psychodynamically different from ASPD. The latter may refer to behaviours which violate social norms, but without displaying the features described by Cleckley.

In DSM-III the hysterical personality was renamed 'histrionic', describing the emotionally shallow but flamboyant, self- dramatizing, attention-craving person. Some psychoanalysts have used the term 'histrionic' to describe a borderline level of functioning person, with a vulnerable sense of self (what the psychoanalyst Elizabeth Zetzel described as the 'bad' hysteric), while retaining the term 'hysterical personality' for a better-integrated patient whose anxiety is largely confined to expressions of sexuality in relationships (Zetzel's 'good' hysteric).

The resulting clusters of personality disorders agreed upon in the DSM-III were Cluster A (odd or eccentric): paranoid, schizoid, and schizotypal; Cluster B (dramatic, emotional, or erratic): antisocial, borderline, histrionic, and narcissistic; and Cluster C (anxious or fearful): avoidant, dependent, and obsessive-compulsive. The groupings have persisted in subsequent DSM editions. Amid ongoing controversy, several other types of personality disorder appeared and disappeared in subsequent revisions of DSM. These include the depressive, sadomasochistic, and passive-aggressive personality disorders, terms which clinicians often find useful, but which formal research does not (yet) warrant according the status of distinct categories. Given the overlap between the various personality subtypes, and the lack of a sharp cut-off between normality and psychopathology, current thinking favours a dimensional rather than categorical approach to classification.

Psychoanalysis again

British object relations

Using techniques of play to understand the inner world of children, Melanie Klein concluded that unconscious fantasies of self and other, shaped by innate sexual and aggressive drives, were present from the earliest days of postnatal life. Her contemporary Donald Winnicott emphasized how the thoughts, feelings, and actual behaviour of the mother, particularly her ability to understand and respond appropriately to the baby's needs (what he termed the 'facilitating environment') influenced the baby's personality development.

Although Klein did not address the personality disorders directly, her account of 'positions' (9) helped shed light on the subject as the following clinical vignette illustrates.

> 'Anna', a patient with a BPD, unexpectedly brings her 2-year old son to a psychotherapy session. Calm, almost cheerful, she begins with an anecdote about a recent matter she had handled competently. Then, as she turns to describing her 'empty' depression the toddler begins to fidget, crawls over her chest, partly obscuring her view of me, and begins to whimper. Anna's demeanour changes abruptly; she flushes angrily, heaves the child off her lap and dumps him roughly on the floor beside her armchair. 'You're a pest, Charlie, Charlie bad boy!', she hisses, then, turning to me apologizes 'I'm sorry, doctor' (she usually calls me Ed), 'I should have fed him before coming, or left him somewhere, but I couldn't find a sitter, I'm sorry.'
>
> Anna seems to be experiencing her child as totally bad, and does not understand his behaviour. She also feels a failure, and 'knows' (via projection) that I judge her accordingly. Instantaneously, therapy has been transformed into a kangaroo court, with the three participants 'trading' perceptions of victim and victimizer. Anna's emotionally charged judgment is total, totally bad, with little room for shades of grey. Klein referred to this as a part-object experience, where a partial view of self or other becomes the whole.
>
> I also feel a tension in myself. I feel protective towards Charlie and have an urge to ask Anna not to be so harsh, since his trivial misbehaviour probably reflects his sensitivity to her distress. Yet, if I say this, she might feel unfairly judged or criticized. If I say nothing, I collude with her hostility and unfair criticism of him.

Klein described how such recursive intersubjective experiences are caused by projective identification. In projective identification one person in a relationship unconsciously splits off and projects an unacceptable or painful aspect of themselves into a recipient who receives it and feels a subjective impulse to respond unthinkingly so as to rid himself of the projected feeling. So, Anna struggles with her sense of innocence, and vulnerability; unconsciously, she splits off and projects her sense of badness into Charlie and into me. This creates my countertransference discomfort.

If her husband has a Cluster B personality disorder, he might, via projective identification, experience Anna's distress and anger as criticism, and feel that she expects him to act decisively on her behalf. He might also perceive Charlie as 'all bad' for having upset Anna, for devaluing his status as a caring husband, and causing their marital tension, whereupon he might punish Charlie severely. Anna and her husband might thereby re-establish an idealized sense of goodness about themselves as individuals and as a couple, and locate the badness outside their relationship, in 'guilty' Charlie (or in me, if they believed I judged them unfairly). Such family dynamics often underpin marital violence and child abuse, and failures of therapy.

Instead of either trying to protect Charlie or ignoring the situation so as not to upset Anna, I try to 'mentalize' my experience (i.e. I try to bear the feelings and reflect upon their nature and possible significance for both Anna and me). I try to offer Anna a way of understanding herself, Charlie, and me in this context in a way that differs from her emotionally fraught, judgmental, 'all good' vs 'all bad' way. I say:

> 'Anna, when Charlie interrupted you, I think he made you angry. Maybe he made you feel that that you're not worthy of care. It's as if you feel Charlie takes over and says that you don't matter because you did something wrong.' Anna became tearful, and talked about her intolerance of mistakes, and self-blame following even trivial errors. She began to realize that blaming Charlie was a defence against feelings of self-blame and unworthiness that dominated her view of herself.

Klein described the switches between these all-good vs all-bad states of mind as characteristic of the paranoid–schizoid position. The 'positions' are not stages of personality development but configurations of a person's experience of self and others which recur throughout life. In the paranoid–schizoid position the defences are pathological denial, splitting, projection, and toxic projective identification. Together with extremes of idealization or denigration of oneself or others, they are typical of the BPD.

In the depressive position, Klein posited that more mature defences enable a person to develop a capacity to tolerate emotional 'shades of grey' in himself and others, and to bear his own mixed feelings towards others. He also recognizes that he lacks the valuable qualities the other offers, and for which he is genuinely grateful, without recourse to envy, false humility, contemptuous devaluation, or omnipotent control. These latter characteristics constitute what Winnicott termed the manic defence (10).

Instead of genuine grief, loss in the paranoid–schizoid position, according to Klein, is defended by denial, contempt for self-weakness, scornful devaluation of others, and 'entitled' anger. Rosenfeld (11) called this 'malignant narcissism'. It is manifest in many severe forms of personality psychopathology, and may be particularly relevant to the dynamics of the suicide risk of a person for whom such an act may appeal as the last-ditch expression of self-assertiveness and self- validation. Winnicott (12) proposed the notion of the 'false self', wherein the child unconsciously modifies its developing ways of knowing and being in order to conform to the expectations and needs of parental figures. Personality disorders reflect one possible outcome of this experience. They are prone to 'basic anxieties', which include the fear of falling forever, going to pieces, having no relationship to the body, having no orientation in the world, and a sense of total isolation. Such agonizing fears are difficult to express in words, perhaps corresponding to what the philosopher Søren Kierkegaard called 'nameless dread'. The British psychoanalyst Ronald Britton (13) noted that the metapsychology of personality pathology implied by the formulations of Klein and Winnicott could be translated into the respective meta-theologies of the English poets John Milton and William Blake. Milton viewed intrinsically flawed human nature as striving towards an ideal self (God), but subverted by Satan (malignant narcissism, intrinsic pride/envy). Blake saw the true self (the innocence of the child's innate primary narcissism, the beautiful/divine) as subverted by worship of the false self imposed by the demands of the external world (the god of organized religion/external authority/societal norms).

Translated into clinical practice, the Miltonian patient (the hostile-dependent Borderline, with all the badness inside) desperately needs the idealized other (lover or therapist) to save her from the tyranny of her inner world, without which she is overcome by rage, wounded pride, revenge, and despair. Conversely, the Blakean patient (the help-rejecting Narcissist, with the all the goodness inside), believes that total control over oneself, expressed as arrogant self-sufficiency, is a necessary bulwark against the inevitable humiliation and abandonment by untrustworthy others. Rosenfeld (14) similarly distinguished between what he termed the thin-skinned and thick-skinned narcissist respectively. These formulations are part of a more general vulnerability seen in patients with personality disorders which Balint termed the 'basic fault' (15).

These ideas were developed by John Bowlby (16); in his attachment theory he hypothesized that a child's sense of secure attachment to its mother, or lack thereof, could have major effects on the child's development throughout life. Based on Mary Aisnworth's descriptions of specific attachment patterns, and measured by Mary Main's Adult Attachment Interview Scale (16), researchers showed how attachment patterns shape the content and form of adults' autobiographical narratives, and influence parenting styles, including attunement and responsiveness to their own children.

Fonagy and colleagues (16) have shown that an adult with BPD often had a disorganized attachment style in early childhood, resulting in difficulty in mentalizing. Fonagy (17) further demonstrated that childhood abuse has specific damaging effects on the brain's attachment system, resulting in the subjective experience of an 'alien self', an experience so intolerable, that unless it is externalized via projective identification into another person, self-attack or suicide may feel like one's only option. The other, into whom such projections and projective identification occurs, is then experienced by the patient as a dangerous, alien other. This may explain some of the subjective and interpersonal difficulties of patients with BPD.

American object relations

Claiming affinity with the ideas of Wilhelm Reich and Anna Freud (though, curiously, omitting any mention of his contemporary, Winnicott), Heinz Kohut (18) argued that the personality trait of narcissism has a separate line of development throughout life, parallel to the capacity for object relations. Narcissism may be healthy and normal, rather than a stage in normal development to be resolved in order for the child to develop the capacity for mature love relations in adulthood. Rather than conflicts about unconscious sexual and aggressive drives as described by Freud and Klein, Kohut suggested that the narcissistically vulnerable person suffers from a deficit in his sense of self, caused by a failure of adequate parental mirroring of, and empathy for, the young child's states of mind.

Otto Kernberg's (19) formulation of BPD integrates Kleinian and Freudian approaches in a model where a patient's unconscious representations of self and other, and the affective link between them, are activated by the patient's relationship with the therapist and with significant others. Kernberg emphasizes unconscious aggression (which may have a genetic predisposition) expressed in the patient's affects, and split-off in relationships. He proposes three levels of personality organization. The *psychotic level* includes schizoid and schizotypal personality disorder, and is a partially expressed form of psychosis. The *borderline level* includes BPD and severe narcissistic personality disorder, and utilizes defences of the paranoid–schizoid position. At the milder end of severity, the split is between sensual and affectionate feelings rather than with the whole self. The *neurotic level* displays an integrated, stable but conflicted sense of self, conforming to Klein's depressive position. While at first glance it may appear difficult to reconcile Kernberg's psychodynamically based system with the Kraeplenian-influenced DSM, it is possible that Kernberg's model may describe endophenotypes, while the DSM describes their phenotypic manifestations.

Neurobiology aspects

The role of genetic, epigenetic, and other biological factors in the genesis of personality disorders have become the subject of burgeoning research in recent decades. Children who go on to develop BPD have a high prevalence of learning difficulties and attention deficit hyperactivity disorder (ADHD), and a tendency to dissociative states when emotionally aroused. This suggests that a neurodevelopmental defect may contribute to or amplify the failed empathy and destructive interpersonal relationships such children experience, leading to insecure attachment (20).

Animal studies have shown that disruptions of early maternal handling, grooming, and attachment cause abnormalities in the corticotrophin stress response, the oxytocin–vasopressin system, and the genes that codes for serotonin (5HT) transport. This increases the reactivity of the anterior cingulate–amygdala circuitry, creating a neurobiological vulnerability to BPD (21).

In psychopathic personality disorder a gene–environment interaction has been demonstrated between maltreatment in childhood and activity of the monoamine oxidase A (*MAOA*) gene, such that a child with low-level activity of *MAOA* is more susceptible to the adverse effects of childhood maltreatment (22). Children and adults with a psychopathic (callous–unemotional) personality profile have been found to have a reduced amygdala response to what normal subjects experience as frightening or distressing imagery. This reduced response may account for the high failure of psychological therapies with such patients.

Treatment considerations

Seven treatment models of proven effectiveness currently exist for the treatment of BPD: mentalization-based therapy (MBT), transference-focused psychotherapy (TFP), the conversational model (influenced by Kohut), cognitive analytic therapy (CAT), cognitive behaviour therapy or schema-focused therapy(CBT/SFT), dialectical behaviour therapy (DBT), and a general psychiatric model utilizing principles common to all these models (23). I shall concentrate on the psychodynamically informed models with which I am most familiar in my clinical practice.

The demands patients with personality disorders make on their clinicians are considerable. As Gabbard (24) perceptively documented, boundary violations often occur when a therapist feels impelled (by projective identification and the dynamics of the transference–countertransference relationship) to believe that only he can cure the patient's distress or save them from suicide. The resultant boundary violations may range from inappropriate disclosure by the therapist of personal information to the patient, or out-of-hours social meetings with the patient, to sexual relations. By contrast, according to Winnicott, appropriate psychotherapy is akin to offering the patient the 'good-enough' parenting he may not have had (or, from Klein's perspective, that he may have 'spoiled' because of this own innate aggression and envy). The therapist creates a 'holding environment' in which the patient feels psychologically 'held', understood, and gradually learns to recognize and understand himself the way the therapist does.

Kohut advocated that in psychotherapy with narcissistic personality disordered patients, the therapist should adopt a stance of empathic mirroring (therapist as a 'self object'), rather than interpreting the patient's conflicts in the transference. In this way, he would foster a strong (albeit temporary) idealization of the patient's self and the therapist. This is the natural response of the young child to feeling understood and validated by a powerful parental figure. When experienced in a therapy context this repairs the patient's sense of self, and reduces the need for the narcissistic defences the patient has been unconsciously using to protect himself against the consequences of parental empathic failure.

Kohut's concept of empathy is intuitively appealing for many practitioners, though he did not describe how the capacity for empathy actually develops in a person. It is probably based on projective identification and the resulting processes of attunement, reverie, holding (in mind), and primary maternal preoccupation, as described in detail by British Kleinians and object relations clinicians (although they did not use the term 'empathy'). Its neurobiological foundations may be the system of mirror neurons in the brain, specialized nerve cells which fire in anticipation of one's own actions or upon observing or imagining the behaviour of others. This may form part of the neurological substrate of understanding the meaning of another's behaviour (25). Two forms of empathy and their anatomical correlates have been described (26). The inferior frontal gyrus (Brodman's area 44) is involved in an emotional form of empathy (a prereflective, prelinguistic form of affective recognition or 'emotional contagion'), while the ventromedial areas of the cortex (Brodman's areas 10 and 11) subtend a cognitive form of empathy (perspective-taking, mentalizing, and having a 'theory of mind'). The controversy between the two broad approaches to the psychodynamic psychotherapy of personality disorders (interpretation/insight vs empathy/reflection) may reflect the relation between these two neurobiological systems.

Bateman, Fonagy, and colleagues' model of MBT (27) has been devised to help patients improve their reflective function by developing an understanding of their affects and cognitions, and a corresponding understanding of the mind of others. Kernberg has criticized the model because while it modifies both the patient's experience of the 'alien' (victimized) self, and the 'alien' other by whom the patient feels persecuted or betrayed, it does not adequately challenge the split-off victimizing or persecuting aspect of the patient and its consequences for the other who is the recipient of such unacknowledged aggression from the patient. Kernberg's TFP (28) aims to integrate the split-off parts of the personality, particularly aggression, arguing that without this, the patient may improve symptomatically, and therapy might be mutually gratifying for therapist and patient, but the latter's relationships outside therapy may remain dominated by splitting, self-idealization, and destructive forms of projective identification. Such criticism also applies to CBT and related therapies. Although Kernberg offers anecdotal evidence in support of such criticism, this has not yet been systematically tested.

Kernberg's approach has in turn been criticized because if the patient experiences interpretations as highlighting reprehensible or shameful aspects of his personality, he is likely to feel attacked or judged by the therapist, resulting in iatrogenic retraumatization. One possible solution emerging from the clinical experiences of skilled psychotherapists offering longer-term therapy for patients with BPD is that the initial (supportive/reflective) phase of therapy seeks to repair the patient's sense of self, using the therapist's empathy, 'holding', and reflective function, so that the vulnerable patient learns to mentalize. In the later (expressive/interpretive) phase of therapy, judicious interpretation may address those split-off, emotionally charged aspects that Kernberg warns are avoided in the first phase.

Alternatively, it may be possible to do both concurrently. The therapist's prefatory remarks and tentative way of offering an interpretation minimize its judgmental quality and conveys the therapist's genuine concern for the patient. For example, 'I have an impression . . .', 'Is it possible that you might be feeling . . . ?', 'I wonder if . . .' . Then, if the patient does feel blamed or judged, this may be explored further, using both empathy and judicious interpretation.

The above controversy highlights the universal difficulty any person has in simultaneously understanding both his own states of mind and those of others, though it is much more difficult for people with personality disorders. Some therapies (e.g. Kohut's) emphasize the former, Kernberg's the latter. Recognizing that the transference straddles both, John Steiner differentiated between patient-focused interpretations (i.e. what the therapist thinks the patient is feeling about himself) and therapist-focused interpretations (what the therapist thinks the patient is feeling about the therapist).

Group, milieu, and family therapy

Alternative or supplementary forms of therapy to the patient–psychotherapist dyad are group therapy, pioneered by W. Bion, and the therapeutic community of Maxwell-Jones, in the 1950s and 1960s, and applied by Main (29) to inpatient care of patients with BPD and other disorders. These approaches, which have been adapted to day hospital and outpatient settings, recognize that the patient may either project into or become the receptacle for the projections *of* others, including other patients and staff. Attention to these dynamics reduces the behaviour escalation, rejection, and scapegoating which are often enacted within the group or ward by patients and staff. These principles are relevant for all psychiatric patients. Family therapy, involving psychoeducation and exploration of family dynamics, including traumas, secrets, and losses, has also been applied.

Although their contribution is often modest, psychotropic medications, including antidepressants, low-dose antipsychotics, and mood stabilizers are sometimes effective in treating BPD, especially those patients with pervasive anger or marked affective instability. Low-dose serotonin reuptake inhibitors (SSRIs) or a monoamine oxidase inhibitor (MAOI) may be useful in treating the Cluster C avoidant personality disorder, which may reflect the latter's neurochemical links with social anxiety.

A psychiatrist working alone may offer both psychotherapy and medication, provided that considerations about the latter do not dominate treatment sessions. Where treatment is divided between two or more clinicians, their respectful, regular collaboration and clear delineation of responsibilities will help avoid rivalry, unconscious splitting, and destructive projective identification.

Comorbidities commonly occur between personality disorders and Axis I disorders, including anxiety disorders, major depression, and alcohol and substance abuse. The presence of one or more personality disorder often increases the severity and reduces the effectiveness of treatment of the Axis I disorder (30). However, when effective, treatment of the Axis I disorder may improve the personality disorder, and vice versa.

Given the complexity, heterogeneity, and comorbidities of BPD, it is unlikely that of the psychotherapy models shown to be effective, one will prove superior for all patients. A rationale for matching patient and model or a flexible, integrated model are needed. Much less is known about the nature and treatment of other personality disorders.

Beyond DSM-IV

Criticisms abound of the DSM Axis II. Experienced clinicians have claimed that it does not adequately represent the realities of clinical practice, particularly the unconscious meaning of the patient's interpersonal difficulties. For example, anger in a person with BPD may signify fear of rejection; in a narcissistic personality disorder, anger may reflect challenges to self-worth; in a dependent personality disorder, fear of rejection might lead initially to anxiety rather than anger, so anger is not mentioned as a diagnostic feature. However, in the course of therapy, the patient may recognize that anger unconsciously fuels his anxiety. In clinical practice such themes defy a clear taxonomy.

Including a particular personality characteristic in more than one diagnostic category leads to one or more comorbidities, while excluding it is inconsistent with clinical reality. The Sheldon–Westen Assessment Procedure (SWAP) (31) addresses this problem in terms of a patient's resemblance to a prototype along several dimensions. For example, the characteristic 'lacking in empathy' appears differently in different prototypes of personality disorders. The narcissistic personality disorder does not readily recognize the needs of others (SWAP describes this as the internalizing mode), the antisocial recognizes the needs of others but may try to exploit them (SWAP's externalizing mode), while the borderline cannot understand others when he is overwhelmed (SWAP's borderline mode).

The DSM does not rate the severity of personality disorders. Many patients may not meet all the DSM criteria for a diagnosis of a personality disorder, yet suffer deeply and also cause great distress to others. For example, patients with BPD who attempt suicide have a suicide rate of approximately 1% per year, which means tragically, that over the course of a decade, 10% of such patients, most of them young adults, will have killed themselves. Many others do not commit suicide, but lead lives of recurrent chaos, anger, and desperation.

Another criticism levelled against the DSM is its neglect of clinically useful psycho-dynamic constructs, such as defences, unconscious guilt, and transference patterns, in favour of relatively naïve Kraeplinian descriptions of observed behaviour.

People do not live in a social vacuum. DSM ignores contextual (particularly family), cultural, racial, gender, socioeconomic, and historical factors which influence person-ality development. Behaviour or attitudes deemed pathological in one culture may be considered normal or desirable in another. For example, a woman's constant deference to her husband might be considered appropriate in a traditional Japanese or Middle Eastern family, but deemed submissive or dependent in Western society. The diagnosis of a personality disorder may be particularly questionable in a member of a group in society which is marginalized, oppressed, or disenfranchised. However, recognizing the effects of physical and psychological trauma on personality development may mean that the person receives effective therapy rather than a punitive judicial response.

Another question concerns the stability of personality disorders over time. By defini-tion, they are 'enduring' or 'lifelong'. However, longitudinal studies, including Vaillant's study of Harvard medical students and studies of BPD (32), indicate that, notwith-standing fluctuations, a trend towards amelioration of personality dysfunction often occurs over time, usually years. Relationships with emotionally significant others have been found to be a factor in this improvement, though the direction of causality is unclear. However, patients who experienced childhood physical and sexual abuse and have PTSD-like experiences have a poorer prognosis, and usually need longer-term psychotherapy.

What is to be done?

These considerations suggest that integrating Axis I with Axis II on a continuum of se-verity better reflects clinical reality. One resulting classification is derived from Robert Cloninger's Temperament and Character model (33) which describes two domains of personality structure: *Temperament*, based on associative or procedural learning, and *Character*, based on insight learning. Temperament, which may be genetically based (the *DRD4* and *SLC6A4* genes are implicated), consists of four dimensions, each linked to a ge-netically influenced neurotransmitter function: harm avoidance (serotonin and GABA), novelty seeking (dopamine), reward dependence(noradrenaline and serotonin), and persistence (glutamate and serotonin). Character, the result of social learning or life ex-perience, consists of three activities: self-directedness, cooperation, self-transcendence. In this model, Cluster B personality disorders, which include BPD, narcissistic personal-ity disorder, and histrionic personality disorders, are low on self-directedness and coop-erativeness, and high in novelty seeking. Cluster C personality disorder patients, which include dependent and avoidant personality disorders, are high in harm avoidance.

Another model, using behavioural genetics, describes how the component traits of a personality disorder (e.g. affective instabilty and impulsivity in the BPD) are exaggera-tions of traits found in normal personalities (34).

In the DSM-V, personality disorders are described as dimensionally arranged traits rather than distinct categories, reflecting a person's ability to fulfil basic life tasks: for example, having a coherent and adaptive internal working model of self and others, capacity for long-term intimate relationships, and capacity for stable employment. 'Middle America's' values underpin these criteria, and psychodynamic constructs are still omitted.

Beyond nature vs nurture

The transmission of personality psychopathology across the generations lies at the heart of the historic nature–nurture debate. Today, we can better understand this.

Some predisposition to and transmission of psychopathology are genetically mediated to varying degrees (35), sometimes for specific personality disorders (schizotypal personality has abnormalities in dopamine metabolism, BPD has abnormalities in serotonin); while in others familial psychopathology (e.g. anxiety) acts as a genetically mediated but non-specific predisposition to an array of psychiatric disorders, including personality disorders. Both patterns are nature's contribution.

Equally, parents with a psychiatric illness (including personality disorder) or physical illness may be impaired in their ability to empathize with and respond supportively to their child (36). This constitutes the faulty nurture dimension. Twin studies demonstrate that the picture is further complicated by the fact that children have genetically influenced capacities to elicit, to be affected by, and to report positive and negative patterns of parental behaviour (37,38).

Defective nurture influences neurobiological processes in the child; for example, the disturbed parent uses primitive defence mechanisms when relating to their child. These defences which may include toxic projective identification, may result in neurobiologically mediated, non-genetic, insecure attachment patterns in the child, negative identifications, a fragile or deficient sense of self, and a hypersensitive readiness to 'fight–flight' responses in relationships. All this may predispose to the development of BPD in early adulthood.

Conclusion

The study of personality disorders arose from the belief that some fundamental process makes us who we are—unique as individuals, yet sharing characteristics which lead us to relate, for better or worse, to one another. Many disciplines have searched for these foundations—clinical psychiatry, psychoanalysis, neuroscience, poetry, literature, philosophy, history, and political science. In addition to the privilege of practicing a medical specialty, the delight of being a psychiatrist for me is the freedom to explore how these differing disciplines contribute to the study and treatment of personality disorders.

References

1 **Burton, R.** (1932). *The anatomy of melancholy.* London: J. M. Dent and Sons, Vol. 1, p. 39.
2 **Millon, T. and Davis, R.** (1995). Conceptions of personality disorder: historical perspectives, the DSMs, and future directions. In: Livesley, W. J. (ed). *The DSM-IV personality disorders*, New York: Guilford Press, p. 5.

3 Millon, T. and Davis, R. (1995). Conceptions of personality disorder: historical perspectives, the DSMs, and future directions. In: Livesley, W. J. (ed). *The DSM-IV personality disorders*. New York: Guilford Press, p. 7.

4 Berrios, G. E. (1993). European views on personality disorders: a conceptual history. *Contemporary Psychiatry* **34**, 14–30.

5 Erikson, E. (1959). The problem of ego identity. In: *Identity and the life cycle*. New York: International University Press, pp. 104–64.

6 Vaillant, G. (1998). *The wisdom of the ego*. Cambridge, MA: Harvard University Press.

7 Cleckley, H. (1955). *The mask of sanity* (2nd edn). St. Louis: C. V. Mosby.

8 Hare, R.D., Harpur, T.J., and Hakstian, A.R. (1990). The revised psychopathic checklist (RPC). *Psychological Assessment* **2**, 228–41.

9 Segal, H. (1980). *Melanie Klein*. New York: Viking Press.

10 Winnicott, D. (1958). The manic defense. In: *Collected papers: through paediatrics to psychoanalysis*. London: Tavistock Publications, pp. 129–44.

11 Rosenfeld, H. (1971). A clinical approach to the psychoanalytic theory to the life and death instincts: an investigation into the aggressive aspects of narcissism. *International Journal of Psychoanalysis* **52**, 169–78.

12 Winnicott, D. (1965). Ego distortion in terms of the true and false self. In: *The maturational process and the facilitating Environment*. London: Hogarth Press, pp. 140–52.

13 Britton, R. (1998). *Belief and imagination: explorations in psychoanalysis*. London: Routledge, pp. 166–77.

14 Rosenfeld, H. (1987). *Impasse and interpretation*. London: Routledge.

15 Balint, M. (1968). *The basic fault: therapeutic aspects of regression*. London: Tavistock.

16 Holmes, J. (1993) *John Bowlby and attachment theory*. London: Routledge.

17 Fonagy, P., Gergely, G., Jurist, E. L., and Target, M. (2002) *Affect regulation, mentalization and the development of the self*. New York: Other Press.

18 Kohut, H. (1977). *The restoration of the self*. New York: International University Press.

19 Kernberg, O. F. (1975). *Borderline conditions and pathological narcissism*. New York: Aronson.

20 Judd, P. H. and McGlashan, T. H. (2003). *A developmental model of borderline personality disorder: understanding variations in course and outcome*. Washington, DC: American Psychiatric Press.

21 Gabbard, G. O. (2005). Mind, brain, and personality disorders. *American Journal of Psychiatry* **162**, 648–55.

22 Caspi, A., McClay, M., Moffitt, T. E. et al (2002). Role of genotype in the cycle of violence in maltreated children. *Science* **297**, 851–4.

23 deGroot, E. R., Verheul, R., and Trijsburg, R. W. (2008). An integrative perspective on psychotherapeutic treatments for borderline personality disorder. *Journal of Personality Disorders* **22**, 332–52.

24 Gabbard, G.mO. and Wilkinson, S. (1994). *Management of countertransference with borderline patients*. Washington, DC: American Psychiatric Press.

25 Gallese, V. (2003) The roots of empathy: the shared manifold hypothesis and the neural basis of intersubjectivity. *Psychopathology* **36**, 171–80.

26 Shamay-Tsoory, S. G., Aham-Peretz, J. and Perry, D. (2009). Two systems for empathy: A double dissociation between emotional and cognitive empathy in inferior frontal gyrus versus ventro-medial pre-frontal lesions. *Brain* **132**, 617–27.

27 Bateman, A. and Fonagy, P. (2004). *Psychotherapy for borderline personality disorder: mentalization-based treatment.* New York: Oxford University Press.

28 Clarkin, J. F., Yeomans, F. E., and Kernberg, O. F. (2006) *Psychotherapy for borderline personality: focusing on object relations.* Washington, DC: American Psychiatric Press.

29 Main, T. (1957). The ailment. *British Journal of Medical Psychology* 30, 129–45.

30 Diguer, L., Barber, J. P., and Luborsky, L. (1993). Three concomitants: personality disorders, psychiatric severity, and outcome of dynamic psychotherapy of major depression. *American Journal of Psychiatry* 150, 1246–8.

31 Westen, D., Shedler, J., Bradley, B., and DeFife, J. A. (2012). An empirically derived taxonomy for personality diagnosis: bridging science and practice in conceptualizing personality. *American Journal of Psychiatry* 169, 273–84.

32 Zanarini, M. C., Horz, S., Frankenburg, F. R. et al. (2011). The 10-year course of PTSD in borderline patients and axis 11 comparison subjects. *Acta Psychiatrica Scandinavica* 124, 349–56.

33 Cloninger, C.R. (1999). A new conceptual paradigm from genetics and psychobiology for the science of mental health. *Australian and New Zealand Journal of Psychiatry* 33, 174–86.

34 Kendler, K., Meyers, J., and Reichborn-Kjennerud, T. (2011). Borderline personality disorder traits and their relationship with dimensions of normative personality: a web-based cohort and twin study. *Acta Psychiatrica Scandinavica* 123, 349–59.

35 Ebstein, R. P. (2006). The molecular genetic architecture of human personality: beyond self-report questionnaires. *Molecular Psychiatry* 11, 427–65.

36 Hobson, R. P., Patrick, M. P. H., and Hobson, J. A. (2009). How mothers with borderline personality disorder relate to their year old infants. *British Journal of Psychiatry* 195, 325–30.

37 Livesley, W. J., Jang, K. L., Jackson, D. N., and Vernon, P. A. (1993). Genetic and environmental contributions to dimensions of personality disorder. *American Journal of Psychiatry* 150, 1826–31.

38 Kendler, K. S. (1996). Parenting: a genetic-epidemiologic perspective. *American Journal of Psychiatry* 153, 11–20.

Essay 18

Psychopharmacology

Philip B. Mitchell and Dusan Hadzi-Pavlovic

Introduction

It is difficult for us in the early 21st century to comprehend the impact that the introduction of the modern psychopharmacological agents had on psychiatric practice in the 1950s. With psychotropic medications now an integral part of the contemporary medical and social landscape—some 5–10% of the population in many Western countries take antidepressants, and antipsychotics are widely used in both psychiatric and primary care settings—our increasing awareness of the limitations of these agents blinds us to the therapeutic revolution which they introduced.

The sharp distinction between the therapeutic impotence of the era prior to the introduction of these first 'modern' psychotropic agents—here termed the *premodern era*—and the dramatic advent of the first agents (particularly chlorpromazine, imipramine, and lithium) is the starting point for this essay. We will then describe what we view as the three eras of modern psychopharmacology.

The first epoch, which we term *the era of discovery, expectation, and promise*, dated from the late 1940s to the mid-1960s. It was during this period that most of the seminal psychotropic drug discoveries were made, and the basic pharmacological actions of some of these agents elucidated. This era was also characterized by a seismic shift in paradigms of mental illness, with the astounding impact of these new biological treatments upon previously intransigent illnesses challenging the dominant zeitgeist of psychoanalytic explanatory models. This was the 'golden era' of psychopharmacology, or in the words of Frederick Goodwin, the beginning of the 'psychopharmacological revolution' (1).

The second phase, which we term *the era of expansion and consolidation*, extended from the mid-1960s to the early 21st century. During this time there was a dramatic increase in the number of new psychopharmacological agents and incremental growth in understanding of the underlying basic pharmacology. However, the majority of these new treatments were to varying extents derivative in nature, being either variations of existing molecules, novel molecules with the same pharmacological action as pre-existing compounds, or new indications for pre-existing medications; for example, the application of drugs initially developed for schizophrenia or epilepsy to the treatment of bipolar disorder.

The third phase, which has insidiously and frustratingly become apparent over the last decade, we term *the era of disillusionment and retreat*. This era has been characterized by a dawning recognition of the profound limitations in the efficacy and effectiveness of these agents, to some extent only becoming apparent with our painful awareness of the failure of the pharmaceutical industry to publish many negative trials. Another hallmark of this era has been the growing scientific impasse of our failure to identify the underlying pathophysiology of the various psychiatric disorders, thereby precluding the possibility of aetiologically targeted and tailored therapies. As a consequence, the very same pharmaceutical companies which were at the vanguard of the scientific advances of the first and second eras have now rapidly retreated from the field of psychiatric research, meaning that no new novel psychotropic agents are on the immediate clinical horizon.

We finish with some observations on the current situation, and view recent confirmations of genes involved in some of the major psychiatric disorders (such as Alzheimer's disease, schizophrenia, and bipolar disorder) and advances in brain imaging technologies as grounds for a cautious optimism. We believe that we will ultimately see the development of scientifically rational and targeted (and thereby more effective) therapies within the lifetime of at least some of the readers of this discourse.

Terminologies

Before starting with an account of the premodern era, a brief overview of some of the terms in this field is apposite here. The term 'psychopharmacology' predated the modern era and originated with David Macht in an article in 1920 in the *Bulletin of the Johns Hopkins Hospital*. It is defined by the *Oxford English Dictionary* as 'the study of the effects of drugs on the mind and behaviour'. The term 'psychotropic' has been ascribed to Ralph Waldo Gerard (1900–1974). The *Oxford English Dictionary* defines this as referring to drugs or plants which are psychoactive or 'affect the mind', and details its usage first appearing in the mid-1950s.

As the science of clinical psychopharmacology progressed, the need to develop accurate terminologies and to categorize the rapidly expanding numbers of medications became apparent. Delay and Deniker coined the term 'neuroleptic' for the effect of chlorpromazine, to indicate the action of this class of drugs in 'reducing, but not paralysing' nervous activity (2). The word comes from the Greek term 'leptikos' meaning accepting and assimilative. Later in the 1950s, the term 'tranquillizer' came into popular usage. While the origin of this term dates back to 1800, its modern usage arose in the mid-1950s, with one of the first accounts ascribed to Aldous Huxley in 1956. The *Oxford English Dictionary* defines a tranquillizer as: 'any of a large class of drugs in widespread use since the 1950s for the reduction of tension or anxiety and the treatment of psychotic states'. 'Minor tranquillizer' was used to encompass sedative-hypnotics, while 'major tranquillizers' was used for medications for psychosis. The origin of the currently popular terminology 'antipsychotic' is not clear, but it was being used at least as early as 1953.

The premodern era of psychopharmacology

What treatments were used in the premodern era of psychopharmacology? Despite (to the modern observer) a lack of evidence for their efficacy, there was in fact a wide range of medicinal agents, hydrotherapies, bloodletting, and other techniques that were still in day-to-day use in asylum practice at least up to the end of the 19th century, and for some treatments until the 1930s and 1940s. Some techniques were introduced in the first half of the 20th century, including fever therapy, primitive psychosurgical procedures, insulin coma, and the early convulsive therapies.

The medicinal agents used in psychiatric practice in the premodern era of the 19th and early 20th centuries were myriad. Opioids were widely used as sedatives until their addictive properties became apparent in the late 19th century. Opium had been freely employed to treat a wide variety of conditions and diseases from the 18th century by both the laity and medical professionals. Morphine was first used in medicine in 1827 and heroin in 1898. The first report of the use of opium in psychiatry was that of Young, who described dramatic improvements in both mania and melancholia, in fact being so impressed that he felt it specifically active for these disorders. He attributed its benefit to stopping the patient worrying, relaxing 'tense nerves', and 'resting agitated particles of his nervous fluid'. The English psychiatrist Henry Maudsley was impressed by the value of opium in the treatment of specific phases of mania: '. . . in that state of mental hyperaesthesia which so often precedes an outbreak of insanity' and 'when the acute symptoms of mania have subsided, and a gloomy and morose mood of mind comes on . . .' (3, p. 439) Likewise, the eminent German psychiatrist Emil Kraepelin commented positively upon its role in melancholia: 'If there is great agitation, opium in increasing doses is often given with benefit' (4).

Other compounds were also frequently used as sedatives. Alkaloid plant extracts that were employed included hyoscine, scopolamine, and atropine. Variants of the former (hyoscyamus or hyoscyamine) appear to have been widely used in mania; Kraepelin noted, 'If the bath is not available, the use of hysoscin hydrobromate hypodermically, or by mouth, is the best remedy for subduing the intense psychomotor activity' (4). Digitalis, also a plant extract, successfully treated delirium in two patients with heart failure, as described by the English physician and botanist Withering. This dramatic report led to its widespread use in psychiatry, with clinicians not distinguishing delirium from other forms of psychosis. The other perceived benefits of digitalis (in an era during which purgation was valued therapeutically) were that it also caused nausea, vomiting and diarrhoea, sedation, and slowed the pulse. Maudsley stated: 'In cases of great excitement, maniacal or melancholic, where it is advisable to give opium, large doses of digitalis sometimes produce good effects in tranquillizing the patient' (3).

Another commonly employed sedative was camphor. Its use as an antimaniacal remedy was first recorded by Kinnear in 1758. A volatile oil obtained from the camphor tree (*Cinnamomum camphora*) of eastern Asia, it had been firmly established in 17th-century pharmacopoeias as a remedy for all nervous disorders. Kraepelin commented that 'In the very extreme excitement with impending collapse, the administration of whisky or brandy or camphor is necessary . . .' (4, p. 420). It remained in the British pharmacopoeia until the 1940s. Camphor was said to lead to exhilaration or stimulation of the nervous system at lower doses, sedation as the dose increased, and seizures at high doses. The first reports applying its convulsive property therapeutically were attributed to Leopold von Auenbrugger (1722–1809), a physician of Vienna.

Other sedating agents included the bromides (first used in 1857), chloral (1869), paraldehyde (1882), and the barbiturates (1903). Continuous narcosis was first developed by Macleod using bromides, with Klaesi later using the barbiturates for the same purpose. Maudsley was impressed with the bromides, stating, 'Bromide of potassium certainly appears to produce good effects in some cases of insanity . . .' (3, p. 440). Paraldehyde was a bitter-tasting liquid of characteristic and penetrating odour. Also available in injectable form for epilepsy, it was purportedly very efficient in calming states of overactivity and excitement. 'Its free use in mental hospitals advertised itself by the smell which met one at the ward door, if not at the front door' (5).

A desperate clutching for effective therapies by the clinicians of the premodern era is palpable in these accounts. Some, however, such as Tuke (1881) remained optimistic that improved therapies would eventually materialize: 'It must be frankly granted that Psychological Medicine can boast, as yet, of no specifics, nor is it likely, perhaps, that such a boast will ever be made. It may be difficult to suppress the hope, but we cannot entertain the expectation, that some future Sydenham will discover an anti-psychosis which will as safely and speedily cut short an attack of mania or melancholia as bark an attack of ague. (6)'

In 1970, the US psychiatrist Frank Ayd reflected upon the conditions in psychiatric wards towards the end of the premodern era:

> Within the bare walls of isolated, overcrowded, prison-like asylums were housed many screaming, combative individuals whose animalistic behaviour required constraint and seclusion. Catatonic patients stood day after day, rigid as statues, their legs swollen and bursting with dependent edema. Their comrades idled week after week, lying on hard benches or on the floor, deteriorating, aware only of their delusions and hallucinations. Others were incessantly restive, pacing back and forth like caged animals in a zoo. Periodically the air was pierced by the shouts of a raving patient. Suddenly, without notice, like an erupting volcano, an anergic schizophrenic bursts into frenetic behaviour, lashing out at others or striking himself with his fists, or running wildly and aimlessly about. Nurses and attendants, ever in danger, spent their time protecting patients from harming themselves or others. They watched men and women who either refused to eat or gorged themselves. They tube-fed to sustain life. Trained to be therapists, they functioned as guards and custodians in a hellish environment where despair prevailed and surcease by death offered the only lasting respite for their suffering charges (7).

The era of discovery, expectation, and promise: the 'golden age' of psychopharmacology

Major advances in medical science during the first half of the 20th century, identifying the aetiology of some physical illnesses and developing tailored therapies (e.g. thyroid gland extract for cretinism), led to expectations that effective treatments for psychiatric disorders would ensue. A number of successful 'silver bullet' treatments were developed for some medical conditions with prominent psychiatric manifestations, such as penicillin for neurosyphilis (general paralysis of the insane), thiamine (vitamin B_1) for Wernicke–Korsakoff syndrome, and niacin (vitamin B_3) for pellagra, which can manifest as a psychosis. While it clearly became apparent that the pathogenic processes underpinning most psychiatric disorders would not easily yield to the rudimentary scientific technologies available at that time, there were some remarkable serendipitous therapeutic discoveries in the 1940s and 1950s concerning psychotropic effects of chlorpromazine, imipramine, and lithium.

In many ways, the impact of this first era was perhaps best captured in an address in Rome in 1958 by Pope Pius XII to the first congress of the Collegium Internationale Neuro-Psychopharmacologicum (CINP)–the fledgling new international organization which had been established to further the scientific aims of this burgeoning new field:

> ... it is easy to see that you are providing precious services to science and mankind. We have seen that you are able to help much suffering and distress that, only three or four years ago, was beyond the reach of medical science. You are now in a position to restore mental health to many patients, and we sincerely share the joy that this confers (8).

Chlorpromazine—the first antipsychotic

Recognition of the antipsychotic action of the phenothiazine compound chlorpromazine, in the early 1950s, essentially transformed the practice of psychiatry. The phenothiazines had first been synthesized by the German chemist Bernthsen in 1883, but only garnered theoretical interest when their antihistaminic action was discovered in the 1940s by the French pharmaceutical company Rhône-Poulenc. Chlorpromazine was synthesized in December 1950 by the chemist Paul Charpentier. Its pharmacological properties were initially evaluated by Simone Courvoisier, who noted an intriguing effect of this new compound on conditioned reflex behaviour in animals. In conjunction with observations about another phenothiazine compound, promethazine, in agitated patients, the company decided to include psychiatric trials in the first clinical studies with chlorpromazine in April 1951. The first reports were encouraging, suggesting possible benefits treating mania with chlorpromazine.

However, the major thrust to investigate the psychotropic properties of chlorpromazine originated outside psychiatry. A French naval anaesthetist, Henri Laborit, had been collaborating with Rhône-Poulenc in investigating the use of antihistamines in surgical practice. He developed an idiosyncratic theory concerning the potential therapeutic role of antihistamines in preventing surgical shock, and in 1951 began trials with the so-called 'lytic cocktail' (which included pethidine, promethazine, and chlorpromazine) to produce 'artificial hibernation' in his surgical patients. During these trials, Laborit noted a 'euphoric quietude' or 'ataraxia' (Greek for 'undisturbed'), commenting that the new agent 'may produce a veritable medical lobotomy'. In 1952 he was the first to state in print the possibility that this compound may have a therapeutic role in psychiatric practice.

Though he was predominantly concerned with its role in anaesthetic practice, Laborit encouraged both Rhône-Poulenc and colleagues to pursue potential psychiatric applications of chlorpromazine. Two psychiatrists who did so, Jean Delay and Pierre Deniker, are now recognized as undertaking the seminal studies at the St Anne psychiatric hospital in Paris. Three months of an open study of 38 patients with schizophrenia, mania, and confusional states culminated in a presentation to the Société Médico-Psychologique in May 1952, reporting the value of prolonged continuous administration.

In 1970, Deniker commented on his experiences in 1952 with chlorpromazine, observing

> Manic excitation and, more generally, psychotic agitation, which were often resistant to shock or sleep therapy, immediately became indications of choice. This effect of the drug became noticeable in the wards. . . . Agitation, aggressiveness, and delusive conditions of schizophrenics improved. Contact with the patients could be re-established, but deficiency symptoms did not change markedly (2).

Despite such reports, French interest in the psychiatric applications of chlorpromazine was slow to develop. When first marketed in December 1952 its indication for the treatment of psychiatric disorders was one among many uses, including anaesthetic potentiation, antiemesis in pregnancy, and prevention of motion sickness. In fact, the European brand name 'Largactil' referred to the presumed 'large' spectrum of 'activity' of the medication. However, international attention to the psychiatric applications progressed rapidly. The first international symposium on the drug was held in Switzerland in November 1953; reports in the English language literature appeared in 1954, with a Canadian report quickly followed by accounts from the United States, the United Kingdom, and Australia.

It was the introduction of chlorpromazine into the United States, and the subsequent large American controlled studies, that finally confirmed the central role of this compound in psychiatric treatment. The American pharmaceutical company Smith Kline & French—under a commercial agreement with Rhône-Poulenc—began clinical trials in 1952, leading to its introduction into the US market in 1954 as Thorazine. The company had decided in 1953 that its main indication in the United States would be psychiatric, and despite initial resistance from a psychoanalytically dominated profession there was a rapid increase in utilization with 2 million patients receiving chlorpromazine within the first 8 months. Widespread clinical experience and further trials provided better understanding of psychiatric indications and adverse effects.

Chlorpromazine appeared to be most effective in schizophrenia, particularly in the acute rather than chronic form. For the first time, admission rates to US psychiatric hospitals declined; in 1956, there was a 1.3% reduction in the US inpatient population. Although it has been argued that this reduction also coincided with the introduction of liberalized admission and administrative policies, there is little doubt about the significant contribution of chlorpromazine to that process, soon supported by scientific studies. In 1960, one of the earliest meta-analyses of psychiatric treatments confirmed that the medication was more effective than placebo in psychotic, but not in neurotic patients. The effectiveness of the phenothiazine class of antipsychotic medications was definitively confirmed with the publication of the National Institute of Mental Health (NIMH) collaborative study in 1964. This large double-blind controlled trial demonstrated that the phenothiazines were more effective than placebo in the treatment of schizophrenia, and had more profound effects (e.g. decreasing apathy) than merely reducing schizophrenic overactivity.

Perhaps the greatest impact of chlorpromazine was that it introduced a relatively simple compound that was able to ameliorate (though not cure) such a complex disorder as schizophrenia. This opened the door to the modern era of potent psychotropic medication, and the endeavour to characterize the biological disturbances responsible for the functional psychoses.

Reserpine

Reserpine is in many ways the 'forgotten antipsychotic' (9). Soon after the introduction of chlorpromazine, reserpine was also marketed as an antipsychotic. This was only 2 years after Mueller had isolated this active pharmacological principle of the rauwolfia (*Rauwolfia serpentina*) root—reserpine accounts for approximately 50% of its active psychotropic effects. The first paper on the use of rauwolfia in neuropsychiatric conditions was published in 1955 by Nathan Kline, followed within 6 months by the reports of Delay and Deniker, who used reserpine itself. After a short-lived clinical popularity from 1954 to 1957, the use of reserpine and other rauwolfia alkaloids rapidly declined because of the widespread clinical uptake of chlorpromazine.

Imipramine and iproniazid—the first antidepressants

Substantive reports on the first antidepressants—imipramine and iproniazid—appeared in 1957.

Imipramine

The development of imipramine arose from the pharmaceutical industry's interest in early reports about the phenothiazine compound chlorpromazine. Geigy, not wishing to merely develop derivative phenothiazines, targeted other heterocyclic compounds, eventually focusing on iminodibenzyl. This was a tricyclic molecule that had originally been synthesized in 1898 and was used briefly as an intermediate compound in the commercial manufacture of the dyestuff 'Sky Blue'. A major difficulty was iminodibenzyl's poor solubility, so chemists added side chains to the central ring of the tricyclic nucleus and developed 42 different substances, each with antihistaminergic, sedative, and analgesic properties. Geigy initially decided to focus on those with sedative properties as potential hynotics. The company approached the Swiss psychiatrist, Roland Kuhn—described as 'a psychiatrist of the old school, an extremely perceptive clinical observer trained in the psychodynamic and psychoanalytic tradition' (10)—who studied the least toxic compound, G22150, on patients with insomnia. It proved to be of little clinical effect. Geigy then focused on iminodibenzyl products with thermolytic properties, such as G22355, which had low toxicity in animals, was not overly sedating, and was both thermolytic and antihistaminergic.

G22355 was studied in patients diagnosed with schizophrenia in an uncontrolled open trial. Kuhn and the Geigy researchers were surprised and distressed by the outcome, as the clinical effects appeared quite different from those which had been reported with chlorpromazine. Some of the patients became agitated, others hypomanic. The clinical researcher, Broadhurst, described one male patient who '. . . got hold of a bicycle and rode in his nightshirt to a nearby village, singing lustily, much to the alarm of the local inhabitants'. Attempting to make sense of these unexpected behavioural changes, the research staff at Geigy speculated that these adverse responses indicated a stimulant effect that might benefit depressed patients. (The possibility of medications being 'antidepressant' without a stimulant effect was alien to the mindset of the 1950s.) A trial in depressed patients commenced in 1955, and 'About two-thirds of the patients showed marked reduction in their depressive symptoms' (10). In Broadhurst's words, 'The fact that we might now, for the first time ever, have an effective treatment (for depression) seemed incredible' (10). In 1957 Kuhn published the results of 40 patients trialled on imipramine for a minimum of 18 months. He later stated: 'A particularly good effect is achieved with typically endogenous depressions . . . as far as they present symptoms of vital depression' (11). However, he also observed benefit in those with reactive depressions.

G22355 was subsequently named imipramine, later to be marketed as Tofranil. Within the extraordinarily short period of 3 months of Kuhn's report, imipramine was marketed by Geigy in Switzerland and 6 months later in a number of other European countries. Despite the dramatic nature of Kuhn's report, imipramine only became established as a widely used antidepressant by 1960, possibly reflecting slow acceptance by the clinical community of the concept of antidepressants, and/or the low profile and idiosyncratic philosophical focus on 'vital depression' of the rural Swiss psychiatrist Roland Kuhn. The first controlled trial was undertaken in the United Kingdom by Ball and Kiloh in 1959.

Iproniazid

While the first major reports of the antidepressant effect of the MAOI iproniazid have been credited to Nathan Kline in 1957, there is much historical evidence to indicate that other researchers and clinicians (including Delay and Deniker in France, and Crane, Saunders, and Loomer in the United States) also contributed substantially to the ultimate demonstration of its antidepressant properties (12). Developed originally by Roche as an antituberculosis agent, and demonstrated by Zeller in 1952 to be an inhibitor of monoamine oxidase, the hydrazine compound iproniazid was observed to have mood-elevating properties in those being treated for tuberculosis. The later development of non-hydrazine monoaminine oxidase inhibitors (MAOIs), phenelzine and tranylcypromine, confirmed that the inhibition of MAO was the critical antidepressant action.

Lithium—the first antimanic agent

Prominent among the psychopharmacological advances of the 20th century was John Cade's discovery of lithium's effectiveness in the treatment of mania. At the time of his seminal report, he was a 37-year-old medical officer working in a war veterans' repatriation hospital for chronic psychiatric illnesses in an outer suburb of Melbourne, Australia. Cade had recently returned from 3 years' incarceration in the Changi prisoner-of-war camp in Singapore. There he had found that many of his patients with psychiatric illness who had died (and were examined post-mortem) had some significant causative medical pathology. This observation impressed upon him the strong likelihood of an underlying physical cause for manic-depressive illness.

In 1947 (13), Cade hypothesized that manic-depressive insanity was analogous to states of hyper-and hypothyroidism, with mania being 'a state of intoxication of a normal product of the body', while 'melancholia is the corresponding deprivative condition'. With the limited investigative techniques of the day—his laboratory was a converted wooden shed in the grounds of the hospital—he began his search for the hypothesized 'toxic agent' in the urine of manic patients. The fact that he was undertaking animal studies in a psychiatric hospital in the 1940s was remarkable in itself.

To examine for the pharmacological effect in animals of any such toxin, he injected guinea-pigs intraperitoneally with the urine of patients with mania, schizophrenia, and melancholia, as well as that of normal subjects. He found that the urine of manic patients was particularly toxic, animals being killed by much lower amounts than by urine from patients with other disorders. Cade then injected the animals with pure forms of the main nitrogenous constituents of urine to identify the specific lethal compound. He found that injections of urea led to exactly the same mode of death as observed with whole urine. He was, however, unable to explain the greater toxicity of the urine of manic patients in terms of higher concentrations of urea. Thus, began his search for substances that could modify the toxic effect of urea, either by diminution or by enhancement. Cade noted in his 1947 article that uric acid appeared to have a 'slightly enhancing' effect on the toxicity of urea.

His 1949 paper (14) described the fruition of the research presaged in his earlier work. He had continued the search for the postulated compound that enhanced the toxicity of urea; however, further study of uric acid was difficult as it was relatively insoluble in water. To overcome this problem, he fortuitously chose lithium urate, the most soluble of the urates. To Cade's surprise, when he injected the guinea-pigs with lithium urate in conjunction with urea, the toxicity was reduced rather than enhanced, suggesting that the lithium could have been protective. Cade further explored this lead by injecting the guinea-pigs with lithium carbonate in conjunction with urea, and once more observed reduced toxicity. He concluded that lithium itself provided a protective effect against the action of urea. This belief then caused him to wonder whether lithium itself would have an effect on his guinea-pigs. Injecting them with large doses of lithium carbonate, he found them to become lethargic and unresponsive.

Cade then decided to exploit this apparent sedative effect therapeutically. After testing the lithium on himself and finding it to be safe, he treated 10 patients with mania, 6 with schizophrenia, and 3 with melancholia in an open-label uncontrolled study. The effect on the patients with mania was dramatic: the first patient to be given lithium had long been the most troublesome on the ward, but he settled down within 3 weeks and was able to leave hospital 12 weeks later. In contrast, there was no benefit for those with schizophrenia or melancholia, suggesting that lithium had a specific effect on mania.

International interest in lithium was slow to develop, only beginning after a Danish academic, Strömgren, read Cade's report in the early 1950s, and encouraged the young psychiatrist Mogens Schou to investigate it further. In addition, 1949 was not a propitious year for Cade's paper to appear, as it coincided with accounts from the United States of deaths caused by lithium toxicity in cardiac patients. The final acceptance of lithium as an effective treatment for bipolar disorder was largely due to the determined research of Schou and his co-worker Poul Christian Baastrup. It was not until 1970 that lithium was approved by the US Food and Drug Administration (FDA) for the treatment of mania.

A number of accounts of the use of lithium salts in psychiatric conditions preceded Cade's paper. This older use of lithium was derived from the 19th century concept of the 'uric acid diathesis' whereby it was believed that many maladies, including those of a mental nature, resulted from a physiological imbalance of uric acid. Consequently, as lithium salts were able to dissolve uric acid crystals *in vitro*, they were employed in the treatment of gout and other conditions also considered due to excess uric acid, such as mania. The term 'mania', as used in the 19th century, described any form of overactive or excited psychosis, namely schizophrenia or bipolar disorder in the current nosology. The English physician Garrod, who originally proposed the use of lithium for gout, also recommended it for mania and depression. While Cade refers to Garrod's use of lithium for 'gouty manifestations' in his 1949 paper, he does not appear to have been aware of its use for psychiatric conditions.

William Hammond, a former US Surgeon General, reported successful treatment of acute mania using lithium bromide, though it is difficult to determine in retrospect whether it was the lithium or the bromide that was the critical agent. It is also of interest to note that Cade recounted that lithium bromide was reputed to be the most hypnotic of all the bromides, which were (as detailed above) then in widespread use as non-specific sedative agents in psychiatry. The Danish brothers Carl and Fritz Lange also used lithium compounds for 'periodical depression', basing their practice on the uric acid theory. These experiences with lithium were, however, quickly lost from the mainstream of psychiatric thought and practice—presumably because of the discrediting of the uric acid diathesis hypothesis. It is indeed ironic, therefore, that uric acid also led Cade to lithium, albeit by a different path.

In what light should history consider Cade's report? Although there had been sporadic accounts of the use of lithium in the late 19th century, these were lost in the mists of time, possibly because of the discrediting of the theory of uric acid diathesis. Cade's paper could easily have suffered a similar fate. Published by an unknown researcher in a little-known journal from a country outside the influential American–European medico-scientific axis, in the year in which lithium became anathema because of deaths in cardiac patients, its chances of success must have been regarded as poor. Without Schou's work, Cade's article would probably have been ignored; in many ways the relationship between Cade and Schou should be regarded as synergistic.

Meprobamate and chlordiazepoxide—the first modern sedative-hypnotics

Though poorly documented in later historical accounts of the early years of psychopharmacology, in fact the most commonly used psychotropic agents at that time were meprobamate and the benzodiazepines—the first of the latter class developed being chlordiazepoxide (15). Meprobamate was developed as a safer alternative to the barbiturates. It was synthesized by Frank Berger and marketed by a small US company called Wallace Laboratories. Although widely used in the United States, it was rapidly overtaken by the benzodiazepines, and like its barbiturate predecessors was eventually found to cause physical and psychological dependence. Chlordiazepoxide—the first of the benzodiazepines—was synthesized by Leo Sternbach at Hoffman-LaRoche in 1958, initially in a research programme to identify a new neuroleptic agent. It was found to have anti-anxiety properties, confirmed in controlled trials by Irvin Cohen in the United States, and was marketed in 1960. Chlordiazepoxide was followed by diazepam (marketed in 1963) and oxazepam (in 1965).

Basic psychopharmacological research on the new psychotropic agents

One of the hallmarks of this 'golden era' of psychopharmacology was the rapid advance in understanding relevant basic pharmacology of a number of these agents. The scientific platform for such research was the discovery in the 1920s and 1930s that chemical neurotransmission, rather than electrical processes, was the means of neuronal communication. The initial seminal finding was reported in 1921 by the German Otto Loewi who demonstrated that acetylcholine was released by stimulation of the vagus nerve in frog heart; along with Henry Dale he received the Nobel Prize in 1936. In 1946, the Swedish pharmacologist Von Euler discovered that noradrenaline acted as a neurotransmitter; along with Julius Axelrod he received the Nobel Prize in 1970.

The major research in basic psychopharmacology after World War II was undertaken at the US National Institutes of Health—initially at the National Heart Institute and later at NIMH. In the words of Sulser, 'It is hard to convey the excitement that permeated the NIH campus in the early 1960s. The laboratories of Bernard Brodie and Julie Alexrod were truly Meccas of psychopharmacology. . . . Data generated in these laboratories in the early 1960s catalysed the concepts of the clinically relevant catechol and indoleamine hypotheses of affective disorders' (16).

Brodie led the critical technological advance that enabled the work of others. He invented the first spectrophotofluorimeter in the 1950s, which permitted the chemical study of the monoamines, their precursors, and metabolites in the brains of animals; this had previously been impossible due to their very low concentration in brain tissue. The reports from France of the exciting therapeutic discoveries with schizophrenia led Brodie to redirect the focus of his research into basic psychopharmacology.

Julius Axelrod, under the inspirational intramural directorship of Seymour Kety at NIMH, discovered catechol-O-methyl transferase (COMT) as a critical metabolizing enzyme for adrenaline and noradrenaline. In 1961 he made the dramatic discovery of the active uptake mechanism for noradrenaline into sympathetic neurons. In 1964, with Glowinski, he demonstrated that tricyclic antidepressants blocked the neuronal reuptake of noradrenaline in the brain. Coyle later reported that these medications inhibited dopamine uptake while Snyder and Carlsson demonstrated their effect on serotonin uptake. Around this same time Brodie discovered that reserpine depleted brain levels of serotonin and noradrenaline. As reserpine was known to cause suicidal depression, these findings implicated noradrenaline and serotonin in psychiatric disease for the first time, leading to the amine hypothesis for the affective disorders.

Arvid Carlsson, who joined Brodie's lab in 1956, returned to Sweden and subsequently demonstrated that dopamine was present as an agonist in the brain, particularly in the basal ganglia. He was the first to report that the antipsychotics acted by blocking receptors for dopamine, and in 2000 received the Nobel Prize with Eric Kandel and Paul Greengard for work on signal transduction in the central nervous system.

Another critical strand of psychopharmacological research in those heady years was the recognition that recreational psychoactive drugs acted via neurotransmitters. For example, Axelrod demonstrated that the hallucinatory effect of lysergic acid diethylamide (LSD) was mediated via its effect on serotonergic neuronal pathways.

The era of expansion and consolidation

The second era of psychopharmacology extended from the mid-1960s to the early 21st century, when psychopharmacology entered, and eventually dominated, mainstream psychiatric practice. This 'biologization' of psychiatry was exemplified by the rapid diminution of psychotherapists among the ranks of leading academic psychiatrists, particularly in the United States, where clinicians with a particular expertise prescribing medications came to be known as 'psychopharmacologists'.

During this period a major expansion in the number of available efficacious psychotropics occurred. By the end of the 1960s, for example, over 80 psychotropics had been studied clinically, and about 50 were marketed in at least one country internationally. There were also substantial refinements in medications, exemplified in particular by the development of antidepressants more selective for acting upon specific neurotransmitter systems (such as the selective serotonin reuptake inhibitors or SSRIs) and antipsychotic medications with an 'improved' side-effect profile.

Perhaps more than the particular scientific developments, the dramatic story of this era was the burgeoning influence of psychopharmacology more broadly on social constructs, with depression and anxiety increasingly viewed as biological or physical illness. This shift in conceptualization was concomitant with an attenuation of the accepted role of psychological and social factors in the causation and treatment of these conditions. This process perhaps reached its zenith with the proposition of 'cosmetic psychopharmacology' (analogous to cosmetic surgery), with fluoxetine (Prozac) and other agents being touted as a means for improving personality and resilience even in those without a formal depressive or anxiety disorder.

Unlike the experience in most other fields of medicine whereby newly introduced medication classes generally replace the old without altering the size of the market, there was a distinctly different experience with the new antidepressants as there was a dramatic increase in the total market. Now 5–10% of adults in the Western world are prescribed antidepressants—a profound shift from the 1950s when clinical depression was viewed as a relatively uncommon entity.

Antipsychotic medications

An increasing number of antipsychotics premised on the basic pharmacology of chlorpromazine were developed in the 1960s and 1970s. Now termed 'typical' or 'first-generation' antipsychotics, these comprised various compounds which antagonized dopamine D2 receptors and included a number of distinct molecular classes including phenothiazine, aliphatic, piperazine, butyrophenone, and thioxanthine compounds. A prime example was the first butyrophenone, haloperidol, which was synthesized by

Paul Janssen in 1958. Animal studies found this to cause 'quietness and passivity' and an antagonism of amphetamine-induced behaviour. It was approved in 1967 by the US FDA for the treatment of schizophrenia.

While similarly effective in their antipsychotic potency (with Carlsson demonstrating that potency correlated strongly with blockade of dopamine D2 receptors), they differed subtly in terms of adverse effect profile. However, all shared a propensity to cause extrapyramidal symptoms, such as akathisia; Parkinson-like tremor, rigidity, and shuffling gait; and, most worryingly, tardive dyskinesia—an often permanent and disfiguring writhing movement of tongue and other facial muscles.

Perhaps the most substantive development in antipsychotic medications during this era was the advent of the 'atypical' or 'second-generation' antipsychotics, a new class premised on the pharmacology of clozapine. Clozapine was a relatively old antipsychotic originally developed in the 1960s but withdrawn from the market because of deaths due to the serious haematological complication of agranulocytosis. Interest in the compound resurfaced in the late 1980s when the US psychiatrist John Kane, in a controlled trial, confirmed widespread clinical impressions that this antipsychotic was more efficacious than 'typical' agents, such as chlorpromazine. As clozapine also had the advantage of a lesser propensity to cause extrapyramidal side effects (and perhaps a greater therapeutic effect on the 'negative' symptoms of schizophrenia such as impaired drive and motivation), other compounds were developed to mimic its pharmacological blockade of both serotonergic and dopaminergic receptors. While some have argued against the scientific validity of a sharp distinction between typical and atypical antipsychotics, a major shift occurred in the development of antipsychotic medications from the early 1990s based on the postulated advantages of this new class. Led by pharmaceutical industry research programs with olanzapine and risperidone, there is now a wide range of atypical antipsychotics. They dominated the market in the developed world, and increasingly so in the developing world as they come off patent and thereby become more affordable.

Unsurprisingly it has become apparent that they are not without limitations. Most significant is their propensity to cause the 'metabolic syndrome', which includes obesity, diabetes, and high lipid levels. This has led to major legal cases between consumers and pharmaceutical companies, as well as settlement payments of hundreds of millions by some firms. Furthermore, the marketing strategy to differentiate products switched from the advantages of atypicals over typicals, to that of which of the atypicals was the least likely to cause such metabolic complications.

Antidepressant medications

As with the antipsychotic medications, there was a rapid increase in the number of different tricyclic antidepressants (and to a lesser extent MAOIs) marketed from the late 1960s to the early 1980s. During that time there was considerable research interest in the relative efficacy and adverse effect profiles of the tertiary tricyclics (such as imipramine) and their active metabolites (such as desipramine), but such distinctions have turned out to be of minimal clinical significance.

The major shift in antidepressant development during this era was the rise of the SSRI antidepressants. The discovery that tricyclic antidepressants inhibited the uptake of both noradrenaline and serotonin led to a search for compounds that were specific inhibitors of either of these neurotransmitters. As serotonin-specific agents were associated with less serious side effects, the focus of antidepressant development turned particularly to discovering compounds selective for serotonin uptake inhibition. The first SSRI found to possess clinical antidepressant efficacy was the Astra compound zimelidine which was discovered to inhibit serotonin uptake in animal studies in 1972 and marketed in 1982. However, it was withdrawn from the market soon afterwards as it caused Guillain–Barré syndrome, albeit uncommonly. Soon afterwards fluoxetine was marketed in the United States. Since then other SSRI antidepressants have been developed, with this class rapidly overtaking the tricyclics as the most prescribed antidepressants in most Western countries. There were a number of likely reasons for this (apart from the very active marketing campaigns): the SSRIs were innocuous in overdose, less likely to cause cardiac complications, and designed (unlike the tricyclics) to contain an effective dose for most patients in one single tablet. These factors led to increasing popularity of the SSRI antidepressants among general practitioners, with specialist prescribing representing an increasingly small proportion.

A growing recognition of limitations in the clinical efficacy of the SSRIs (and perhaps industry attraction to yet another new marketing opportunity) led to the development of compounds which (like the tricyclics) inhibited uptake of both noradrenaline and serotonin, without the inherent cardiac and sedative complications of the tricyclics. These more recent antidepressants included the serotonin-noradrenaline reuptake inhibitors (SNRIs) such as venlafaxine and duloxetine, and serotonin and noradrenaline receptor antagonists such as mirtazapine.

The dramatic increase in antidepressant prescribing (particularly SSRIs) has led to major professional and public discussion about the appropriateness of this shift, in terms of potential public health advantages or complications. A major focus was a possible link between these antidepressants and suicidal or aggressive behaviour. While there has been growing evidence that the SSRIs may increase suicidal thought in children and adolescents, the relationship has not been convincingly confirmed in adults. Rather, studies of national datasets in Scandinavia, Australia, and the United States have demonstrated in contrast that greater use of antidepressants is associated with reductions in suicide rates.

As this era of expansion and consolidation progressed, there was also some return of balance to the relative roles of pharmacological and psychological approaches in the treatment of depression and anxiety. A number of scientifically validated short-term psychological treatments for these conditions (such as cognitive behavioural therapy and interpersonal therapy) were developed and widely promulgated. Increasing research demonstrated the benefit of combining antidepressants with such psychological therapies, particularly for patients with chronic depression. Further, it became more apparent that milder forms of depression benefited more from psychological treatments, moderate forms were similarly responsive to both drugs and psychotherapy, whereas for more severe depressions antidepressants were of most benefit and psychotherapy less so.

Medications for bipolar disorder ('mood stabilizers')

At the beginning of this era, there was only one accepted treatment, lithium, for bipolar disorder, though *de facto* the typical antipsychotics were widely employed in clinical practice, despite a lack of strong evidence for their use. By the end of this era, there existed a wide range of new efficacious and approved therapies, though all had been originally developed for either epilepsy (carbamazepine, valproate, and lamotrigine) or schizophrenia (the atypical antipsychotics). No novel treatments were developed specifically for bipolar disorder.

During the 1980s the term 'mood stabilizer' came into widespread usage, though definitions and interpretations have differed widely. The purist definition for a mood stabilizer of 'proven acute and prophylactic efficacy for both mania and depression' would not be fulfilled by most of the agents commonly listed under this rubric.

Anticonvulsant mood stabilizers

Carbamazepine Carbamazepine was the first anticonvulsant to be found effective in patients with bipolar disorder. While the initial reports on its efficacy in bipolar disorder arose from the open data of Okuma in Japan in the 1970s, the first controlled studies were undertaken by Ballenger and Post at NIMH in the 1980s. Further randomized controlled trials from the United States and Europe confirmed its efficacy in the acute treatment of mania, but it was not approved for this indication by the FDA until 2004. While there are some limited data on its prophylactic efficacy, it has never received FDA approval for this indication. In general, carbamazepine has not been widely used for bipolar disorder, perhaps related to the delay in FDA approval, and its tendency to be associated with more marked adverse events than other treatments for bipolar disorder.

Valproate The first report of a potential role for the antiepileptic agent valproate in bipolar disorder was that of Lambert in France in 1966. A series of controlled studies from Europe and the United States, culminating in the pivotal trial of divalproex by Bowden in 1994, led to FDA approval for the indication of acute mania in 1995. As for carbamazepine, there has been no evidence for the prophylactic benefit of valproate and no FDA approval for this (despite its widespread clinical use as a maintenance treatment).

Lamotrigine The first suggestions of psychotropic effects of lamotrigine arose in the 1990s, with reports of a potential antidepressant effect in those with epilepsy. The first controlled trials in the late 1990s were undertaken in bipolar I disorder patients while currently depressed. The first published reports suggested strong effects in bipolar depression, but later trials were negative, though subsequent meta-analyses have suggested some moderate efficacy. The most persuasive data was for prophylactic potency, particularly for prevention of depressive relapse. Lamotrigine was approved by the FDA in 2006 for prevention of relapse in bipolar I disorder.

Antipsychotic mood stabilizers

In the 1970s and early 1980s, a number of controlled comparisons of lithium and antipsychotics in acute mania were published, demonstrating a consistent superiority for lithium, though the neuroleptics were either of equivalent or superior potency for the clinical features of motor hyperactivity and agitation. No controlled studies of typical antipsychotics in the prophylaxis of bipolar disorder were undertaken, and none of the typical antipsychotics were approved by the FDA for the indication of bipolar disorder. The first reports suggesting that the atypical antipsychotics had potential mood-stabilizing properties arose from open-label trials with clozapine in the 1990s. Subsequent experiences during the controlled trials of olanzapine in patients with schizophrenia were consistent in suggesting mood effects of this class of medications. These observations encouraged the relevant pharmaceutical companies to undertake controlled trials of the atypical antipsychotics in subjects with bipolar disorder. The first reports were from the olanzapine trials, demonstrating acute efficacy for mania (in 1999) and later for prophylaxis. Similar findings have emerged for all the other atypical antipsychotics; each has been found to have acute antimanic actions and most also prevent manic relapse. Two (olanzapine and quetiapine) also have acute and preventive effects on bipolar depression.

Sedative-hypnotic (anxiolytic) medications

A short comment on sedative-hypnotics in this era is important. The benzodiazepines rapidly became the most widely used psychotropic agents internationally until conclusive evidence of their dependence potential in the early 1980s led to a dramatic and continuing decline in their use. An important legacy of research into this class of medications was the basic pharmacological discovery of benzodiazepine receptors in the brain.

The era of disillusionment and retreat

The last decade or so has provided a sobering reality check to the field of psychopharmacology for a number of reasons. First, there has been compounding evidence of the limited efficacy and effectiveness of the psychotropics, prompting a crisis of confidence in these medicines, in medical professionals and in the general community. Second, there has been a failure to clarify the pathophysiology of the major psychiatric disorders, and thereby identify targets for tailored and improved drug therapies. Third, the pharmaceutical industry has retreated from the psychiatry/central nervous system arena—overtly due to the expense of new drug development in psychiatry, but undoubtedly also related to the lack of new drug targets. Finally, there have been major blows to the integrity of the relationship between the psychiatric profession and the pharmaceutical industry, with very public exposés of opaque and questionable professional and industry behaviour (17,18).

A number of highly publicized meta-analyses of the efficacy of antidepressants have appeared in recent years. The major reports have been those of Kirsch et al. in 2008 and Fournier et al. in 2011 (19,20). While the latter could be viewed as a more 'antidepressant friendly' analysis of the data, both were consistent in identifying that there is only a distinct benefit for antidepressants over placebo for those with more severe levels of depression. The importance of recognizing the high placebo response rates in antidepressant trials was highlighted nearly half a century ago by Klerman and Cole, who wrote:

> Many skeptics doubt that any of the so-called antidepressant drugs are 'really' effective therapeutic agents, and argue that what clinical efficacy these drugs have is mediated by

socio-psychological mechanisms . . . Partial substantiation of this viewpoint is found in the high rate of placebo response in depressed patients reported in many controlled clinical trials (21).

For those with mild to moderate levels of depression, the benefit is either non-existent or negligible. Adding weight to these results was the fact that unlike prior meta-analyses, the authors had access to unpublished data provided in company sub-missions to the FDA for regulatory approval. Such reports have added to growing evidence from other sources of a failure of the pharmaceutical industry to publish on the outcomes of many negative trials, leading to an inflation of the apparent effect size for antidepressants. This lack of transparency has bolstered the cynicism of 'anti-drug' advocacy groups, and engendered despair among clinicians and consumers.

A number of large US NIMH-funded effectiveness (pragmatic clinical setting) trials have also confirmed the limited benefit of a number of the different psychotropic classes. First, the STAR*D Trial (Sequenced Treatment Alternatives to Relieve Depression Trial) comprised the largest ever trial of depression treatment, involving almost 3000 patients with major depression, and incorporating antidepressant and cognitive behavioural therapy options—as monotherapy or in combination, using a stepped algorithm approach. The study found that only 30% of patients remitted with initial treatment, and that over 40% failed to obtain benefit from two or more treatments (22).

The other major effectiveness trial was the CATIE (Clinical Antipsychotic Trials of Intervention Effectiveness) trial in patients with chronic schizophrenia. This was the largest trial for this condition, enrolling almost 1500 subjects who were randomized to perphenazine (one of the typical antipsychotics) and a number of the atypical agents (olanzapine, quetiapine, risperidone, and ziprasidone). The essential findings of this trial were that there were no differences in effectiveness between the typical and atypical antipsychotics. A high proportion (up to 74%) of patients on all antipsychotics had their treatment discontinued (because of either failure to respond or significant adverse events) with the median time to discontinuation being only 6 months (23). The main differences between the medications were in terms of side effects, with the atypicals being associated with higher rates of weight gain and elevated cholesterol and triglyceride levels. Similar findings were reported in the CUtLASS trial (24). Intriguingly, although the major findings of these reports were published in 2005 and 2006 with much public fanfare, there has been minimal resulting change in antipsychotic prescribing practice, with continued high usage of the new and expensive atypical agents.

Dramatic changes in the working relationship between the psychiatric profession and the pharmaceutical industry between the first and later eras are also worthy of mention here. Whereas the first era was largely characterized by a joint venture in scientific discovery between industry and leading academic psychiatrists, the second and particularly third eras were characterized by an increasingly intimate relationship between the so-called 'key opinion leaders' of academic ranks and the marketing (rather than research) departments of pharmaceutical companies. It has been clear that there has been a lack of transparency and accountability in this relationship to both the general and clinical communities. Some of the more flagrant cases have been paraded in the headlines of leading US news outlets, though undoubtedly there has been much similar behaviour that has occurred less publicly. The response to this has been legislative change mandating transparency over financial relationships, in particular the recently enacted 'Sunshine' Act in the US Congress. Associated with this change in relations between psychiatrists and industry has been an increasing critique (largely arising from figures outside medicine) of 'disease-mongering'–the medicalization of 'normal' human behaviour and experience—by industry and senior medical figures. Examples include labelling sadness as 'major depression' and premenstrual tension as 'premenstrual dysphoric disorder'. Some of this critique has been justified, though undoubtedly much has also been ideologically driven.

Final reflections

Despite the travails of the last decade, we view the period as a necessary 'healthy correction' for the field. There is no denying that the advent of the modern psychotropic medications has made an enormous difference to individuals suffering from mental illness and to their families. The initial recounting of life in the asylums before the 1950s at the beginning of this essay bears testament to that. However, it is now very clear that there are major limitations to our present therapeutic armamentarium—particularly in terms of efficacy and effectiveness, but also in terms of tolerability and safety. It is now apparent that we have overplayed our hand in touting the benefits of these agents to the public.

Rather than wallowing in despair and acceding to those ideologically opposed to physical therapies, we must squarely face up to these limitations and embrace the challenge of elucidating the pathophysiology of these conditions which will allow for more effective and targeted treatments. We agree with the philosophy of the past and current directors of the US National Institutes of Health who believe that truly effective therapies can only be developed once the responsible aetiologies are elucidated—be this for psychiatric or other medical illnesses.

We believe that there are grounds for cautious optimism. For example, recent replicated reports elucidating responsible molecular genetics processes—involving both rare structural and common genetic variations—in Alzheimer's disease, schizophrenia (25), and bipolar disorder (26) are beginning to pinpoint specific causative genes, suggesting particular biochemical pathways. These will ultimately provide targets for new drug development, with the promise of more effective and personalized treatments. We have no doubt that the identification of such targets will re-engage the pharmaceutical industry in this shared endeavour. The challenge is to move forward in the collaborative spirit of discovery epitomized by that first era of modern psychopharmacology— our patients should demand nothing less of us.

Conflict of interest declaration

Neither Philip Mitchell nor Dusan Hadzi-Pavlovic have received remuneration from pharmaceutical companies or have been members of industry advisory boards over the last 3 years.

Acknowledgements

Some of the material included in this essay has been adapted and modified from these previous publications of the authors:

Mitchell, P. (1993). Chlorpromazine turns forty. *Australian and New Zealand Journal of Psychiatry* **27**: 370–3.

Mitchell, P. B., Hadzi-Pavlovic, D. (2000). Lithium treatment for bipolar disorder. *Bulletin of the World Health Organization* **78**, 515–20.

Mitchell, P. B. and Kirkby, K. (2006). Biological therapies before the introduction of psychotropic drugs. In: Lopez-Munoz, F. (ed.) *History of psychopharmacology* (2nd edn). [*Historia de la psicofarmacologia. Las terapias biologicas antes de la introduccion de los modernos psicofarmacos.* Madrid: Médica Panamericana].

References

1 Goodwin, F. K. and Ghaemi, S. N. (1999). The impact of the discovery of lithium on psychiatric thought and practice in the USA and Europe. *Australian and New Zealand Journal of Psychiatry* 33 (suppl.) S54–S61.

2 Deniker P. (1970). Introduction of neuroleptic chemotherapy into psychiatry. In: Ayd F. J., Blackwell B. (eds.) *Discoveries in biological psychiatry*. Philadelphia: Lippincott.

3 Maudsley, H. (1867). *The physiology and pathology of the mind*. London: Macmillan.

4 Kraepelin, E. (1907). *Clinical psychiatry: a textbook for students and physicians* (adaptation by A. R. Diefendorf of 7th edition of *Lehrbuch Der Psychiatrie*). New York: Macmillan.

5 Jones, W. L. (1983). *Ministering to minds diseased: a history of psychiatric treatment*. London: William Heinemann Medical Books.

6 Tuke, D. H. (1881). Presidential Address, delivered at the Annual Meeting of the Medico-Psychological Association, held at University College, London, August 2nd, 1881. *Journal of Mental Science* 27, 305–42.

7 Ayd, F. J. (1970). The impact of biological psychiatry. In: Ayd F. J., Blackwell B. (eds.) *Discoveries in biological psychiatry*. Philadelphia: Lippincott.

8 Extract from the Address of Pope Pius XII to the First CINP Congress in Rome (1998). In: Ban, T. A., Healy, D., and Shorter, E. (eds.) *The rise of psychopharmacology and the story of CINP*. Budapest: Animula Publishing House.

9 Lehmann, H. E. and Ban, T. A. (1997). The history of the psychopharmacology of schizophrenia. *Canadian Journal of Psychiatry* 42, 152–62.

10 Broadhurst, A. D. (1998). The discovery of imipramine from a personal viewpoint. In: Ban, T. A., Healy, D., and Shorter, E. (eds.) *The rise of psychopharmacology and the story of CINP*. Budapest: Animula Publishing House.

11 Kuhn, R. (1998). History and future of antidepressants. In: Ban, T. A., Healy, D., and Shorter, E. (eds.) *The rise of psychopharmacology and the story of CINP*. Budapest: Animula Publishing House.

12 Healy, D. (1997). *The antidepressant era*. Cambridge, MA: Harvard University Press.

13 Cade, J. F. J. (1947). The anticonvulsant properties of creatinine. *Medical Journal of Australia* 2, 621–3.

14 Cade, J. F. J. (1949). Lithium salts in the treatment of psychotic excitement. *Medical Journal of Australia* 2, 349–52.

15 López-Muñoz, F., Alamo, C., and García-García, P. (2011). The discovery of chlordiazepoxide and the clinical introduction of benzodiazepines: half a century of anxiolytic drugs. *Journal of Anxiety Disorders* 25, 554–62.

16 Sulser, F. (1998). From imipramine to desipramine. In: Ban, T. A., Healy, D., and Shorter, E. (eds.) *The rise of psychopharmacology and the story of CINP*. Budapest: Animula Publishing House.

17 Nutt, D. and Goodwin, G. (2011). ECNP Summit on the future of CNS drug research in Europe. *European Neuropsychopharmacology* **21**, 495–9.

18 Mitchell, P. B. (2009). Winds of change: growing demands for transparency in the relationship between doctors and the pharmaceutical industry. *Medical Journal of Australia* **191**, 273–5.

19 Kirsch, I., Deacon, B. J., Huedo-Medina, T. B. et al. (2008). Initial severity and antidepressant benefits: a meta-analysis of data submitted to the Food and Drug Administration. *PLoS Medicine* **5**(2), e45.

20 Fournier, J. C., DeRubeis, R. J., Hollon, S. D. et al. (2010). Antidepressant drug effects and depression severity: a patient-level meta-analysis. *JAMA* **303**, 47–53.

21 Klerman, G. L. and Cole, J. O. (1965). Clinical pharmacology of imipramine and related antidepressant compounds. *Pharmacological Reviews* 17, 101–41.

22 Valenstein, M. (2006). Keeping our eyes on STAR*D. *American Journal of Psychiatry* **163**, 1484–6.

23 Lieberman, J. A. and Stroup, T. S. (2011). The NIMH-CATIE Schizophrenia Study: what did we learn? *American Journal of Psychiatry* 168, 770–5.

24 Jones, P. B., Barnes, T. R., Davies, L. et al. (2006). Randomized controlled trial of the effect of Quality of Life of second- vs. first-generation antipsychotic drugs in schizophrenia. Cost Utility of the Latest Antipsychotic Drugs in Schizophrenia Study (CUtLASS 1). *Archives of General Psychiatry* **63**, 1079–87.

25 Schizophrenia Psychiatric Genome-Wide Association Study (GWAS) Consortium (2011). Genome-wide association study identifies five new schizophrenia loci. *Nature Genetics* **43**, 969–76.

26 Psychiatric GWAS Consortium Bipolar Disorder Working Group (2011). Large-scale genome-wide association analysis of bipolar disorder identifies a new susceptibility locus near ODZ4. *Nature Genetics* **43**, 977–83.

Essay 19

Convulsive and non-convulsive treatments in psychiatry

Max Fink

Introduction

At the ringing of bells heralding the 20th century, the understanding and treatment of mental illness was negligible. Little was known of causes and even less of helpful interventions. No classification of psychiatric syndromes was accepted, although European psychopathologists had defined the clinical features of dementia praecox, manic-depressive illness, catatonia, and hebephrenia. Treatments were ineffective and often invasive. The asylums had grown into massive institutions with ever-larger numbers of severely ill patients who were cared for by physicians experienced mainly in neuropathology.

In this bleak landscape, sprigs of progress emerged. Dementia paralytica (a consequence of syphilis) was a much-feared disorder but its pathology was soon described, the chemical treatment arsphenamine shown to be effective, and fever therapy introduced in 1917—a treatment considered so valuable that the Austrian neuropsychiatrist Julius Wagner-Jauregg received the Nobel Prize in Medicine in 1928.

Vitamin deficiencies as causes for delirium and dementia were identified, and dietary changes and supplements developed that largely eliminated these disorders from the Western world. Discoveries of hormones led to an understanding of the roles of insulin and thyroid in behaviour. The introduction of electroencephalography in 1929 and phenytoin in 1938 markedly improved the understanding and treatment of the epilepsies.

The enthusiasm for Freud's theories diverted interest away from the psychoses and mood disorders to the neuroses and personality problems. This psychoanalytic focus divided practitioners into the physicians caring for the hospitalized mentally ill and the psychology-minded catering to people treated in the community. In succeeding decades, new forms of psychological therapies were developed, many by people trained in psychology, social work, and nursing, dividing the care of the mentally ill among the disciplines.

And then, in a single decade, insulin coma (1933), chemically induced seizures (1934), frontal lobotomy (1936), and electroconvulsive therapy (1938), treatments directed at the brain, were launched and widely adopted. Over the next 30 years these treatments curbed the growth of the mental hospitals through deinstitutionalization, a process that was speeded up by the introduction of psychopharmacological agents:

amobarbital in 1930 for catatonia, chlorpromazine in 1954 for psychosis, meprobamate in 1955 for anxiety, imipramine in 1957 for depression, and lithium in 1966 for mania. By the 1970s the cornucopia of psychoactive drugs offered much for the treatment of psychiatric patients. The application of insulin coma and lobotomy ceased, but electroconvulsive therapy (ECT) continued to be the main non-pharmacological treatment in psychiatry (1–3).

In this essay I shall focus on the non-chemical brain treatments and their vicissitudes in practice (see Mitchell and Hadzi-Pavlovic, this volume, pp. 335–44, for an account of the history of medications in psychiatry).

Novel interventions—1933–1938

Insulin coma treatment (ICT), induced grand mal seizures (ECT), and lobotomy were introduced and adopted as principal treatments for the severely mentally ill. At the time governments maintained ever-larger, underfunded hospitals, offering their patients little more than custodial care. The treatments dramatically relieved manic excitement and frenzy, brightened mood and the gloom in which suicidal thoughts festered, and ended oppressive thoughts in patients that others sought their harm or that the world was coming to an end. The flood of increasing numbers of hospital beds ebbed (1–3).

In time we understood that inducing a seizure was the essential feature of each intervention, with speed of recovery determined by their number, frequency, and intensity. In ECT, grand mal seizures are induced directly. In insulin coma, seizures occurred in about 10–20% of comas. When coma alone failed to yield benefit, electrically induced seizures were added, improving clinical outcome (4). Lobotomy was an even less efficient method, with seizures occurring late in the course of treatment as a result of brain scarring.

Insulin coma treatment

When Manfred Sakel first administered insulin to psychiatric patients, it was to promote the appetite of those experiencing anorexia and malaise during opiate dependence withdrawal. Dosing resulted in stupor followed by a reduction in agitation and restlessness, similar to the benefits of deep sleep. In Sakel's next post in Vienna he needed a way to reduce the excitement and belligerence of psychotic patients. Recalling his experience with insulin, he applied increasing doses of the hormone, observed benefit, and reported his findings in 1933. He published his technique in 1937 (5). His best results were in patients with a recent onset of illness, especially those with delusions and disturbances in mood. Of 50 patients treated, 70% remitted completely. His method was soon widely adopted.

With more experience, light comas were shown to have less benefit; insulin doses were increased, leading to deeper and longer comas. Spontaneous grand mal seizures became more frequent. Some physicians combined the treatments and soon insulin dosages were administered to induce ever deeper and longer comas (with loss of deep tendon reflexes and loss of pupillary response to light) lasting at least an hour. Comas were ended by glucose administered intravenously or by lavage (a tube to the stomach).

Prolonged comas occurred, persisting after glucose was administered, and patients remained unresponsive for hours. Ways to treat these comas were lacking, and patients died, with mortality rates up to 5%. While the understanding of the mechanism of ICT is poor, it is best regarded as an inefficient form of seizure therapy (4).

When chlorpromazine was shown to improve psychosis it was logical to compare it to ICT. My own randomized controlled trial (RCT) at Hillside Hospital in New York City tolled the death knell for ICT when we found that chlorpromazine reduced psychosis equally effectively, at much less risk, with fewer persistent side effects and at less cost in professional staffing (6). By 1960 ICT was abandoned in most psychiatric centres. It persisted longer in the Soviet Union and China, and then in Israel as Soviet physicians brought their experience to that country.

An interesting sidelight concerns the treatment of John Nash, the 1994 Nobel Prize winner for economics. Following his doctoral studies at Princeton he developed a florid paranoid psychosis. He was first treated at the Harvard-affiliated McLean Hospital but quickly relapsed and was admitted to Trenton State Hospital in New Jersey. His friends, seeking to optimize his treatment, prevailed on the medical director to include Nash in its ICT programme, the hospital's best staffed service. Nash responded to ICT well and was discharged with prescriptions for chlorpromazine. His story has been brilliantly told by Sylvia Nasar in *A Beautiful Mind*, and also turned into a prizewinning film (7).

Lobotomy (leucotomy, psychosurgery)

Surgical ablation of the frontal lobes of chimpanzees was undertaken at Yale University by the physiologist John Fulton. The animals are notoriously aggressive when handled, but they became peculiarly docile after surgery. A demonstration of two animals managed outside their cages at an international neurology conference in 1935 led Egas Moniz, a Portuguese neurologist, to suggest that similar ablations in humans might similarly alter the behaviour of severely afflicted patients. In 1936 he reported that cutting the frontal lobes indeed did so. Despite a high rate of death, stroke, and recurrent seizures, frontal lobotomy became popular to reduce aggression, then widespread in mental hospitals (8). Moniz was awarded the 1949 Nobel Prize for Medicine for this work.

An American neuropsychiatrist, Walter Freeman, perhaps the staunchest advocate of lobotomy in its history, used an ECT seizure to induce loss of consciousness and then inserted a simple metal device into the brain via the orbital plate. His enthusiasm led him to offer treatments at hospitals throughout the United States. His indiscriminate use of lobotomy offended public opinion and cast a shadow over all brain interventions in psychiatric patients (9). The introduction of chlorpromazine soon replaced lobotomy, which was regarded as exceedingly risky as well as inefficient.

Convulsive therapy

In the 1930s, Ladislas Meduna, a Hungarian neuropathologist, found concentrations of glial cells in brain tissue to be relatively sparse in patients with psychosis and in surfeit in those with epilepsy. Parallel observations found that the incidence of seizures in schizophrenic patients was lower than expected. Schizophrenic psychosis also seemed to improve in patients suffering from seizures following head injury or infection. Perhaps inducing seizures would have a beneficial effect in schizophrenic patients generally?

Since seizures followed the intramuscular injection of camphor in animals, Meduna injected the agent into six chronically ill psychotic patients in early 1934. Over the next several weeks he extended the number of treated patients and numbers of treatments for each patient (2,3). Half the patients benefited, with two sufficiently improved to leave the hospital. An examination of the hospital's records later showed that 9 of the first 11 patients treated were catatonic, 6 requiring parenteral feeding to sustain them. By 1937 Meduna had treated over 100 patients, reporting a 50% recovery rate in whom seizures had been chemically induced, using either camphor or pentylenetetrazol (10).

Meduna's results were soon replicated but in 1938 a more efficient electric induction of seizures replaced the chemical method. Relief from manic-depressive syndromes was also reported. By the mid-1940s ECT was widely applied and hailed as a miraculous treatment (1–3).

From the 1940s to the late 1960s, ECT was commonly offered to the severely mentally ill. Treatments were accompanied by unwanted risks such as fractures, fear, and confusion. The introduction of the muscle relaxant succinylcholine in 1953 became an essential part of the procedure, together with an intravenously administered sedative (amobarbital, methohexital). These modifications significantly reduced the fear of the treatment and the risk of fractures, making ECT a much safer and acceptable procedure.

In the early 1960s, comparisons of ECT and the newly introduced antidepressants and antipsychotics found the drugs to be effective and they were hailed as replacements for ECT. Within two decades, however, growing evidence of the failure of medications in a substantial proportion of patients encouraged the resurrection of ECT (1–3). Active anti-ECT and anti-psychiatry movements severely impeded its renewed acceptance (11).

Research on ECT was similarly subject to criticism. Rather than looking at the remarkable benefits and seeking to understand the mechanisms of change, most research efforts were devoted to fiddling with the electrical parameters of the stimulus in the mistaken belief that electricity was the cause of the side effects on cognition and memory. A calculus of the electrical stimulus that would erase these side effects became the holy grail of ECT studies. To justify this work, investigators trumpeted the erroneous idea that seizures lead to persistent memory impairment.

However, many did pursue the question as to whether the electric current or the seizure was the therapeutic mechanism. Subconvulsive stimulation, the passage of a current insufficient to provoke a seizure, was tested. In our own study at Hillside Hospital in New York, 51 patients referred for ECT were randomly assigned to either convulsive or subconvulsive conditions. In 24 patients in whom seizures were induced, 17 improved. In 27 who received subconvulsive treatment, only 4 benefited. When the non-responders received seizure-induced ECT, most improved. Subsequent studies comparing sham and non-sham treatments confirmed the centrality of the seizure (12).

In the 1950s and 1960s, various electrode positions were examined in an effort to learn more about the role of current pathways in influencing outcome and producing side effects. ECT had customarily been administered with an electrode applied to each temporal region. Other locations were then tested. Applying the electrode unilaterally on one side of the head appeared to be effective and was associated with less immediate confusion. In several RCTs, however, the benefits of unilateral electrode placement were inferior to those generated by bilateral placement. Although unilateral treatment was accompanied by less immediate confusion and lesser slowing of the electroencephalogram (EEG), it was used clinically less frequently since the patients referred for ECT were severely ill and had failed many other treatments (13).

In the 1980s, however, the furore over the reintroduction of ECT and the brouhaha about persistent memory impairment prompted investigators to mount further comparisons between unilateral and bilateral applications. Controlled studies of energy dosing and electrode placement found that unilateral ECT administered at six times the energy levels of bilateral ECT produced seizures which were equally effective and with equivalent disturbances in cognition. Although unilateral ECT does produce seizures, these are inefficient, confirming our understanding that the efficacy of ECT lies in the intensity of the induced seizure.

Confirming the role of the seizure through research

In studies of relapse rates following ECT, two large collaborative studies known as CORE (Collaborative Research in ECT) and CUC (Columbia University Consortium) examined patients with unipolar depression referred for ECT (14–16). Virtually all had failed to respond to trials of several antidepressants and many diverse psychotherapies. Diagnoses, severity of symptoms, frequency of treatments, and outcome measures were similar in the two studies, except that the Columbia group opted for treating the patients with unilateral ECT and the CORE group applied bilateral ECT. The results confirmed clinical experience. To achieve the same level of improvement the unilaterally treated patients required an average of 10 treatments over 4 weeks compared to only 7 in 3 weeks in the bilateral condition. The immediate effects on memory were less with unilateral treatment, but a few weeks after the last treatment this advantage had evaporated. The unilateral group had the temporary advantage of less immediate cognitive impairment, but at the cost of additional anaesthesia inductions and seizures and an extra week of illness with its associated costs and risks. The studies supported the long-established clinician's judgement that bilateral electrode placement is the better way of applying ECT (16).

From its introduction in the 1930s to its replacement by medications in the 1960s, ECT was widely used in psychiatrists' private offices and clinics, treatment continuing until full remission (1,2). ECT was reintroduced in the 1970s as a hospital-based intervention with fixed numbers of treatments becoming the norm. Relapse rates steadily rose. The CUC and CORE collaborative studies assessed different continuation programmes in their patients. After an ECT schedule leading to remission, patients in CUC were randomized to continuation with placebo, nortriptyline alone, or the combination of nortriptyline and lithium. In the CORE study the patients were randomized to either continuation ECT or the same nortriptyline and lithium combination. At the end of 6 months, four of five patients receiving placebo continuation had relapsed; three out of five with nortriptyline alone, and two out of five with the combination of lithium and a tricyclic, and the same with ECT (14,15). These findings encourage the use of either continuation ECT or continuation of the lithium–tricyclic combination until remission is solidly established.

Other brain physical treatments

Transcranial magnetic stimulation (TMS) has been developed and tested in depressed patients in the belief that magnetic pulses have less adverse effects on the brain than electric currents. Rapid pulses of magnetic energy are delivered through a figure-of-8 field electrode placed over the scalp. Using various positions and frequency of pulses, a 20% decrease in symptoms, albeit transient, has been reported (17). When sham and active pulses are compared, however, there is no difference in effects, suggesting that the 'clickity-clack' of the active pulses is responsible for the limited positive outcome (18).

An RCT comparing TMS and ECT in depressed patients showed no effect for TMS and a significant benefit for ECT. The advantage of ECT was recorded even though the ECT patients were treated with unilateral electrode placement and twice weekly treatment, an inefficient form of ECT (19).

Magnetic seizure therapy (MST) is a modification of TMS in which high magnetic energy currents are used to induce seizures (17). Seizures have been successfully provoked but with great difficulty, discouraging clinical use. Effects on cognitive function have also been minimal. Considering the high cost of TMS devices and the complexity of the induction process, it is unlikely that MST will supplant ECT in the foreseeable future.

Vagus nerve stimulation (VNS) involves the insertion of a pacemaker (akin to a cardiac pacemaker) under the skin of the patient's chest wall (17). Electrodes are snaked to the left vagus nerve in the neck. Stimulation does not lead to seizures but is thought to tickle the brainstem by energies that pass up the vagus. Enduring effects on depressed mood or cognition have not been found. Cough and change in voice, as well as the cost of surgical implantation (and removal), inhibit the application of VNS.

Despite the absence of demonstrable benefits, as well as risks and expense, the manufacturers of the device corralled sufficient testimonies from prominent academics to facilitate its marketing. However, interest in VNS has dissipated given that it is generally viewed as an expensive placebo therapy.

Deep brain stimulation (DBS) originated with the implantation of electrodes in brain nuclei associated with Parkinson's disease; repetitive low-energy currents under the patient's control ameliorates rigidity, tremor, and dystonia sufficiently to improve quality of life. When the manufacturer of the DBS device sought to expand its market, the substantial number of depressed patients who fail to respond to antidepressant treatments were considered a potential target group. Based on a highly imaginative theory, certain brain loci were suggested as targets for stimulation and limited trials launched. The benefits are idiosyncratic, suicide rates persist, and yet this experimental technology arouses interest in the search for a specific brain locus for severe depression (17).

The mechanism of action of induced seizures

Although we are capable of inducing grand mal seizures safely and effectively and identifying the clinical conditions that remit, we have scanty knowledge of the brain and systemic mechanisms that are involved. This failure is an unacknowledged challenge to psychiatry and to neuroscience (20). As our understanding of the causes of many psychiatric disorders remains limited, and effective interventions are still elusive, it is profligate to dismiss ECT as a treatment and to disregard the mechanism by which it affects brain function and mental states. A sound theory must take the known facts about the treatment into account (12,20,21). The repeated induction of seizures regardless of the method, whether chemical or electrical, is the essential element for the changes in behaviour. All attempts to produce equivalent benefits without a seizure have failed.

A single seizure rarely offers sustained relief, and seizures administered weekly are also inefficient. Treatment frequency, depending on the patient's diagnosis and the severity of the illness, ranges from two to three seizures under one anaesthesia to daily, and to alternate days. For optimal results, seizures are induced two or three times a week. To sustain the benefit and preclude relapse, ECT continues as often as needed for as long as needed, much like continuation treatment for lithium and other psychoactive agents or like insulin in patients with diabetes (12,13).

Reports of elevated blood cortisol in depressions of the melancholic type and thyroid dysfunction in retarded depression turned the attention of researchers to neuroendocrine functions (22,23). Cortisol levels were high when patients were severely depressed, returned to normal when treatment was effective, and went up again in the case of a relapse.

We now know that each seizure is associated with the release of hypothalamic and pituitary peptides (e.g. prolactin, growth hormone, and endorphins) into the cerebrospinal fluid (CSF) and blood. CSF and blood calcium levels fall as calcium is absorbed into glandular cells to replace the discharged hormones. Since the integrity of the blood–brain barrier is compromised with repeated seizures, substances readily shift between CSF and blood (12,20).

How do these observations relate to the clinical changes? Immediately following the seizure, hypothalamic peptides are released into the CSF and blood. Levels rise over the next minutes to hours, and fall to new basal levels as additional seizures are precipitated. Cortisol is not the only hormone released. Serum prolactin increases rapidly following each seizure. The extent of release varies with seizure-inducing strategies: the dose of electrical energy, the form of stimulus, electrode placement, and frequency of inductions. These variables reflect a direct impact of the stimulus on centrencephalic structures. Greater endocrine releases accompany seizures induced with higher energies and bilateral electrode placement and are accompanied by greater and more rapid clinical benefit. Bilateral electrode placement is more efficient than unilateral as the electrical energies stimulate greater hypothalamic peptide release through the direct effect of the current. The cortisol findings in ECT compel our interest, since they provide the most coherent account of seizure physiology.

The evidence that peptide functions are abnormal in melancholia and that seizures release peptides argues for endocrinal dysfunction in the aetiology of the condition. Like the drive in physics and chemistry to fill out the missing elements in the Periodic Table, we are required to seek a neuroendocrine abnormality as the basis for syndromes that respond well to ECT. Research into neuroendocrine functions has fallen out of fashion, a result of the poor definition of unipolar and bipolar depressive illnesses and the difficulty of distinguishing bipolar disorder from schizophrenia. When cortisol function was examined in relation to these diagnoses as defined in the third edition of the *Diagnostic and Statistical Manual* of the American Psychiatric Association (DSM-III), associations were poor. Rather than examining and revising DSM-III diagnostic criteria, investigators rejected the role of neuroendocrine testing. This rise and fall of the neuroendocrine hypothesis is documented in detail in the book by Edward Shorter and Max Fink, *Endocrine psychiatry: Solving the Riddle of Melancholia* (22).

An ethical dimension

ECT, insulin coma therapy, and frontal lobotomy were initially hailed as remarkable treatments in relieving the plight of the severely psychiatrically ill (24). ECT became widely available as an outpatient procedure, but challenged neurologists whose goal was to suppress seizures, as well as a sizable proportion of psychiatrists who adhered to the psychological theories of mental illness. The tensions between the 'biological' and the 'psychodynamic' camps came to a head after World War II as the psychoanalysts mounted drumbeat attacks highlighting the risks of seizures and the use of electricity, and defended their faith that the causes of mental illness lay in the unconscious and could only be dealt with through psychotherapy (2,12). The enthusiasm for new psychoactive substances in the 1950s pushed these arguments aside. Two decades later, when psychotropic medications were no longer considered a panacea, the place of ECT was recalled, albeit accompanied by a fresh anti-ECT movement (1,2,11).

Stories of ECT abuse were depicted in films (e.g. *One Flew over the Cuckoo's Nest*); the Church of Scientology used an anti-ECT protest as a rallying cry to entice new members; and psychologists' preoccupations with their mantra that ECT induced memory loss coalesced to suppress the treatment's use. Tractable legislators passed restrictive legislation that persists to this day in many jurisdictions in the United States and in some other countries. These anti-ECT efforts are detailed in a book by Jan-Otto Ottosson and Max Fink, *Ethics in Electroconvulsive Therapy*.

As with all aspects of physician–patient interaction, the application of ECT calls for consent by a competent patient who is informed about the risks and benefits of the treatment (in some centres with the aid of a DVD, before voluntarily giving their consent) (12,25). In some jurisdictions (e.g. State of Victoria, Australia), involuntary patients may be given ECT without their consent if the psychiatrist regards the treatment as an essential part of treatment; it may be given with a court approval in American states. Contemporary ECT treatment offer benefits that far exceed risks, satisfying the ethical principles of beneficence and non-maleficence. But practice fails the ethical principle of justice. The availability of ECT is severely restricted by legislative actions, so precluding patients who need the treatment from obtaining it. Many psychiatric hospitals forego the treatment by not supporting an equipped facility and trained personnel. The training of staff does not reach a standard to assure maximal safety or effective treatment delivery. These impediments are paradoxically unrelated to medical knowledge, but attributable to internecine arguments within the psychiatric profession and between it and the public.

The future of physical brain treatments

What can we anticipate for these treatments in the future? ICT and lobotomy will not be revived. Neuro-stimulation methods result in so little benefit that society is unlikely to support such ineffective treatments despite the financial encouragement of the companies and the support of accommodating physicians.

ECT, the principal effective treatment of those covered in this essay, may not survive given the stigma and proscriptions that disrupt its use. Economic forces already have an adverse effect inasmuch as reimbursement rates, at least in the United States, are inconsistent with the time that trained physicians, anaesthesiologists, and nurses expend to provide a safe and effective service. The anti-ECT position of many psychiatrists, neurologists, and psychologists, and ignorance about the safety and efficacy of ECT of physicians and other health professionals, dominate every consideration of its potential use.

The Food and Drug Administration (FDA), a statutory body in the United States that is responsible for assessing the efficacy and safety of medications and the safety of medical devices, is reviewing the classification of ECT devices. ECT devices have been classified as 'safe' under the rule that those in use in the 1950s and 1960s when the FDA first reviewed equipment for safety were approved, so-called 'grandfathered'. In the several decades that electricity has been applied to induce seizures, ECT techniques have improved substantially so that the devices offer no direct hazards and include EEG, electromyography (EMG), and heart rate monitors that further protect patients. But repeated public calls by scientologists and others for formal studies of safety have stimulated regulatory authorities to review the classification, possibly calling for extensive studies to allow approval for marketing of ECT devices. The risk of these being proscribed as currently devised is small but worrisome. Practitioners and patients face the experience that marked abortion before the US Supreme Court's decision in Roe vs Wade; namely, that ECT will be available to patients able to travel to other jurisdictions or carried out by doctors willing to challenge legal restrictions.

Another factor potentially derailing the use of ECT is the poor training of psychiatrists. Training in ECT is commonly perfunctory, usually limited to a single lecture or demonstration in medical school or demonstration of treatments during residency training. Psychiatrists seeking the requisite skills often attend specific programmes; the snag is that a one-day workshop without hands-on experience is often considered sufficient. In the United Kingdom, criticism of past treatment programmes led to an ECT accreditation service whose charge is to evaluate treatment facilities and staff for safety and efficiency. Treatment sites not meeting adequate criteria have been closed. No such accrediting body has been established in the United States or in other countries (26).

Clinicians interested in ECT have been tempted into taking responsibility for industry-sponsored non-convulsive treatments such as TMS, VNS, and DBS. So active has this drive become that the single society in the United States dedicated to ECT, the Association for Convulsive Therapy, changed its name to include 'neuro-stimulation'. Similarly, the American Psychiatric Association changed its ECT Task Force to one covering other forms of neuro-stimulation.

Notwithstanding that ECT is safe, effective, even lifesaving, it remains the most stigmatized intervention in medicine and poorly defended by the profession. That it has continued to be used universally is testimony to its remarkable efficacy and safety. But its future is bleak, with economically based discrimination and an erroneous association with ineffective forms of neuro-stimulation serving as new hurdles to its retaining a place in psychiatric practice.

References

1 Shorter, E. (1997). *History of psychiatry*. New York: John Wiley and Sons.

2 Shorter, E. and Healy, D. (2007). *Shock therapy: a history of electroconvulsive treatment in mental illness*. New Brunswick, NJ: Rutgers University Press.

3 Dukakis, K. and Tye, L. (2006) *Shock*. New York: Penguin.

4 Fink, M. (2003). A beautiful mind and insulin coma: Social constraints on psychiatric diagnosis and treatment. *Harvard Review of Psychiatry* **11**, 284–90.

5 Sakel, M. (1938). *The pharmacological shock treatment of schizophrenia*, translated by J. Wortis. New York: Nervous and Mental Disease Publishing.

6 Fink, M., Shaw, R., Gross, G., and Coleman, F. S. (1958). Comparative study of chlorpromazine and insulin coma in the therapy of psychosis. *JAMA* **166**, 1846–50.

7 Nasar, S. (1998). *A Beautiful mind*. New York: Simon and Shuster.

8 Shutts, D. (1982). *Lobotomy: resort to the knife*. New York: Van Nostrand Reinhold.

9 El-Hai, J. (2005). *The lobotomist*. New York: Wiley.

10 Meduna, L. (1937). *Die Konvulsionstherapie der Schizophrenie*. Halle: Karl Marhold.

11 Fink, M. (1991). Impact of the anti-psychiatry movement on the revival of ECT in the U.S. *Psychiatric Clinics of North America* **14**, 793–801.

12 Fink, M. (1979). *Convulsive therapy: theory and practice*. New York: Raven Press.

13 Fink, M. (1999). *Electroshock: restoring the mind*. New York: Oxford University Press.

14 Kellner, C. H., Knapp, R. G., Petrides, G. et al. (2006). Continuation ECT versus pharmacotherapy for relapse prevention in major depression: a multi-site study from CORE. *Archives of General Psychiatry* **63**, 1337–44.

15 Sackeim, H. A, Haskett, R. F., Mulsant, B. H. et al. (2001). Continuation pharmacotherapy in the prevention of relapse following electroconvulsive therapy: a randomized controlled trial. *JAMA* **285**, 1299–307.

16 Fink, M. and Taylor, M. A. (2007). Electroconvulsive therapy: Evidence and challenges. *JAMA* **298**, 330–2.

17 Lisanby, S. H. (ed.) (2004). *Brain stimulation in psychiatric treatment*. Washington, DC: APPI Press.

18 George, M. S., Lisanby, S. H., Avery, D. et al. (2010). Daily left prefrontal transcranial magnetic stimulation therapy for major depressive disorder. A sham-controlled randomized trial. *Archives of General Psychiatry* **67**, 507–16.

19 Eranti, S., Mogg, A., Pluck, G. et al. (2007). A randomized controlled trial with 6-month follow-up of repetitive transcranial magnetic stimulation and electroconvulsive therapy for severe depression. *American Journal of Psychiatry* **164**, 73–81

20 Fink, M. (2000). Electroshock revisited. *American Scientist* **88**, 162–7.

21 Bolwig, T. G. (2011). How does electroconvulsive therapy work? Theories on its mechanism. *Canadian Journal of Psychiatry* **56**, 13–18.

22 Shorter, E. and Fink, M. (2010) *Endocrine psychiatry: solving the riddle of melancholia*. New York: Oxford University Press.

23 Davies, B., Carroll, B. J., and Mowbray, R. M. (1972). *Depressive illness: some research studies*. Springfield, IL: C. C Thomas.

24 Taylor, M. A. and Fink, M. (2006) *Melancholia: the diagnosis, pathophysiology and treatment of depressive disorders*. Cambridge: Cambridge University Press.

25 Ottosson, J.-O. and Fink, M. (2004). *Ethics of electroconvulsive therapy*. New York: Brunner-Routledge.

26 Fink, M. and Kellner, C. H. (2007). Belling the cat: ECT practice standards in the United States. *Journal of Electroconvulsive Therapy* **23**, 3–5.

Essay 20

Cognitive theory and therapy: past, present, and future

Aaron T. Beck and David J. A. Dozois

Introduction

From its inception in the early 1960s (1–3) the formulation of a coherent theoretical framework has preceded the development of cognitive therapy (CT) interventions. Specifically, Beck's objectives for deriving and evaluating this system of psychotherapy has involved an overall plan to construct a comprehensive theory of psychopathology that maps clearly onto the treatment approach, to investigate scientific support for the theory and to test the efficacy of therapeutic interventions (3,4). Cognitive theory and therapy were first developed for depression (1,2) and later systematically applied to suicide (5), anxiety disorders (6), personality disorders (7), substance abuse (8), and, finally, schizophrenia (9).

CT, often labelled as cognitive behaviour therapy (CBT), has grown exponentially as evidenced by its ubiquitous presence in training programmes in psychology, psychiatry, medicine, social work, nursing, and other allied health professions that value evidence-based practice (10). CT and CBT have been described as 'the fastest growing and most heavily researched systems of psychotherapy on the contemporary scene' (11, p. 332). In this essay we outline the historical development of both the theory and the therapy. After this recapitulation, we present an overview of the conceptual, practical, and empirical aspects of CT and highlight the core concepts and the empirical research pertaining to cognitive theory. General treatment strategies are outlined and a brief review of the efficacy of the approach is provided. We conclude with recommendations for future research.

The origins of cognitive therapy

Observations and theory (1956–1964)

The evolution of the cognitive model and of CT can best be understood in terms of a biographical note. The therapy did not emerge full-blown but went through many tortuous paths in terms of several phases punctuated by surprises and anomalies.

Beck's first foray into the area of cognition, in 1956, occurred as a result of treating a particular patient. Beck was then practicing psychodynamic psychotherapy. The patient, M, who had been referred with depression, had followed the fundamental rule of psychoanalytic treatment. Like most patients in this form of therapy, he had ostensibly followed instructions of not censoring thoughts that he was concerned about and reporting everything that came to his mind.

While freely associating, M had been criticizing the therapist angrily through much of a session. After a pause, Beck asked him, operating according to the 'book', what he was feeling. 'Guilt', he responded. Beck then interpreted what he thought was the causal sequence: M was feeling angry, expressed the anger, and the anger itself evoked guilt. In other words, hostility led without any intermediary variables to guilt—one emotion directly to another. There was no need to insert any other links into the chain.

Then M shared a completely unexpected observation when he stated that while criticizing the therapist he was aware of another unexpressed stream of thought: 'I said the wrong thing . . . I should not have said that . . . I'm wrong to criticize him. I'm bad . . . I have no excuse for being so mean.' This incident came as a total surprise to Beck and presented him with an anomaly: If M was reporting everything that came to mind, how could he have experienced a conscious flow of associations and not reported it? Furthermore, how could two streams of thought occur simultaneously? The answer to the latter question embodies a key principle: there can be more than one stream of thought running in parallel. The first, more readily expressed, represented the most conscious component. The second, at the periphery of awareness, and not reported, probably corresponded to what Freud had described as 'preconscious'.

Beck's formulation ran as follows: M's self-critical thoughts were intermediate between his expressions of anger and his feelings of guilt. The anger did not directly activate the guilt, but led to self-critical thoughts, and his self-criticism produced the guilt. This notion ran contrary to the psychoanalytic dictum that anger leads directly to guilt. Beck later discovered that self-critical thoughts could lead to guilt and sadness without any preceding anger.

Beck found that many other patients had also experienced this double stream of thinking: reported and unreported thoughts. For the most part, however, they were not aware of the second stream (later labelled 'automatic thoughts'). One could see why they had not previously been communicated. First, they tended to be fleeting. Second, they were just on the fringe of consciousness. Third, they were not the kinds of thoughts that people were accustomed to sharing with others. In order to prime their awareness, Beck asked his patients to note what thoughts occurred immediately before the experience of a particular feeling. When patients focused in this way, they were almost always able to recognize their automatic thoughts.

Beck tested this notion with his next patient, B. She was a sad 25-year-old woman who spent most of the session freely relating stories of her sexual escapades, without any attempt to censor them. B did, however, report anxious feelings during much of the session. Beck developed a standard formulation: the anxiety was possibly due to a sense of shame over exposing herself to the therapist's censure. However, following the lead from M, Beck asked her to focus on thoughts she had had just prior to the anxiety. As B continued to describe her sexual adventures, she also focused on her anxiety and the thoughts most closely linked to it. She then conveyed the following: 'I am not expressing myself clearly. He is bored with me. He probably can't follow what I am saying. This sounds foolish to him. He will no doubt get rid of me.'

After piecing together his observations from the reported automatic thoughts of these two patients (as well as the reports of other patients, his own introspective explorations, and those of friends and relatives), Beck arrived at the beginnings of a cognitive theory. There are at least two systems of thought. The first, the 'conversational mode', is directed to others and, when freely expressed, comprises the sort of feelings and thoughts commonly divulged. The second system, the 'self-signalling mode', consists of self-monitoring, self-instructions, and self-warnings, and includes the rapid, automatic interpretation of events, self-evaluations and anticipations. Its function is to communicate with oneself rather than with others. As discovered later, the internal dialogue was the source of much of the patient's problems. By tapping into this system, the therapist could better understand patients' difficulties and help to resolve them. Beck also recognized that there were errors in the way the person interpreted experience, made predictions, or formulated plans of action.

As it turned out, B believed that she was boring and inarticulate. She tried to compensate for this by entertaining the therapist but her negative self-evaluation persisted. She continued to regard herself as boring, even though she was actually very articulate. As Beck subsequently realized, her belief that she was boring shaped her interpretation of her behaviour and her expectations of rejection by others. At that point, however, Beck was not aware of how information processing was dictated by fundamental beliefs.

At first, automatic thoughts seemed to be relevant only to the 'transference'; that is, they were concerned with the patient's unconsciously derived ways of relating to the therapist. But it soon emerged that these reactions generalized. B, for instance, believed that she was boring in all situations. Thus, her activated automatic thoughts, not spontaneously reported, could be a fertile area to explore. In contrast, readily available thoughts, namely discussion of sensitive sexual issues, while clinically relevant, did not get to the heart of her problem.

Beck began to 'train' patients to observe and convey their unreported thoughts, thus securing a database of rich material, in essence the raw data, for devising a new approach to psychopathology and psychotherapy. To paraphrase Pasteur, 'In the field of observation, the rewards go to the person who is prepared to hear'. Perhaps, Beck was unwittingly influenced by the beginning of the 'cognitive revolution' in psychology (see reference 12).

The negativity of depression permeated patients' internal communications, such as self-evaluation, attributions, expectancies, inferences, and recall; they were manifest as low self-esteem, self-blame and self-criticism, pessimistic predictions, negative interpretations of experiences, and unpleasant recollections. In ambiguous situations, depressed patients were particularly prone to making a negative interpretation when a positive one seemed more appropriate; they would not only magnify their own unpleasant experiences, but also either blot out or label as negative experiences that others would consider positive.

Beck also noted a variety of errors inherent in depressive thinking—selective abstraction, overgeneralization, dichotomous thinking, and exaggeration of negative aspects of one's experiences (these errors are outlined later in this essay). Furthermore, patients predicted negative outcomes from tasks they might undertake as well as long-range, bad outcomes more generally. A high degree of negative expectations ('hopelessness') appeared to predict suicide. These phenomena were universal across all types of depression.

The negative themes in depression seemed to fit into what was later termed the 'negative cognitive triad'. Patients were in the grip of a negative view of themselves, their personal world, and their future. Whether they looked back or ahead, all they could see was failure, frustration, and inadequacy (2).

To account for the specificity of negative thinking in depression, Beck postulated a 'negative cognitive shift'; that is, he observed that persistent negativity occurred only while the patient was dejected. According to this thesis, as the patient enters a state of depression, cognitive organization changes so that much relevant positive information is filtered out or disqualified, whereas negative self-referential information is amplified (cf. 13).

Beck was in for another set of surprises. He had made it a practice to inquire from his patients who returned for booster sessions months or years after completing therapy what they had learned from their psychoanalytic experience. He expected them to make comments such as 'I learned that I had made my wife into a mother figure', 'I worked through my sibling rivalry', or 'I overcame my oral fixation'. In contrast, they made statements like, 'I learned to think before I acted', or 'I realized that I exaggerate too much', or 'I learned that I always saw the gloomy side of things'. Almost uniformly, they said that therapy had taught them to 'think straight'.

Early research (1959–1962)

Beck was determined to test selected psychoanalytic hypotheses regarding depression. Research on this topic seemed like a fertile field since the hypotheses were well elaborated, generally accepted, and seemingly testable. Depression was also an obvious state to investigate given its high prevalence in patients. The most prominent psychoanalytic hypothesis at the time remained what Freud purported in his 1917 essay *Mourning and Melancholia*, that depression was a manifestation of hostility directed to oneself (see 14).

The research objectives were twofold: (1) determine where to look for such internalized hostility and (2) ascertain how to measure it. Freud had stated that dreams were the 'royal road to the unconscious'. Perhaps this type of ideational material would lend itself to investigation. If people with depression were filled with covert hostility then presumably it could be identified by analysing the content of their dreams. The theory of hostility turned inwards had a plausible ring. First, one could observe that patients with depression—at least those with severe depression—seemed to have less conscious hostility and reacted less than did non-depressed individuals to situations that might be expected to arouse hostility. Second, various depressive symptoms (e.g. self-criticism, loss of enjoyment, images of themselves as depraved, and, ultimately, the wish to kill themselves) seemed consistent with the formulation of hostility directed to the self.

Using existing scales of hostility, Beck measured this variable in the dreams reported by depressed and non-depressed individuals. In a pilot study, depressed patients showed less hostility in their dreams than did the non-depressed group. Although depressed individuals had fewer dreams in which they played a hostile role, they did have a preponderance of dreams in which they felt thwarted, deprived, victimized, or disappointed. One patient, for instance, described the following dream: 'I was tremendously thirsty. I put my last nickel in a Coke machine, and all I got was fizz—no Coke or liquid'. A man dreamt that he was late for a formal dinner and discovered that the shoes he was planning to wear were both for the left foot. A third patient had a dream that she was calling her therapist at a time of considerable desperation. All she got was a recording of the therapist's voice—no direct contact.

The depressed individuals all showed the same themes (albeit less dramatically) in their waking experiences. In contrast to non-depressed patients, they viewed themselves as the subject of an unpleasant event. They also saw themselves as 'losers' in every sense of the word: they had lost something of great value, and felt defeated, deficient, and extruded from society.

Beck was engaged in two other projects to test these findings more systematically. In the first, the initial 20 dreams reported by 6 depressed and 6 non-depressed patients were reviewed. Beck then still adhered to the psychodynamic model of internalized hostility but shifted the conceptualization as follows: since depressed patients turned their hostility inwards, it could be experienced only indirectly and would manifest in self-punishment or other expressions of a need to suffer. By suffering, they were punishing themselves; that is, inflicting hostility against themselves. This 'masochism' would show as self-criticism, courting rejection, and suicidal wishes.

Thus, the 'loser' dreams were labelled 'masochistic'. A manual, with examples of how to score the dreams, was prepared. A colleague, who was blind to the patients' diagnoses, scored the dreams. A significant difference between the groups emerged. All the depressed individuals had substantially more masochistic dreams than did the non-depressed patients. In order to substantiate this finding, a replication study was conducted on a much larger sample (210 hospitalized and ambulatory patients) and with more refined instruments. The investigators developed a system to achieve reliable diagnoses and to measure depression using clinical ratings and self-report (the latter evolved into the Beck Depression Inventory; 15,16).

A severely depressed group reported many more masochistic dreams than did their non-depressed counterparts—consistent with the original findings. Although the psychoanalytic theory of depression seemed to have been confirmed, at least preliminarily, it was necessary to approach the hypothesis from other vantage points and using different techniques. The next study involved a controlled experiment applying a verbal reinforcement interpersonal reward–punishment paradigm. The experimenter subtly expressed approval or disapproval of the research participant for using certain words in response to a questionnaire. The hypothesis was that, since the depressed patients had a 'need to suffer', they would quickly learn responses that were 'punished' and be slower in learning rewarded responses. Contrary to expectations, the depressed patients were particularly sensitive to feedback. They learned more rapidly than did non-depressed patients which responses were rewarded but did not recognize the responses that were 'punished' any more readily than the rewarded responses—a total reversal of what had been expected.

Other studies also failed to support the 'masochism' hypothesis. Could it be that the manifest content of dreams, instead of being an expression of a deep-seated need for punishment or self-directed hostility, reflected the way patients actually viewed

themselves and their experiences? In examining patients' descriptions of their thinking during the waking state, Beck noted a consistency in the content of two diverse
phenomena: dreams and automatic thoughts. That is, the latter thoughts represented a
negative distortion of reality, as did their dreams. Continuity of content and themes in
these two types of ideation also emerged. In waking life, the person might respond to
an event with a thought, 'I'm lonely' (and feel bad). In his or her dreams, this would be
graphically dramatized and probably exaggerated by a pictorial representation of being
entirely alone, perhaps in a bombed-out area, shut in a closet, or in a hospital, dying.
Among the depressed people, were automatic thoughts such as, 'nobody likes me', 'I'm
worthless', 'I've lost everything', 'nothing ever works out for me'. By understanding the
connection between their negative concepts and their symptoms, the depressive episode became less mysterious and more manageable.

Therapy phase (1965 onwards)

The next question was how to intervene therapeutically. If the depressed person has a
pervasive negative outlook, what can therapists do about it? Can they alleviate the distress by modifying the negative constructions of reality? To describe this next step, we
need to reiterate what patients believed they had learned from psychoanalytic therapy:
(a) not to take their thoughts at face value, (b) to think reflectively before they acted,
(c) to recognize their exaggeration of the significance of events, and (d) to appreciate
that they frequently misinterpreted the motives of others.

As the switch to CT emerged, strategies were incorporated that were being promoted
in behaviour therapy:

1 Engage patients' interest in viewing their negative interpretations not as reality
   but as hypotheses that could be (a) evaluated in terms of positive and negative
   evidence, logical deductions from the evidence, and alternative explanations; and
   (b) subject to empirical testing. Thus, a patient who concluded that nobody cared
   for her would be questioned regarding the basis of this judgement. Then if she
   had misinterpreted an event, she would be asked to look for evidence to support
   or refute the hypothesis, set up criteria, and logically analyse the data.

2 By encouraging patients to examine their automatic thoughts, their thinking
   shifted from an absolutist mode ('my conclusions are absolutely correct') to a
   questioning mode ('are my conclusions correct?').

3 The approach, one of 'collaborative empiricism' in which rapport, mutual trust,
   and sensitivity were established (17), involved the patient working *together* with
   the therapist to investigate the validity of his or her beliefs.

4 In the mid-1960s, Beck specifically operationalized each procedure of CT. For
   instance, problem-solving was applied to all the patient's difficulties—whether
   it was a problem in their thinking (e.g. cognitive distortions), other depressive
   symptoms (e.g. lack of energy, sadness, suicidal wishes), or 'external problems' at
   work and at home. A behavioural strategy, 'graded task assignment', was deployed
   to deal with feelings of anergia, anhedonia, and apathy. As patients successfully
   completed one step towards a goal, they would be encouraged to take the next—
   more difficult—step. The goals of each task, specific steps for reaching them, and

criteria for their attainment were defined in advance; provision for feedback was facilitated. Other features included, (a) setting an agenda at the beginning of each session, (b) providing for feedback from the patient (e.g. ensuring that patients understand the rationale; inquiring about how they perceived therapy to be proceeding) at specific intervals during, and at the end of, the session, and (c) assigning 'homework' (e.g. reading handouts on CT, completing daily activity schedules, and filling in dysfunctional thought records).

As this approach was developed, patients began to improve almost immediately, many becoming symptom-free by the seventh or eighth session. By the twelfth session, enough ground had been covered to terminate therapy—with the proviso that patients return for 'booster sessions' at monthly, then semi-annual intervals. As more patients showed remission following this regimen, it was obvious that an effective, short-term therapy for depression had crystallized.

Over the years, more emphasis was placed on conceptualizing each case than on techniques. The rationale was that if therapists could prepare a coherent formulation about their patients they could then individualize relevant techniques. The formulation was later based on a further elaboration of the original theory (2) and stresses the role of core beliefs (for example, 'I am stupid'), conditional beliefs (e.g. 'if people knew the real me, they would reject me'), and compensatory strategies ('if I am funny and entertaining, they will accept me'). The task of the therapist was to show how core beliefs mould the patients' reactions to situations and make them vulnerable to particular types of stress.

Early trials of cognitive therapy

A key question as to whether the positive results in applying CT represented an idiosyncratic phenomenon or could be replicated using other therapists was the next challenge. Consequently, an intensive outpatient study was undertaken at the University of Pennsylvania with the goal to assess the efficacy of CT compared to antidepressant medication; CT was found to be the more effective of the two (18).

The techniques of CT were specified in a manual, later published as a book (17). Therapists were supervised weekly by experienced clinicians. By the end of active treatment, both treatment groups showed statistically significant decreases (p <0.001) in depressive symptoms according to self-reports, observer evaluations, and therapist ratings. The response rate to both pharmacotherapy and CT exceeded the reported ranges for placebo response in depressed outpatients. Of the CT patients, almost 80% showed marked improvement or remission by the end of therapy, whereas only 20% of those who received medication showed a similar degree of response. Follow-up of the completers 1 year after the end of treatment revealed that, although many patients had an intermittently symptomatic course, both groups maintained their gains. However, self-rated depressive symptoms were significantly lower in the CT group and the medication patients relapsed twice as frequently (19).

This was the first controlled outcome study to show the superiority of any psychological intervention over antidepressants in moderate to severely depressed outpatients. A later study compared the effect of CT alone with a combination CT and antidepressant medication. Both groups improved substantially, including at follow-up. Adding an antidepressant, however, did not increase the efficacy of CT.

Many randomized controlled trials of CT in depression have been conducted since the above work. In addition, other applications of CT have indicated that this treatment is effective for a host of psychiatric and medical conditions.

Further evolution of cognitive theory and therapy

To qualify as a system of psychotherapy, it must satisfy three criteria (a) a conceptual or theoretical framework and empirical data to support this, (b) a set of therapeutic strategies that articulate with the theory, and (c) evidence of efficacy (3). We will highlight these matters in the remainder of this essay.

Cognitive theory

CT is based on the premise that information processing is crucial for effective adaptation. Without the ability to process information from the external world, synthesize it, and formulate a plan for dealing with it, we would not survive. Information processing is intricately tied to emotional, motivational and behavioural systems. Each of these systems serves specific functions and also operates in synchrony applying coordinated goal-oriented strategies (e.g. approaching pleasure, avoiding pain) (20). The fight–flight response, for instance, is made up of cognitive (perception of threat), emotional (feelings of anxiety or anger), motivational (the impulse to confront or flee the threatening stimulus), and behavioural (the action itself) systems. The onset of a condition (e.g. panic disorder) occurs when these systems shift from a quiescent state to a highly activated one. In the example above, this might take place when the fight or flight response is routinely activated by 'false alarms' (e.g. misperceiving bodily sensations as harmful). Cognitive theory suggests that psychopathology is characterized by the activation of a conglomerate of related dysfunctional beliefs, meanings, and memories that operate in coordination with emotion, motivation, behaviour, and physiological responses. Different conditions are associated with specific biases that influence how an individual incorporates and responds to new information.

According to the model (17), the *cognitive appraisal* of internal and external stimuli influences and is, in turn, impacted by the other systems. Thus, although cognition plays a key role (i.e. the assignment of meaning is crucial to understanding maladaptive behaviour), mental health problems involve a complex interplay among a number of diverse and interrelated systems.

Different levels of cognition, ranging from surface thoughts to 'deeper' cognitive schemas, occur within the cognitive system (21). The latter are organized structures of stored information that contain individuals' perceptions of self and others, goals, expectations, and memories. These elements within the cognitive structure influence the screening, coding, categorizing, and interpreting of incoming stimuli and retrieval of stored information. Schemas are adaptive insofar as they afford efficient processing of information; however, when they become negatively biased, maladaptive, rigid, and self-perpetuating, they contribute to psychopathology.

Maladaptive cognitive schemas develop initially during early childhood and become increasingly consolidated and organized as new experiences are assimilated into the existing belief structure (3,17). Poor early attachment experiences and other adverse events (e.g. childhood maltreatment), for example, may contribute to the development of a maladaptive belief system. Cognitive theory is essentially a diathesis–stress model. In other words, it is possible to have maladaptive beliefs and not exhibit symptoms so long as the cognitive schema (and related systems) is not activated. Once triggered (e.g. by external events, drugs, endocrine factors, and the like), however, a cascade of information processing biases—represented as attention, memory, or interpretational—is initiated (17,21,22). For instance, individuals with anxiety disorders perceive themselves as vulnerable and the world as dangerous. Such individuals attend selectively to threat-pertinent information at the expense of data that are inconsistent with threat or which suggest that one has sufficient resources for dealing it (6). A person vulnerable to depression may have an underlying belief that he or she is unlovable; this may become salient when adverse circumstances activate an underlying negative schema. Such an individual may then attend selectively to and recall information that is consistent with this negative view of self (e.g. paying attention to cues that suggest being unloved and minimizing information that is inconsistent with that belief).

Activation of a maladaptive cognitive schema and the ensuing information processing biases are also apparent in more surface-level cognitions or what are referred to as automatic thoughts. The latter refer to the stream of positive and negative thoughts that run through a person's mind unaccompanied by conscious deliberation. Although the thoughts are more superficial and proximal to a given situation than are other levels of cognition, they are functionally related to deeper beliefs and schemas and arise associatively as different aspects of a core belief system are activated.

Cognitive schemas have a variety of characteristics such as breadth, intensity, and, most importantly, an energy level. As a result, there are various degrees of activation. When schemas are activated, as in depression, they are not only identifiable but also influence information processing, as manifested by cognitive biases. This negative thinking, in turn, exacerbates depressive symptoms. When a depressive episode remits, negative schemas are deactivated (or vice versa).

Another aspect of the model is *content-specificity* (22). That is, different emotional experiences and forms of psychopathology are related to a unique cognitive profile or set of beliefs. To illustrate, depression is related to thoughts and beliefs of personal loss, deprivation, and failure (17). People with marked anxiety overestimate the probability of risk while simultaneously underestimating their resources for coping with possible threats. Their thoughts focus on the self as vulnerable, the world as dangerous, and the future as potentially catastrophic (6). A person with dependent personality disorder, in contrast, views him- or herself as weak, helpless, and incompetent (7).

The empirical literature has provided considerable support for various aspects of cognitive theory (see 21,22 for review). In an early unpublished review of over 200 studies (23), the vast majority supported the model in terms of the cognitive triad, schemas, and cognitive processing. The closer the studies related to clinical observations, the greater their support for the theory; for example, research involving student participants were less supportive than those of clinically depressed patients (see 22).

Hundreds of studies have demonstrated that people filter information and respond to stimuli in a way that is consistent with their pre-existing beliefs and assumptions. Research has also found that negative cognitive biases precede the emergence of anxiety and depressive symptoms. Distinctive levels of cognition work in synchrony to affect emotional and behavioural responses and emotional experiences or clinical disorders can be characterized by a specific set of beliefs and automatic thoughts (i.e. content-specificity; see 21,22). Support has been found in the empirical literature for schema organization (see 21) and activation (e.g. 24). Moreover, research evidence suggests that cognitive variables contribute to the onset of psychiatric disorders (e.g. 25).

Cognitive therapy

CT rests on three main propositions: (a) *the access hypothesis*—with appropriate training, motivation, and attention, people can become aware of their thinking; (b) *the mediation hypothesis*—the way in which people think about, interpret, and construe events influences their emotional and behavioural responses; and, (c) *the change hypothesis*—people can become more functional and adaptive by intentionally modifying their cognitive and behavioural responses to the circumstances they face (12). CT is a structured, collaborative process that helps people to consider both the accuracy and usefulness of their thoughts through exploring (determining one's idiosyncratic meaning system and maladaptive beliefs), examining (reviewing the evidence for and against a belief and considering alternative interpretations), and experimenting (testing the validity of a belief system) (26). This approach is used initially to target more proximal and surface cognitions (e.g. automatic thoughts, dysfunctional attitudes) and later in therapy to modify deeper cognitive structures and core beliefs.

CT does not aim to replace negative thoughts with positive ones; rather, it seeks to help shift maladaptive cognitive appraisals to evidence-based, adaptive ones. Patients learn how to become scientists of their own thinking—to treat thoughts as hypotheses rather than as facts and to put them to the test. Framing a belief as a hypothesis provides an opportunity to test its validity, consider alternative explanations, and gain distance from a thought thereby facilitating greater objective scrutiny (10). Patients then can modify their thoughts making them congruent with existing evidence. When thoughts are aligned with evidence, but negative feelings persist, the therapist helps patients to deal with emotional sequelae by introducing coping strategies, fostering skill development (e.g. teaching assertiveness or other social skills) and/or problem-solving.

Cognitive therapists assist patients to explore, examine, and experiment using collaborative empiricism, guided discovery, and Socratic dialogue. *Collaborative empiricism*, described earlier, involves patient and therapist becoming co-investigators both in terms of ascertaining treatment goals and investigating the patient's thoughts. *Guided discovery* permits patients to test their own thinking through personal observations and experiments rather than being subject to cajoling or persuasion. This process enables patients to shift from 'a conviction mode to a questioning mode' (27, p. 216). In addition, by collaboratively designing new experiences to try out (behavioural experiments) patients can acquire a different perspective on themselves and their circumstances (20). *Socratic dialogue* is one method of guided discovery in which the therapist asks carefully sequenced questions to define problems, assists in the identification of thoughts and beliefs, examines the meaning of events, or assesses the ramifications of particular thoughts or behaviours.

CT is time-limited—the average course of treatment is between 12 and 24 sessions. The initial sessions focus on enhancing the therapeutic alliance, identifying the specific problem(s) that brought someone into treatment, socializing the patient to the cognitive understanding of psychopathology, and obtaining symptom relief via behavioural strategies. The therapist plays a more active role than the patient during this phase. As therapy progresses, the emphasis shifts from symptom amelioration to examining and modifying patterns of thinking of the patient who assumes a more active role (identifying problems and solutions and developing and conducting homework assignments). Towards the end of treatment, sessions are usually more widely spaced so enabling the patient to consolidate gains and acquire confidence in applying newly learned skills. Booster sessions are often scheduled 1–2 months after termination.

Because the therapeutic hour constitutes only a small proportion of the week, homework assignments (or *action plans*) are an essential component; they provide opportunities to enhance mastery and to transfer learned skills to the 'real world', thereby augmenting outcome.

CT techniques vary depending on the disorder being treated and the formulation although they typically include (a) establishing the therapeutic relationship; (b) behavioural change strategies; (c) cognitive restructuring strategies; (d) modifying core beliefs and schemas; and (e) preventing relapse or recurrence. Given that it not possible to describe the science and art of CT in this brief essay (see 28), we provide instead a capsular summary of these components.

The therapeutic relationship is a key ingredient of all psychotherapies; CT is no exception. There appears to be a bidirectional relationship between the patient's perception of the therapeutic alliance and outcome such that the connection between patient and therapist may facilitate change; and symptom change, in turn, enhances the bond between patient and therapist (10). Many basic interpersonal variables common to other forms of psychotherapy (e.g. warmth, accurate empathy, unconditional positive regard) serve as a major foundation for change. However, as Beck et al. note, these features 'in themselves are necessary but not sufficient to produce an optimum therapeutic effect' (17, p. 45).

Behavioural strategies are used to test and alter automatic thoughts and assumptions and to facilitate new learning. In a behavioural experiment, for instance, a patient may predict an outcome based on his or her automatic thoughts and beliefs, conduct an agreed-upon behaviour, and evaluate the evidence in the context of the experiment. A related approach is hypothesis testing, which has both cognitive and behavioural components. A doctor in training who insists 'I am not a good doctor', for example, can be asked to generate a list of criteria that constitutes good 'doctoring' (e.g. ability to establish rapport; knowledge; capacity to make decisions under pressure). The experiment would involve collecting data by monitoring his or her behaviour and seeking input from colleagues and supervisors which may modify this conviction (e.g. 'I am a good doctor for my level of experience and training') (20). Other behavioural techniques are used to alter one's reinforcement schedule (thereby increasing pleasure or mastery), habituate to feared stimuli (exposure), relax (progressive muscle relaxation), or prepare for upcoming situations (behavioural rehearsal). Given that these techniques are used to foster cognitive change, the therapist routinely assesses the patient's perceptions, thoughts, and conclusions after each experiment (20,28).

Cognitive restructuring strategies are also used to help patients identify and test the validity of their cognitions. One technique to elicit and evaluate negative automatic thoughts is the *daily record of thoughts* (DRT). The DRT is made up of columns which represent the situation encountered, the emotion or symptoms experienced, and associated thoughts. Once patients are able to identify the automatic thoughts that carry the greatest emotional charge, the process of answering back to these thoughts (or putting them on trial) can begin. This process often involves writing down the evidence that pertains to a particular belief and developing an alternative thought that incorporates the facts that bear on the belief. By writing down an activating event, the mediating thoughts, and the ensuing emotional response, the DRT fosters more objectivity about one's thoughts. The evidence pertaining to a particular belief is then examined using guided discovery and collaborative empiricism.

Specifically, patients are asked a number of questions including: 'What is the evidence for or against this belief?' 'What are the alternative ways to think about this situation?' 'If my best friend or loved one knew that I had this thought, what would he or she say to me?' 'What would it mean about me even if this particular thought was true?' (28). Following this analysis, patients are taught to generate alternative thoughts that incorporate the evidence and lead to a shift in their emotional experience. If a thought is inconsistent with the weight of evidence that bears on the subject matter (e.g. 'I am unlovable'), the therapist helps the patient to alter and realign the thought so that it is evidence-based and, consequently, more adaptive. Collecting more information or conducting a behavioural experiment may also be used to test a certain belief.

After a number of sessions using the DRT, therapist and patient may note a consistent pattern in the types of automatic thoughts elicited. This is because such thoughts and cognitive distortions (e.g. 'If I fail at X, then I am not worthwhile') are functionally related to deeper core beliefs and schemas. Modifying core beliefs and schemas results in change that generalizes and contributes to the prevention of relapse (29). 'Deeper' beliefs are tested and reconfigured using Socratic dialogue and guided discovery, role plays, behavioural experiments, and other change strategies.

The final sessions focus on consolidating skills learned and on preventing relapse/recurrence. This includes a gradual titration of sessions and extending the interval between them, reviewing strategies that were applied and proved most helpful, creating a plan for the future, discussing feelings about termination, preparing for setbacks, identifying any triggers of relapse, and ensuring that the patient recognizes that he or she was the agent of treatment change.

Empirical evidence for cognitive therapy

CT is one of the most researched psychotherapies (30) and has received empirical support for a host of conditions. We focus first on depression as this has been the most extensively studied.

Over 75 clinical trials and numerous meta-analyses have been conducted on CT for depression (30). CT is comparable to other bona fide psychological treatments and antidepressants for an acute episode, with each superior to placebo (see 31). Earlier findings (32) suggesting that CT was not effective for severe cases have generated considerable controversy. The perception that CT is ineffective for severe cases has persisted despite compelling data to the contrary (see 10 for review). DeRubeis et al. (33), for example, conducted a mega-analysis in which they pooled the data from four related trials and found that CT was as effective as antidepressants in treating severe cases. Other studies have also demonstrated similar benefits from the two types of treatment (34,35).

CT also carries an advantage over antidepressants in reducing the rate of relapses. Gloaguen et al. (36), for instance, reported that the average relapse risk (based on a 1–2 year follow-up) was 25% following CT, compared to 60% for antidepressants. Patients who receive CT alone are no more likely to relapse after treatment than those who continue to receive medication (37). Hollon et al. (35) found equivalent outcomes for medication and CT in the acute phase of treatment but a lower relapse rate for CT compared to continuance medication.

Consistent with these findings are studies that have examined potential mechanisms for the prophylactic benefits of CT. It appears as though CT and antidepressants may both change certain aspects of negative thinking (such as information processing, automatic thoughts, dysfunctional attitudes) but that CT may further modify 'deeper' cognitive structures (e.g. reduced activation of negative thinking following a negative mood manipulation in CT relative to medication) that give rise to relapse and recurrence (e.g. 29). Several studies have also assessed neuroimaging changes in CT. Goldapple et al. (38), for example, examined neurobiological responses to CT (in unmedicated depressed patients) and compared these findings to an independent sample of individuals treated with SSRIs. Differential pre- vs post-treatment changes in the metabolic activity (measured using PET) were obtained in individuals treated with CT compared to those treated with antidepressants. These researchers proposed that a top-down (cortical-limbic) mechanism may be active with CT, whereas a bottom-up (limbic-cortical) mechanism may be active with antidepressant treatment.

CT for other psychiatric disorders

Butler et al. (30) reviewed meta-analyses of outcome for CT for a number of disorders. Rigorous meta-analyses covering almost 4 decades of trials and involving 10,000 participants were examined. The review focused on effect sizes that compared outcomes of CT with outcomes for control groups, providing an overview of the efficacy of CT. Large effect sizes were obtained for unipolar depression, generalized anxiety disorder, panic disorder, social anxiety, and childhood internalizing problems. Moderate effect sizes were found for couple distress, anger, childhood somatoform disorders, and chronic pain. Small effect sizes were obtained for sexual offenders. CBT also showed promising results as an adjunct to medication for schizophrenia (9).

Epp and Dobson (31) have reviewed outcomes for CT and summarized the meta-analytic data according to absolute efficacy (the extent to which CT demonstrates favourable outcome to no treatment, wait list controls, or treatment as usual), efficacy relative to medication, and other forms of psychotherapy. Considerable support has accumulated for the efficacy of CT. For certain disorders (e.g. some anxiety disorders, bulimia nervosa), the evidence is compelling enough to suggest that CT should be considered the treatment of choice. CT is at least as effective as medication for a range of problems, although direct comparisons are not found for some disorders (e.g. bipolar disorder, psychosis) for which CT is used adjunctively (28).

CT for physical conditions

CT is also effective for the treatment of anxiety and depression that accompanies medical states (e.g. 39). In addition, benefits have been found for a range of physical illnesses including chronic pain, back pain, functional impairment related to cancer, rheumatoid arthritis, chronic fatigue syndrome, fibromyalgia, irritable bowel syndrome, hypertension, tinnitus, headaches, sexual dysfunctions, and various neurological conditions. For some of these, systematic reviews and meta-analyses have demonstrated various biopsychosocial benefits from CT.

Future directions

In 1976, Beck posed the question, 'Can a fledgling psychotherapy challenge the giants in the field—psychoanalysis and behaviour therapy?' It appears that four and a half decades of research support the cognitive model for a variety of health problems. Moreover, the model has been expanded to incorporate evidence from experimental cognitive science and the neurosciences (22,40,41). Several reports in the United Kingdom and the United States have recommended the use of CT for a number of psychiatric conditions (4). Notwithstanding, CT is not a panacea and the necessity of testing and modifying cognitions has not gone unquestioned. For example, behaviourally based interventions tend to perform as well as CT for depression and anxiety. It is important to point out, however, that behavioural interventions have always been part of CT (17). In addition, cognitive theory states that whatever treatment is used so that the patient improves (or if improvement occurs via spontaneous remission), the negative beliefs must also normalize. Indeed, Harmer et al. (42) found that antidepressants modulate emotional processing in depressed people prior to shifts in symptoms, supporting the primacy of cognitions in change. However, CT also alters 'deeper' levels of cognition (29); targeting these deeper thoughts may account for its reduced relapse rates relative to medication.

What of future directions for the field? Since the 1990s, many longitudinal studies have supported the diathesis–stress model of cognitive vulnerability (21). Researchers have also achieved a better understanding of gene–environment interactions in the context of psychopathology. For example, a relationship has been found between negative cognitive processing and the short version of the serotonin transporter gene (41). Further work is necessary to elucidate the complex relationships among genetic, neurophysiological, environmental, and cognitive vulnerabilities in the study of psychopathology and to understand the intricate connections between cognitive, affective, motivational and behavioural systems.

Future research will no doubt clarify the key mechanisms of change in CT. Studies have suggested that cognitive change is a relevant mediator of symptomatic improvement (e.g. 10, 29) but we need more studies to ensure that the finding is robust and, if so, to determine which strategies (and what therapeutic doses) lead to the most stable cognitive change. Enormous strides have been made in understanding, evaluating, and refining CT. We are confident that similar progress will be made in improving our knowledge base of cognitive vulnerability and optimizing the delivery of CT.

Acknowledgements

This essay represents the amalgamation of two earlier manuscripts: (1) Beck, A. T. (1988) *Cognitive therapy of depression: a personal reflection*. The Malcolm Miller Lecture in Psychotherapy, University of Aberdeen, Department of Mental Health, Aberdeen, UK: Scottish Cultural Press; (2) Beck, A. T. and Dozois, D. J. A. (2011). Cognitive therapy: Current status and future directions. *Annual Review of Medicine*, **62**, 397–409. The authors are grateful for the permission to reproduce portions of this material.

References

1 Beck, A. T. (1963). Thinking and depression .1. Idiosyncratic content and cognitive distortions. *Archives of General Psychiatry* **9**, 324–33.

2 Beck, A. T. (1964). Thinking and depression. 2. Theory and therapy. *Archives of General Psychiatry* **10**, 561–71.

3 Beck, A. T. (1976). *Cognitive therapy and the emotional disorders*. New York: International University Press.

4 Beck, A. T. (2005). The current state of cognitive therapy: a 40-year retrospective. *Archives of General Psychiatry* **62**, 953–9.

5 Beck, A. T., Resnik, H. L. P., and Lettieri, D. J. (eds.) (1974). *The prevention of suicide*. Bowie, MD: Charles Press.

6 Beck, A. T., Emery, G., L., and Greenberg, R. L. (1985). *Anxiety disorders and phobias: a cognitive perspective*. New York: Basic Books.

7 Beck, A. T., Freeman, A., Davis D., and associates. (1990). *Cognitive therapy of personality disorders*. New York: Guilford Press.

8 Beck, A. T., Wright, F.D., Newman, C. F., and Liese, B. S. (1993). *Cognitive therapy of substance abuse*. New York: Guilford Press.

9 Beck, A. T., Rector, N.A., Stolar, N., and Grant, P. (2008). *Schizophrenia: cognitive theory, research, and therapy*. New York: Guilford Press.

10 DeRubeis, R. J., Webb, C. A., Tang, T. Z., and Beck, A. T. (2010). Cognitive therapy. In: Dobson, K. S. (ed.) *Handbook of cognitive-behavioral therapies* (3rd edn). New York: Guilford Press, pp. 277–316.

11 Prochaska, J. O. and Norcross, J. C. (2010). *Systems of psychotherapy: a transtheoretical analysis* (7th edn). Belmont, CA: Brooks/Cole.

12 Dobson, K. S and Dozois, D. J. A. (2010). Historical and philsophical bases of the cognitive-behavioral therapies. In: Dobson, K. S. (ed.) *Handbook of cognitive-behavioral therapies* (3rd edn), New York: Guilford Press, pp. 3–38.

13 Dozois, D. J. A. and Dobson, K. S. (2001). Information processing and cognitive organization in unipolar depression: specificity and comorbidity issues. *Journal of Abnormal Psychology* **110**, 236–46.

14 Dozois, D. J. A. (2000). Influences on Freud's *Mourning and Melancholia* and its contextual validity. *Journal of Theoretical and Philosophical Psychology* **20**, 167–95.

15 Beck, A. T., Ward, C.H., Mock, J., Mendelsohn, M., and Erbaugh, J. (1961). An inventory for measuring depression. *Archives of General Psychiatry* **4**, 561–71.

16 Beck, A. T., Steer, R. A., and Brown, G. K. (1996). *Beck Depression Inventory-II manual.* San Antonio, TX: Psychological Corporation.

17 Beck, A. T., Rush, A. J., Shaw, B. F and Emery, G. (1979). *Cognitive therapy of depression.* New York: Guilford Press.

18 Rush, A. J., Beck, A. T., Kovacs, M., and Hollon, S. D. (1977). Comparative efficacy of cognitive therapy and pharmacotherapy in the treatment of depressed outpatients. *Cognitive Therapy and Research* 1, 7–37

19 Kovacs, M., Rush, A. J., Beck, A. T., and Hollon, S. D. (1981). Depressed outpatients treated with cognitive therapy or pharmacotherapy: a one-year follow-up. *Archives of General Psychiatry* **38**, 33–9.

20 Beck, A. T. and Weishaar, M. E. (2011). Cognitive therapy. In: Corsini, R. J. and Wedding, D. (eds.). *Current psychotherapies* (9th edn). Belmont, CA: Brooks/Cole, pp. 276–309.

21 Dozois, D. J. A. and Beck, A. T. (2008). Cognitive schemas, beliefs and assumptions. In: Dobson, K. S. and Dozois, D. J. A. (eds.) *Risk factors in depression.* Oxford: Elsevier/Academic Press, pp. 121–43.

22 Clark, D. A., Beck, A. T., and Alford, B. (1999). *Scientific foundations of cognitive theory and therapy of depression.* New York: John Wiley and Sons.

23 Ernst, D. (1985). Beck's cognitive theory of depression: a status report. Unpublished manuscript.

24 Segal, Z. V., Gemar, M., and Williams, S. (1999). Differential cognitive response to a mood challenge following successful cognitive therapy or pharmacotherapy for unipolar depression. *Journal of Abnormal Psychology* **108**, 3–10.

25 Alloy, L. B., Abramson, L. Y., Whitehouse, W. G., and Hogan, M. E. (2006). Prospective incidence of first onsets and recurrences of depression in individuals at high and low cognitive risk for depression. *Journal of Abnormal Psychology* **115**, 145–56.

26 Hollon, S. D. and Dimidjian, S. (2009). Cognitive and behavioral treatment of depression. In: Gotlib I. H. and Hammen C. L. (eds.) *Handbook of Depression* (2nd edn). New York: Guilford Press, pp. 586–603.

27 Padesky, C. A. and Beck, A. T. (2003). Science and philosophy: Comparison of cognitive therapy and rational emotive behavior therapy. *Journal of Cognitive Psychotherapy* **17**, 211–24.

28 Dobson, D. and Dobson, K. S. (2009). *Evidence-based practice of cognitive behavioral therapy.* New York: Guilford Press.

29 Dozois, D. J. A., Bieling, P. J., Patelis-Siotis, I. et al. (2009). Changes in self-schema structure in cognitive therapy for major depressive disorder: a randomized clinical trial. *Journal of Consulting and Clinical Psychology* **77**, 1078–88.

30 Butler, A. C., Chapman, J. E., Forman, E. M., and Beck, A. T. (2006). The empirical status of cognitive-behavioral therapy: a review of meta-analyses. *Clinical Psychology Review* **26**, 17–31.

31 Epp, A. and Dobson, K. S. (2010). The evidence base for cognitive-behavioral therapy. In: Dobson, K. S. (ed.) *Handbook of cognitive-behavioral therapies.* New York: Guilford Press, pp. 39–73.

32 Elkin, I., Shea, M. T., Watkins, J. T. et al. (1989). National Institute of Mental Health Treatment of Depression Collaborative Research Program. General effectiveness of treatments. *Archives of General Psychiatry* **46**, 971–82.

33 DeRubeis, R. J., Gelfand, L. A., Tang, T. Z., and Simons, A. D. (1999). Medications versus cognitive behavior therapy for severely depressed outpatients: Mega-analysis of four randomized comparisons. *American Journal of Psychiatry* **156**, 1007–13.

34 DeRubeis, R. J., Hollon, S. D., Amsterdam, J. D. et al. (2005). Cognitive therapy vs medications in the treatment of moderate to severe depression. *Archives of General Psychiatry* **62**, 409–16.

35 Hollon, S. D., DeRubeis, R. J., Shelton, R. C. et al. (2005). Prevention of relapse following cognitive therapy vs medications in moderate to severe depression. *Archives of General Psychiatry* **62**, 417–22.

36 Gloaguen, V., Cottraux, J., Cucherat, M., and Blackburn, I. M. (1998). A meta-analysis of the effects of cognitive therapy in depressed patients. *Journal of Affective Disorders* **49**, 59–72.

37 Dobson, K. S., Hollon, S. D., Dimidjian, S. et al. (2008). Randomized trial of behavioral activation, cognitive therapy, and antidepressant medication in the prevention of relapse and recurrence in major depression. *Journal of Consulting and Clinical Psychology* **76**, 468–77.

38 Goldapple, K., Segal, Z., Garson, C. et al. (2004). Modulation of cortical-limbic pathways in major depression: treatment-specific effects of cognitive behavior therapy. *Archives of General Psychiatry* **61**, 34–41.

39 Sensky, T. (2004). Cognitive-behavior therapy for patients with physical illnesses. In: Wright J. (ed.) *Cognitive-behavior therapy: review of psychiatry.* Arlington, CA: APA Publishing, pp. 83–121.

40 Beck, A. T. (1996). Beyond belief: A theory of modes, personality, and psychopathology. In: Salkovskis, P. M. (ed.) *Frontiers of cognitive therapy.* New York: Guilford Press, pp. 1–25.

41 Beck, A. T. (2008). The evolution of the cognitive model of depression and its neurobiological correlates. *American Journal of Psychiatry* **165**, 969–77.

42 Harmer, C. J., O'Sullivan, U., Massey-Chase, R. S. et al. (2009). Effect of acute antidepressant administration on negative affective bias in depressed patients. *American Journal of Psychiatry* **116**, 1178–84.

Psychodynamic psychiatry—rise, decline, revival

Jeremy Holmes

Introduction

This essay tracks the varying fortunes of psychodynamic psychiatry (PP) from its 1960s heyday, through sharp decline in the 1980s and 1990s 'decade of the brain', to retrenchment and revival in the 21st century. I start by exploring of what is meant by the term 'psychodynamic', mentioning some of the key psychodynamic ideas that have entered into everyday psychiatric thinking and vernacular. The discussion then shifts to an historical account of the rise and fall of PP in the United Kingdom and the United States, followed by a brief worldwide survey. Moving to a possible future role for PP, I consider its evidence base, its contribution to the understanding and treatment of the principal psychiatric disorders, and its role in the expanding fields of neuropsychoanalysis, neurogenetics, and developmental psychopathology.

What is psychodynamic psychiatry?

Prejudice is rife in psychiatry. Mental illness is stigmatized, as are its sufferers and, to an extent, its practitioners. Within psychiatry itself psychoanalytic psychotherapists are sometimes characterized as antediluvian 'Freudians', clinging to outdated ideas and impervious to evidence-based theory and practice. In the course of this essay I hope to bust some of these myths.

Psychodynamic psychiatry must be differentiated from its parent discipline of psychoanalysis, although they are often mistakenly viewed as synonymous; here we shall be concerned with the role of psychoanalysis only insofar as it has impacted on PP. The term 'psychodynamics' predates Freud (first used in 1874), but traditionally refers to a multimodular mind in which the various forces considered to comprise the psyche—consciousness and 'the' unconscious, id, ego, and superego—are in states of dynamic equilibrium. There is an implicit contrast with 'psycho-static', 'medical model' categories of mental illness with their specific aetiologies and treatments.

The brain/mind can be visualized as a dynamic system comprising two principal circuits, one intrapsychic, the other interpersonal. The former corresponds to the classical account, in which the basic affective mesolimbic primary processes—panic/grief, rage, care, seeking, lust and play—are subject to continuous appraisal and regulation (mentalizing) by cortical functions (1). The interpersonal circuit links these cortical functions, especially in the right hemisphere, to emotional interchange with significant others, actual (parent, spouse, combat 'buddy') or symbolic (i.e. an internal representation of the other) in an individual's immediate and developmental environment. A large body of evidence now supports the view that, at least in infancy and early childhood, intrapsychic equilibrium is moderated by this interpersonal environment (2). John Donne's assertion that no man is an island is now an evidence-based statement. This relational view found early champions in the United States in the Washington School of psychiatry under the leadership of Harry Stack Sullivan, and in the United Kingdom through the group of psychiatrists and psychoanalysts associated with the Tavistock Clinic in London.

The umbrella term 'psychodynamic psychiatry' thus implies both a developmental and interpersonal perspective on the origins of psychological distress and dysfunction, together with specialist expertise in the psychotherapeutic treatments able to alleviate them. A number of PP concepts and approaches have been incorporated into the psychiatric mainstream. Here I shall touch on three.

First is the view that psychiatric symptoms—depression, anxiety, addiction, delusions, etc.—need to be viewed not merely at face value, but as manifestations of underlying dynamic processes, the resultant of the interplay between affects and the various defences needed to modulate and regulate them. A psychodynamically informed 'formulation' aims to tease out, say, the precipitating loss events that have triggered a depression, together with pre-existing vulnerabilities dating back to childhood. The latter might be associated with a 'narcissistic injury' in which a loved parent was herself depressed and therefore unable to provide the validation and unconditional delight children need if they are to acquire the store of self-esteem required to mitigate life's later vicissitudes. Or, to take another example, deliberate self-harm might be viewed as an misplaced attempt at self-soothing in someone whose opportunities for comfort when distressed are compromised, both at a physiological level due to adverse early childhood experience, and contemporaneously through social isolation or problematic relationships.

Implicit in the above is the affect–defence model of psychic function. Paradoxically, depression in the first instance becomes a defence against experiencing the unbearable pain of loss and failure; in the second self-harm is viewed as a way of avoiding feelings of abandonment and rage at those who have let the sufferer down. These processes have been studied and developed by George Vaillant (2) who classified defence mechanisms (a term originally developed by Anna Freud) as mature (e.g. humour), neurotic (e.g. intellectualization), immature (e.g. passive-aggressive), and pathological (e.g. denial and projection).

Valliant's long-term follow-up studies of men classified originally under those four headings reveal that those with mature defences had better adjustment, happiness, job satisfaction, and friendships; fewer hospitalizations; better overall health, and a lower rates of mental illness. Conversely the presence of 'immature defences' is related to poor adjustment, higher divorce rates and marital discord, less satisfactory friendship patterns, higher incidence of mental illness, greater number of sick leave days taken, and poorer health generally. Implicit in this model of psychopathology is the idea that a person's character can be understood in terms of how they negotiate the psychobiological challenges of development—the need to be safe, to reproduce, to be part of a social network, to provide for and rear children, to cope with loss and trauma, etc. 'Defences' represent the largely unconscious strategies and attendant compromises used to balance the internal, relational and social forces to which humans are subject.

A second key psychodynamic theme flows from the affect–defence model. People are most likely to deploy defences in situations that arouse anxiety. Since anxiety is a feature of almost all psychiatric illnesses, and will be evoked by consequent encounters with the mental health system, such defences are likely to be particularly salient in psychiatric settings. The psychoanalytic notion of transference and countertransference apply routinely to psychiatric work in that people suffering from mental illness are often in the grip of these ingrained models of care-seeking/care-giving—often mirrored in the reciprocal responses of mental health professionals. The defences implicated in psychiatric illness derive typically from childhood, and since the majority of psychiatrically ill people will have suboptimal developmental experiences, problematic expectations will be 'transferred' on to the mental health system. Splitting and projection (e.g. 'this *wonderful* psychiatrist, that *appalling* one'), avoidance (inability to comply with arrangements and appointments), clinging (entrenched dependent roles), risky behaviours (life-threatening or sexual), angry outbursts (which trigger instant attention, albeit negative) are common occurrences in mental health work and betoken the emergence of primitive affect–defence patterns enacted in relation to the mental health system.

Psychiatrists need to be able to read and react to such turbulence in terms of transference rather than themselves being sucked into the maelstrom of primitive mental functioning. The pressure and anxiety of psychiatric work likewise may elicit countertransference responses from mental health professionals. These may be manifestations of 'projective identification'; that is, the lodging of the patient's unwanted feelings within the psychiatrist which, if correctly understood, provide a useful guide to the patient's state of mind. Thus, for example, if the psychiatrist feels frightened when interviewing a patient, it is likely that the patient will be terrified too, however overtly threatening he or she may appear.

The notion of countertransference also captures the psychiatrist's own developmental history and how it may be activated in the clinical situation. Effective psychiatric work needs a space and time for self-scrutiny, whether through staff groups, personal analysis, 'mindfulness' training, or simply self-directed fostering of the capacity for reflection. However achieved, without such self-knowledge, the psychiatrist himself may 'act out' in counter-therapeutic ways—becoming a 'compulsive carer'; overworking; being frightened to take the risks needed to empower patients to take responsibility for their own lives; or, in a species of unconscious aggression, subtly blaming and undermining patients for their perversity or failure to improve. A key PP premise is that interactions between mental health professionals and their patients will be coloured by prior developmental experience. Awareness of these processes—at individual and group levels—will militate against reproducing pathological relational (and thereby iatrogenic) patterns in clinical interactions.

A third general point flows from the fact that, compared with non-medical therapists, the psychodynamic psychiatrist is in an unique position to provide an integrative approach to the treatment of psychiatric disorders. The most obvious example is that psychiatrists both prescribe psychotropic medication and provide psychotherapy. But that combination presents particular challenges. The patient may project their anger and disappointment in the psychiatrist by focusing on the 'uselessness' of a prescribed medication; requests for more pills may be a covert way of alluding to deprivation; the psychiatrist may alleviate his own sense of futility and covert narcissism by juggling with the patient's prescription. Prescribing is a 'real-world' action, and thus potentially runs counter to the atmosphere of 'as-if-ness' and free association the psychodynamic therapist wishes to foster; it can easily become an enactment of interpersonal dynamic rather than a rational and logical means to alleviate distress. None of these are insuperable obstacles, but the psychodynamic psychiatrist needs to be sensitive to them, and be prepared to attend to the inevitable mistakes and moments of acting-out on their part when they arise.

Another aspect of integration flows from the fact that psychodynamic whole-person models of the mind and its disorders do not map neatly onto DSM-type diagnostic categories. Psychodynamic therapy is inherently holistic rather than disorder-specific, and has suffered in comparison to cognitive-behaviour therapy (CBT; see Beck and Dozois, this volume, pp. 366–82) because of this. Some of the specialist therapies which have now been developed for borderline personality disorder (BPD), depression, anxiety, and eating disorders to be discussed below exemplify this issue. The psychodynamic psychiatrist needs to be a non-partisan integrative practitioner, bringing the full range of psychotherapeutic expertise to bear on psychiatric illnesses in ways that the evidence suggests is most effective. This applies also across psychotherapeutic modalities: for some conditions (depression and anxiety) CBT is the initial treatment of choice, followed by psychodynamic therapy for non-responders; for others (eating disorders) best is the combination of individual and family therapy, for yet others (BPD) long-term psychoanalytically informed group therapy supplemented by mindfulness training may be the treatment of choice.

In the next sections I look at the ways in which these general principles have played out in the specific historical conditions in various parts of the world.

Psychodynamic psychiatry in the United Kingdom

War is a potent catalyst for social change. World War I raised the profile of psychiatry by drawing on the skills of such outstanding intellects as W. H. Rivers and Henry Head in the understanding and treatment of shell shock (3, 4). In World War II the UK military command needed to identify potential leaders from men outside the traditional officer class. A group of psychoanalytically trained psychiatrists and psychologists, was recruited to the task. They were seen as having expertise in assessing 'character', and, rather than relying on academic or rank, devised methods of selection based on observing people's actual behaviour in group situations. Tapping into a person's psychodynamics in the here-and-now provides a better picture of their aptitudes than a consciously shaped interview performance.

The period 1930–60 saw an upsurge of interest in psychoanalytic approaches in the United Kingdom, and, as we shall see, in the United States. Even before the outbreak of war there had been an influx of psychoanalytic refugees from Nazi Germany to the United Kingdom. Freud arrived in London with his daughter Anna in 1938. Other asylum-seekers included Melanie Klein (invited by Ernest Jones, Freud's first biographer and key pioneer of psychoanalysis in the United Kingdom), Hannah Segal, and Michael Balint.

The Tavistock Clinic in London had been founded by Hugh Crighton-Miller for the treatment of World War I shell shock. After World War II it became a centre of excellence, training a cadre of psychodynamically minded psychologists, psychiatrists, and child psychotherapists; its leaders included Jock Sutherland, John Bowlby, Donald Winnicott, Wilfred Bion, and Michael Balint.

Michael Balint

From the point of view of PP, Balint's contribution was particularly significant. A Hungarian, analysed by Sandor Ferenczi, Balint was a pioneer in the then embryonic field of psychotherapy research, recruiting fellow-analyst David Malan to undertake one of the first outcome studies of brief dynamic psychotherapy. They found that 6 months of weekly therapy for people suffering from depression, anxiety, and mild personality problems could produce significant benefits, sustained at 2-year follow-up. Technical innovations came with time-limited once-weekly therapy. These included: an 'active' therapist; relentless focus on the presenting problem and its psychodynamic meanings; and preparing for termination from the outset, thereby bringing to the fore issues of loss and abandonment, so salient in the origins of neurosis (5).

Balint's enduring contribution was the development of the eponymous 'Balint groups' (6). These were originally conceived as a means of training general practitioners in psychodynamic thinking, enabling them to interact more sensitively and effectively with the considerable psychiatric element in their caseload. The impetus behind the Balint group movement was the realization that high-cost, highly labour-intensive, psychoanalysis could not make a significant impact on the mental health on the general population (but cf. Germany, discussed later). Training front-line workers in psychodynamic thinking, and facilitating the 'small but significant' alteration in personality which flows from a psychodynamic approach, was, Balint maintained, the best way to change a medical and psychiatric culture rooted in instrumentalism, paternalism, and mind-blindness.

Balint groups are innovative in form as well as aim. A group of clinicians meet regularly with a psychoanalytically trained facilitator. Discussion is based around case material brought by one or more of the participants. In contrast to the prevailing psychoanalytic mores, the role of the facilitator is neither pedagogic nor authoritarian. The participants are assumed to be the experts on themselves, their patients, and one another. The facilitator's role is to set the scene, to maintain the boundaries of the group, and to widen and deepen the discussion where necessary, encouraging mute members, while restraining the loquacious.

In the United Kingdom and other Anglophone countries, trainee psychiatrists are required to attend a weekly Balint group, facilitated by a senior psychotherapeutically trained practitioner. This provides an opportunity to examine the impact of working with highly disturbed and suicidal patients, and to begin to identify, respect, and make use of the countertransference reactions that such work evokes. Learning from one another's mistakes, successes, doubts, and uncertainties is integral to the process.

John Bowlby

Another influential figure was John Bowlby, who ranks as one of the best-known and most influential psychoanalyst-psychiatrists of the second half of the 20th century (7). He is credited with being one of the first clinicians to work directly with parents and children together, and hence is a founding father of family therapy. Bowlby's studies of the impact of separation of children from their parents when admitted to hospital, popularized by the films made by James Robertson, led to a radical change in paediatric medicine, leading to hospitals providing open access for parents. Family work in preventing relapse in schizophrenia (see Leff, this volume, pp. 96–116) can also be traced to Bowlby's pioneering spirit.

Bowlby's development of attachment theory, while arising in part from his psychoanalytic roots, created a new psychological paradigm. His trilogy *Attachment, Separation, and Loss* represents the integrative potential of the hybrid discipline of psychiatry at its best. Attachment theory embodies the simple yet profound idea that psychological health depends on the availability of a sensitive and responsive care-seeker/care-giver, and that when such relationships are rigid, insensitive, strained, or severed, adverse psychological consequences follow. The link between loss and depressive illness, first noted by Freud, is consistent with Bowlby's conceptualization. Grief and bereavement, and abnormal grief reactions were studied by Bowlby's colleague Colin Murray-Parkes, and represent an important psychodynamic contribution to mainstream psychiatry (8).

The 1950s saw the establishment of a number of 'therapeutic communities' using psychoanalytically informed individual and group methods for the treatment of mental illness. These were antithetical to the mental hospital setup of the day, challenging a culture based on based on erosion of individuality, patient passivity, and a paternalistic philosophy in which power was located around a hierarchically organized staff structure. Therapeutic communities encouraged patients to be active, to play a full part in maintaining the institution both practically (washing, cleaning, cooking, etc.), and in reflective thinking. Group meetings ensured that the support and challenge from fellow-sufferers was as important as professional expertise. A key part of the philosophy was the trust placed in mentally ill individuals to find their own solutions, placing professionals in a facilitating rather than controlling role.

R. D. Laing

One of the champions of social psychiatry was R. D. Laing, who achieved international renown in the 1960s, especially with his first book *The Divided Self*. Published when he was only 28, it was based on his experiences as an army psychiatrist and trainee psychoanalyst, first in Scotland and then at the Tavistock Clinic. Far removed from the stereotypical psychoanalytic mould of Jewish émigré or upper-middle-class Bloomsbury grouper (although sharing with both a degree of 'outsider-ness' integral to psychoanalytic culture), Laing came from humble Scottish origins to take the psychiatric world by storm. He introduced British readers to Harold Searles and Fromm-Reichman's psychoanalytic models of psychosis, as well as European existential philosophy. *The Divided Self* was on the bookshelf of every would-be 1960s radical. Sadly, Laing's meteoric rise was short lived, burnt out by alcoholism, drug addiction, and success itself.

Despite this tragic denouement, Laing's long-term influence should not be underestimated. He drew attention to the inhumane condition and culture of mental hospitals, detailed also by Goffman and Wing, leading eventually to their closure and replacement with acute hospital units and community-based services. Laing validated the inner world and experience of the severely mentally ill, seeing psychotic phenomena as covert communications, often about traumatic or painful experiences, rather than meaningless manifestations of a dysfunctional brain. He emphasized the family context of psychosis, and although wrong in attributing blame to the parents of psychosis sufferers (family miscommunication is as much a consequence of the stress of living with psychosis as it is a cause of illness), his ideas stimulated research which showed that lowering expressed emotion in families reduces relapse rate in schizophrenia (see Leff, this volume, pp. 96–116). Laing's work helped to destigmatize mental illness, presciently anticipating research showing that psychotic symptoms are relatively common in non-clinical populations, with the mentally ill representing the severe end of a spectrum of widespread non-rational ways of being and seeing (see Bhavsar and Murray, this volume, pp. 45–63).

Psychodynamic innovations in the UK National Health Service

During the 1970s and 1980s there was a rapid expansion in the numbers of psychodynamically-trained psychiatrists in the United Kingdom. Consultant psychiatrists specializing in psychotherapy—almost all psychoanalysts—were redesignated as consultant psychotherapists. Their principal role was to train junior psychiatrists in the basics of PP, and specialist trainees to become consultant psychotherapists. In addition, led by consultant psychotherapists, a small number of tertiary specialist units such as the Cassel Hospital and the Henderson Hospital provided day and inpatient services run along psychodynamic lines for severely disturbed, mainly personality-disordered patients. Being patient- rather than training-focused, these units were necessarily eclectic, employing large and small group therapies, art therapy, and psychodrama. An influential paper from this period was Tom Main's 'The ailment' (9), describing the impact of 'difficult patients' on mental health services, the ramifications of institutional countertransference, and the need for forums in which to think about such dynamics.

This efflorescence was, however, short lived. By the 1990s clinical psychology was beginning to emerge strongly as an independent profession, throwing off the shackles of its handmaiden role. Just as interventional radiology has replaced much of work previously done by surgeons, so clinical psychologists began to become the primary providers of psychological therapies. Enthusiastically espousing the new psychotherapeutic discipline of CBT, their services were now seen by cash-strapped managers as cheaper and more comprehensible than those provided by consultant psychotherapists.

At a political level consultant psychotherapists were fatally handicapped by having no identified client group for whose care they were directly responsible. As the economic situation worsened, managers realized that psychotherapy services could be curtailed without any danger of protest from concerned patients or their families. Refusing to cut their cloth, to develop diagnosis-specific brief treatments, to engage in outcome research, or to embrace a variety of differing psychotherapeutic approaches, psychotherapists became increasingly marginalized. There was a tendency to resort to *ad hominem* 'interpretations' of envy or psychological flaws in their opponents, as a way of bolstering their increasingly precarious status. PP ran the risk of being a desirable yet dispensable 'luxury', concerned mainly with the so-called 'worried well' rather than an integral part of civilized psychiatric practice.

Growth points

There were honourable exceptions to these self-defeating trends. Jonathan Pedder's *Introduction to Psychotherapy* (co-authored with Dennis Brown, and later, Anthony Bateman) remains an excellent introductory text. Bloch's *Introduction to the Psychotherapies* (now in its fourth edition), first appeared in 1977 and was well ahead of its time in bringing together the whole range of psychotherapies rather than merely focusing on one modality. The Jungian analyst Robert Hobson, co-author with Russell Meares of the influential paper, 'The persecutory therapist' (10), developed his 'conversational model' (CM), a brief dynamic therapy emphasizing the here-and-now relationship and the 'minute particulars' of therapist–patient interaction, in preference to putative childhood reconstructions.

CM was ahead of its time in using video recordings of sessions for both research and teaching, and became one of the first psychodynamic therapy models to be tested empirically. David Shapiro and his colleagues in Sheffield showed the efficacy of CM in a head-to-head 16-session study of CBT vs CM in mild–moderate depression, establishing the so-called 'equivalence paradox', or equifinality of outcomes between the two techniques.

Another notable contributor was Anthony Ryle, whose model of brief integrative therapy, cognitive analytic therapy (CAT; 11) contained a number of innovative features: the use of written communications in which the therapist offers the patient a formulation after four sessions, and a 'goodbye letter' in the penultimate one; an explicitly collaborative rather than expert–supplicant milieu; an emphasis on the cyclical self-perpetuating aspects of neurosis and a focus on the search for 'exits' from such vicious circles; and homework tasks aiming to promote benign ones. CAT has been shown in its 24-session form shown to be a promising treatment for BPD (12).

Despite these hopeful signs, two well-intentioned institutions set up by the UK Labour government (1997–2008) contrived to strike fear into the hearts of psychodynamic psychiatrists. NICE, the National Institute for Health and Care Excellence, convenes experts who review research in specific topics, leading to 'guidelines' for evidence-based practice in all branches of medicine, including psychiatry. Laudable as this may be, nowhere does NICE advocate PP as a first-line treatment for psychiatric disorders. Currently pharmacotherapy and CBT out-shine psychodynamics when it comes to published evidence. While absence of evidence does not necessarily equate to evidence of absence, it was initially hard for PP to challenge this bias. Recently a more balanced position is beginning to emerge, as outcome studies favourable to PP have been published, demonstrating the need for long-term PP for patients whose Axis I diagnoses are also associated with a history of childhood trauma and/or neglect.

Another related development has been a Department of Health sponsored Increasing Access to Psychological Therapies (IAPT) programme. The impetus behind this innovation should have benefited PP. Impressed by the evidence from advanced countries that greater economic prosperity does not necessarily equate with increased happiness, the economist Richard Layard persuaded the UK government that investment in psychological therapies would help raise the general level of happiness, as well as reducing the numbers of people suffering from chronic depression and somatization disorders, often living on costly welfare benefits. As with NICE, CBT was seen as the treatment of choice for these conditions, and training programmes were set up establishing IAPT therapists across the country. PP, once again, was out in the cold, although belatedly the IAPT board added a brief dynamic therapy, dynamic interpersonal therapy (13) (see below) to its programme.

With CBT now the first-line treatment for common mental disorders in primary care, the focus and role of PP has shifted, perhaps appropriately, to complex and disturbed cases requiring long-term treatments. A significant development has been the development by Anthony Bateman and Peter Fonagy, psychoanalysts both, the one a psychiatrist, the other an academic clinical psychologist, of a psychodynamically informed treatment for people suffering from BPD. Bateman's clinical base was a psychodynamic day hospital in a deprived area of north-east London. Determined to compete in the mainstream of psychiatry research, he and Fonagy undertook an randomized control trial (RCT) outcome study, with long-term follow-up, in which a particular version of psychodynamic psychiatry, mentalization based therapy (MBT), was compared with treatment as usual (TAU). Their methodology was impeccable and their results remarkable, resulting in a series of acclaimed papers in the *American Journal of Psychiatry* (14). Bateman and Fonagy have shown that a 2-year partial hospitalization programme for BPD sufferers, in which they receive a combination of individual, group, and milieu therapy, outperforms TAU on almost all the important criteria: days in hospital, episodes of deliberate self-harm, medication levels, health and social service resources consumed. Interestingly, differences only begin to emerge strongly 18 months into the programme, which strengthens the PP case that a longer-term perspective is needed if the current 'fast-therapy' culture is to be questioned. Eight-year follow-up shows that these gains are maintained, although the quality of life of BPD sufferers still remains poor. The programme is based on intensive staff supervision and support, and a coherent treatment philosophy. People suffering from BPD are seen as lacking the reflexive (or 'mentalizing') skills needed to negotiate the world of interpersonal relationships ('to see others from the inside and oneself from the outside'; 15), as well as being prone to states of easily triggered hyperarousal incompatible with mentalizing. The core of the programme is to take everyday 'living/learning' (a therapeutic community catchphrase) experiences and to foster the participants' capacity to mentalize the actions and feelings of themselves and others in terms of beliefs, desires and intentions.

The significance of Bateman and Fonagy's contribution is that they have developed and tested a specific model of therapy for a defined client group, for whom PP offers a positive outcome, in contrast to conventional psychiatry which often leads to iatrogenic deterioration in BPD sufferers. The specific skills of the psychodynamic psychiatrist—able to prescribe when needed, manage suicide and deliberate self-harm, as well as offering reflexive psychoanalytically informed therapeutic practice—suggest a future role for PP as the custodian of Axis II clients with complex and difficult problems.

Psychodynamic psychiatry in the United States

Summarizing the discussion so far we can identify a number of themes: the wartime role of psychoanalytic psychiatrists in helping people with combat stress; expansion led mainly by refugees from Europe fleeing fascism; insularity and arrogance of PP practitioners militating against cross-fertilization and research; medical elitism; the inexorable rise of CBT and of the psychology profession; attempts to limit costs incurred in long-term therapies by government and insurance companies.

Despite the very different sociopolitical context of the United States, we see similar forces in evidence. The vicissitudes of US psychoanalysis, and with it PP, has been charted in seminal contributions by Stepansky (16), Paris (17), Luhrmann (18), and Kandel (19). For at least two decades psychoanalysis was 'the only game in town', with psychiatrists in the ascendant. Ignoring Freud's espousal of 'lay analysis', US psychoanalysts insisted that candidates be medically trained. In the 1950s and 1960s heads of psychiatry departments throughout the United States, were to a man (and they were mostly men) psychoanalysts. Three-quarters of posts within the American Psychiatric Association (APA) were held by psychoanalysts. Personal analysis and psychoanalytic candidature were *de rigeur* for psychiatrists who wished to advance in their profession. There were of course tensions. Psychologists felt justifiably envious and excluded. Psychoanalysts of a liberal bent clashed with their more orthodox counterparts. There was nevertheless a sense of a psychoanalytic mainstream—in the mid-1950s Charles Brenner's *Elementary Textbook of Psychoanalysis* sold more than 1 million copies.

But in the mid-1970s things began to change. A number of factors came together to threaten and eventually to replace psychoanalytic hegemony. The oil crisis of 1973 meant that a period of unprecedented economic growth and stability in the United States faltered. Cheaper, more effective, less opaque therapies were required. Insurance companies insisted that only treatments for defined medical conditions would be reimbursed. The IPPS (International Project for the Study of Schizophrenia; see Bhavsar and Murray, this volume, pp. 45–63 and Leff, this volume, pp. 96–116) project found that American psychiatrists' diagnostic practices were far vaguer and more all-inclusive than those in other countries including the United Kingdom (with the ironic exception of the USSR). The APA responded with the third edition of the *Diagnostic and Statistical Manual* (DSM-III), which abolished overnight the psychoanalytic shibboleth of the neurosis–psychosis dichotomy in favour of specific diagnoses required to satisfy highly specific criteria.

The way was open for CBT to produce time-limited packages of treatment for DSM-defined conditions such as depression, anxiety, post-traumatic stress disorder, and bulimia. This was in stark contrast to psychoanalysis's typically unfocused, ill-defined, intensive therapies of uncertain length. Psychopharmacology was also gathering momentum as a scientific force. The catecholamine hypothesis for depression, and the dopamine hypothesis for schizophrenia, while not intrinsically antithetical to PP, shifted the focus from the psyche to the brain. Private insurance companies' 'managed care' paradigm increasingly favoured cheaper psychopharmacological treatments over psychotherapy. In the notorious 'Chestnut Lodge' case, Raphael Osheroff, a neurologist suffering from major depressive disorder, successfully sued the celebrated psychoanalytic inpatient unit, when, after prolonged ineffective psychoanalytic treatment, his family arranged for him to be treated with antidepressants and he recovered in short order.

Faced with this challenge, psychoanalytic psychiatrists responded in a number of ways. Some clung to a fundamentalist mentality, seeing brief therapies and psychopharmacology as manifestations of a fast-therapy degenerate society, with psychoanalysis as guardians of the true faith. Others shifted the focus of psychodynamics away from treating mental illness towards a secular quasi-religious exploration of the Self. Some abandoned psychoanalysis altogether and joined the biological opposition. Others, notably Otto Kernberg (who developed an innovative treatment for BPD)and Robert Wallerstein (a doughty champion of psychoanalytic 'common ground' and integrative perspectives generally) and John Gunderson, belatedly realized that systematic evaluation was needed if PP was to re-enter the scientific mainstream, and initiated programmes of painstaking research.

Another leading figure in the fightback was Glen Gabbard, professor at the famous Menninger Clinic in Kansas (eponymously named after brothers William and Karl Menninger who occupied a dominant position in US psychiatry in the post-war period), itself a victim of the changing fortunes of PP, now relocated to Houston. Gabbard's *Psychodynamic Psychiatry in Clinical Practice*, first published in the 1980s, remains a best-seller, now into its 4th edition. He is a vigorous critic of the funding imbalance between general medicine and psychiatry, and between 'organic' psychiatry and psychotherapy, commenting, with characteristic aphoristic aplomb, 'It is not uncommon for insurance policies to pay in six figures for organ transplants but offer only nickels and dimes for psychotherapy'. In addition to psychoanalytic expertise, Gabbard exudes a persuasive mix of common sense, clinical wisdom, style, and wit. The thrust of Gabbard's approach is not to reject non-psychodynamic methods but to argue for an integrated approach in which psychopharmacology and various forms of psychotherapy, including psychoanalysis, work in concert. The common factor is the doctor–patient relationship; the central contribution of PP its capacity both to both theorize that relationship, and maximize its therapeutic efficacy.

Global perspectives on psychodynamic psychiatry

From a UK and USA perspective, the situation of psychodynamics in the German-speaking world (Germany, Austria, Switzerland) appears paradisal. Psychotherapy, including psychoanalysis, is treated as a medical speciality, equivalent to physical medicine, and is covered by private and government insurance schemes, up to a total of 300 sessions. The historical reasons for this may lie in part in reaction against the shameful Nazi dismantling of the 'Jewish science' in the 1930s (which, ironically, led to the flowering of psychoanalysis in the United Kingdom and the United States); also to the fact that research in psychotherapy outcome was initiated in Germany in the 1950s, some 20 years before the need was felt in the Anglophone world. Today Germany remains at the forefront of both process and outcome studies (20) in psychodynamic psychotherapy.

Psychodynamics are similarly valued in the Scandinavian countries. In the 1970s an interesting development was the development of 'shuttle training', in which a group of UK psychoanalysts and group analysts (including Pedder, mentioned earlier) went regularly to Denmark to 'train the trainers' until a sufficient cadre was established for self-sufficiency. Similar arrangements have more recently been developed in Russia, eastern Europe, and now China, where, following the demise of communism, there has been a hunger for psychoanalytic ideas and therapies. With developments in electronic communication, supervision by services such as Skype helps maintain a psychoanalytic culture in these hitherto deprived regions.

In Europe, France represents something of a special case. Psychoanalysis is divided between the Freudian and Lacanian schools. Lacan, although often hard to understand, brought a useful sociological perspective to PP, arguing that psychological disorders need to be seen in an historical three-generation context in which the very name of the newborn child, let alone assimilated hopes and expectations, represents the continuation of the past into the present. Many psychiatrists are psychoanalytically trained. Empirical approaches, including psychotherapy research, tend to be seen as an Anglo-Saxon aberration, and eschewed in favour of philosophical disputation and Freudian fundamentalism. In the Francophone areas of Canada, however, the concept of mentalizing has been developed, feeding into MBT as developed by Bateman and Fonagy.

As British ex-colonies, Canada and Australia have built on and improved some of the more positive features of the mother country. While not as intensive as in Germany, in both Canada and Australia limited psychoanalytic therapy is are covered by insurance, and training in PP is a mandatory requirement for qualification as a psychiatrist. Both boast centres of psychodynamic excellence. Pre-dating Bateman and Kernberg, Russell Meares in Sydney integrated Heinz Kohut's self-psychology into an evidence-based treatment for BPD. In Canada, Allan Abbass extended Malan and Habib Davanloo's work into a model of intensive short-term dynamic psychotherapy, showing it to be effective in treating depression, post-traumatic stress disorder (PTSD), and BPD (21).

A burgeoning urban middle-class and a post-Catholic culture have made South America a fertile seedbed for psychoanalysis. The early leading figures trained in Europe and then returned to South America to establish their own schools. Argentinian Horatio Etchygoen's *Fundamentals of Psychoanalytic Technique* is a masterly account of Kleinian psychoanalysis. Psychology is a popular undergraduate subject in South America, and the majority of psychotherapists are psychologists, not psychiatrists. Extending psychoanalytic approaches to the wider population remains problematic, although, intriguingly, Peru now has a pioneering indigenous psychoanalyst.

In Africa PP is more or less confined to South Africa. For the non-white and rural population mental disorders are largely treated by traditional healers, but there are now psychodynamically informed outreach projects in the townships, for victims of sexual abuse, for example. An interesting development in Uganda has been an interpersonal therapy (IPT) outreach project in which a controlled study of group therapy for depression facilitated by locally trained therapists has been shown to be effective. Another development has been narrative therapy for victims of war trauma, where controlled studies have been successfully evaluated and found to be helpful.

In Asia, a number of non-theistic religions and psychological disciplines such as Daoism, Shintoism, and Zen Buddhism have been incorporated into professional treatment, raising the possibility of an authentic Asian psychodynamic approach to mental illness and its therapy. There are flourishing psychoanalytic institutes in South Korea and Japan. Takae Doi coined the term *amae* to describe a particular kind of mother–child intimacy unique to Japan, which has thrown new light on the kinds of intimate dependency PP can foster. Salman Ahktar, an Indian psychoanalyst working in the United States, has questioned the neo-Kleinian emphasis on negative emotions such as envy and destructiveness, as opposed to hope, optimism, and humour, and written about the positive influence of the psychoanalyst, illustrating how East–West dialogue in psychotherapy can become a two-way process.

Green shoots for a psychodynamic future

Can PP survive as a significant force within psychiatry? Or is it doomed at best to a role, like osteopathy vis-à-vis mainstream medicine, of 'optimal marginalization'; at worst to be an esoteric backwater yearning nostalgically for a long-gone past? Has psychotherapy effectively been handed over to clinical psychology, with psychiatrists returning to their 19th-century role as neurologists and psychopharmacologists? In this concluding section I survey some signs that psychodynamics may indeed yet recover some of its former glory and play a worthwhile role in the psychiatry of the future.

Neuropsychoanalysis

Neuropsychoanalysis has captured the imagination of leading figures in both psychoanalysis and neuroscience. One of Freud's earliest essays (1895), was the unpublished 'Project for a scientific psychology', attempting to combine—in vain, he later decided—the neurology of the day with his burgeoning psychoanalytic ideas. Over a century on, there has been a tentative rapprochement between psychoanalysis and contemporary neuroscience (22). Analysts in search of scientific credibility have been beguiled by the vivid imagery and circuitry of their neuroscience colleagues, who in turn have found in psychoanalysis meanings that underlie their brain mappings.

There are numerous areas of mutual interest. These include the distinction between the explicit/declarative memory system and implicit/procedural memories, and the ways in which the latter may encode early trauma with far-reaching but largely unconscious effects; parallels between Freud's conscious/unconscious dichotomy and the interplay between cortical and subcortical structures, especially the limbic system; 'mirror neurons' as the basis for empathy in which watching others' actions and emotions trigger equivalent parts of the brain in the observer; neuroplasticity and thus the possible ameliorative impact of psychotherapy; tracking changes in regional blood flow in response to therapeutic interventions. Unexpected support for a rapprochement between neuroscience and psychoanalytic approaches has come from the Nobel Prize winning neuroscientist and psychiatrist Eric Kandel.

Developmental psychopathology

Another growth area concerns links between developmental psychopathology and attachment theory as a science of intimacy. A developmental perspective is indispensable for understanding major psychiatric illness (see Bhavsar and Murray this volume, pp. 45–63). Gene–environment interaction and epigenetic processes are cutting-edge research areas. A now classic example is the finding by Avshalom Caspi and colleagues that only in the presence of the short-allele version of the serotonin transporter gene does childhood adversity predispose to adult depression (see McGuffin this volume, pp. 22–44). Another relevant finding is that another epigenetic locus, the *DRD4* allele, increases biological sensitivity to environmental context, with potential for negative health effects under conditions of adversity, but positive effects when support and protection are available, the latter including psychotherapy (23).

Apart from general validation of PP's emphasis on the importance of early environmental influence and of a developmental perspective, PP has a specific contribution to make to this field in that it focuses on the subtleties of interpersonal interaction that may trigger adverse or beneficial epigenetic processes. The adult attachment interview is a sophisticated instrument for studying the minutiae of intimate relationships: parent–child, spousal—and psychotherapeutic. An example is a study which tracks how in the course of Kernberg et al.'s transference-focused therapy, BPD sufferers' capacity to articulate and reflect on their experience changes in a positive direction (24).

Training

A continuing theme that has kept psychodynamics alive has been the acknowledgement that trainee psychiatrists, whatever their eventual orientation, need basic psychotherapeutic skills, and to be conversant with the theories and practical uses of psychodynamic approaches in the treatment of mental illness. A 'signed-up' case book recording supervised practice in a number of psychotherapeutic modalities, including long- and short-term psychodynamic therapy, is now a precondition for qualification as a psychiatrist in the United Kingdom, the United States, and Australasia.

Another notable recent development has been the establishment of departments of psychoanalysis and psychoanalytic studies within the universities. Rejected by the anti-Semitic culture within the universities of his day, Freud created his own institutions for training and promulgation of psychoanalysis. While this fostered freewheeling creativity, it has also meant that psychoanalysis failed to keep step with many of the intellectual currents of the 20th century: systems theory, observational child development, ethology, structuralist anthropology, linguistics, and philosophy. In particular, psychoanalytic research was confined and constricted by Freud's conception of the individual case study, important though that is, rather than subjecting analytic therapies to the statistical and probabilistic methods of mainstream science.

University College London (UCL) established UK's first chair of psychoanalysis in the 1980s. It was initially held on a short-term basis sequentially by John Bowlby, Joseph Sandler, and the French psychoanalyst Janine Chasseguet-Smirguel. Since the 1990s it has been permanently occupied by the psychologist, psychoanalyst, psychotherapy outcome researcher and child development expert Peter Fonagy. Thanks to Fonagy and his colleague Mary Target, and following incorporation of the Anna Freud Centre (AFC), UCL-AFC has become an international powerhouse for teaching and research in psychoanalysis and PP. In addition to the Psychoanalysis Unit at UCL there are now in the United Kingdom psychoanalytic departments at the Universities of Essex, Sheffield, Birkbeck, and Exeter. A free-standing Psychoanalytic University has been founded in Berlin, and the New School for Social Research in New York has a major psychoanalytic presence. Such departments allow for cross-fertilization between different disciplines (including such diverse areas as philosophy, literary and gender studies, and art history), and encourages psychoanalytic research in its widest sense. Exposing PP to the rigours of academia helps hone its strengths and blow away its fusty anachronisms.

Evidence base for PP

One of the ironies of psychiatry is that although the majority of psychiatrists see themselves primarily as medical experts in diagnosis and prescription, the public consistently stress the need for talking therapies. But hard evidence is needed if governments and insurance companies are to be persuaded to fund psychotherapies. We have seen how PP quixotically gave CBT a 20-year head-start when it came to evidence of efficacy and effectiveness. The merits of psychodynamic therapies are steadily emerging, however, and ways of overcoming the methodological difficulties in evaluating psychodynamic therapies begin to be developed.

But in studying PP, blinding is impossible, randomization undesirable, and funding for long-term therapy hard to obtain. A compromise is to compare active treatment either with 'treatment as usual', or reliance on pre-/post measures. The second half of the 2000s saw a number of meta-analyses of PP in high-impact journals (25), all of which pointed to similar conclusions. First, psychodynamic therapies produce large effect sizes (average 0.8–1.2), comparable to those achieved both by CBT and IPT, and by antidepressants. Second, gains tend to increase even after the period of therapy has finished, in contrast to non-psychotherapeutic treatments. Third, improvements in psychodynamic therapy subjects, although substantial, tend to reveal themselves towards the latter period of therapy, suggesting an initial period of psychological reorganization ('pupation') before enduring change, butterfly-like, can emerge. Fourth, the longer the period of therapy, the greater the gains. This was important since earlier studies claimed a negative logarithmic 'dose–effect curve', these new studies suggest that, with time, effective psychodynamic therapy initiates benign cycles of action and reflection. Finally, psychodynamic therapy, despite being labour-intensive, is cost-effective in that utilization of health and social services after therapy tends to drop dramatically compared with controls.

Another relevant point concerns the mechanism of action of psychotherapies generally. Knowing that a given therapy 'works' in terms of symptomatic improvement and improved social outcomes says nothing about how therapy brings about change. There is some evidence that basic psychodynamic processes may apply to all effective therapies. Two key factors are the establishment of a secure, sensitive, and interactive *working alliance*, and the capacity of the therapist to *facilitate experiencing* of previously avoided painful feelings. It seems that even in CBT, these 'psychodynamic' factors contribute significantly to the outcome variance (26).

Such claims for the efficacy of PP have not gone unchallenged. One criticism is that psychodynamic therapy outcomes have been measured with a heterogeneous collection of patients with a variety of diagnoses and problems. It is therefore it is difficult to determine the precise indications for psychodynamic therapies, as compared with the diagnosis-specific therapies developed by CBT. Another is that head-to-head studies are lacking where psychodynamic therapy can be compared with briefer, cheaper therapies. A third objection centres on the tension between standard psychotherapeutic technique—which for BPD sufferers may be ineffective or produce deterioration—as compared with diagnosis-specific treatments. Thirdly, there is a need for real-world effectiveness studies which can encompass integrative approaches. The latter might well include packages comprising psychopharmacology, social measures, and family therapy in parallel with individual PP.

Recent work has begun to address some of these questions. Anxiety disorders are typically seen as the preserve of CBT, so it is significant that Milrod and colleagues (27) have developed a psychodynamic therapy model for anxiety, concentrating particularly on the avoidance and denial of anger, demonstrating good outcomes in 21 sessions compared with controls, sustained over 6 months follow-up (a short period admittedly, but comparable to CBT studies enamoured of third-party funders and NICE).

A number of evidence-based psychodynamic treatments have now been developed for depression. Brief PP has been found to be as effective as CBT, IPT, or antidepressants (28). An example is dynamic interpersonal therapy (DIT), which has managed to breach CBT's monopoly in the UK Improving Access to Psychological Therapies programme (see above). DIT concentrates on the interpersonal aspects of depression: how recent losses trigger traumatic memories of early childhood separations; how these may be reactivated in therapy (transference reactions to therapist's absences); and fostering the capacity to think about ('mentalize') negative affects rather than being overwhelmed by them.

The complexity and difficulty of the problems posed by people suffering from BPD represents a major problem for psychiatric services. Patients often fail to engage with standard treatments and, as we have seen, when they do, therapy may interfere with the natural tendency of BPD to remission. Two manualized modified psychodynamic therapies, Kernberg's transference-focused therapy (TFT) in New York, and Bateman and Fonagy's MBT in London, have both been shown to produce significant improvements for BPD sufferers compared with treatment-as-usual controls. As mentioned above, MBT combines attachment and psychoanalytic principles, seeing BPD sufferers as deficient in mentalizing skills, and therefore liable to recurrent interpersonal conflict without being able to learn from experience. MBT eschews 'deep' or infancy-oriented interpretations. The latter at best are incomprehensible to people who lack reflexive competence, at worst precipitate feelings of shame and humiliation. MBT, TFP, and indeed non-psychodynamic therapies for BPD such as dialectical behaviour therapy, are optimally delivered in dedicated centres by specially trained and closely supervised and supported groups of therapists. This group of patients—for whom suicide and deliberate self-harm are an ever-present risk—is best treated by psychodynamically sophisticated mental health professionals, among whom psychodynamic psychiatrists play a leading role.

Finally we turn to the controversial role of psychoanalytic approaches to schizophrenia, which illustrate in microcosm the rise, fall, and tentative rebirth of PP charted in this essay. 'Schizophrenia' and related psychoses were, since Freud's account of Judge Schreber's memoir, seen as legitimate subjects for PP, although Freud himself was sceptical about the possibility of analysis with such patients. Pioneering units such as Chestnut Lodge in Maryland were staffed by outstanding analysts including Harold Searles and Frieda Fromm-Reichman who wrote freely about psychoanalytic therapy for psychosis (to be weighed alongside her many virtues, the latter was also responsible for the egregious misnomer 'schizophrenogenic mother'; see Bhavsar and Murray this volume, pp. 45–63). Following Melanie Klein's accounts of manic-depressive psychosis, British analysts including Bion and Herbert Rosenfeld similarly wrote and upheld the view that psychotic illness could be understood and treated psychoanalytically.

The turn away from PP began with the discovery in the 1950s (see Mitchell and Hadzi-Pavlovic this volume, pp. 335–54) of effective drug treatments for psychosis. It became clear clinically that many patients with schizophrenia failed to improve or even deteriorated when treated psychoanalytically. Eventually Tom McGlashan (29) and Gunderson, psychodynamic psychiatrists both, the former a Chestnut Lodge staff member, published a much-publicized follow-up study of schizophrenic patients, showing that psychoanalytic therapy was contraindicated, ironically in line with Freud's caution first expressed nearly a century earlier.

At this stage, it seemed that PP for psychosis was dead and buried. But gradually the picture has begun to change. In Scandinavia a 'needs adapted' approach to schizophrenia was developed whose components include recognition of the value of each patient and their individual life trajectory; minimal medication; intensive family therapy; and establishing a long-term relationship with a key worker (30). Such a relationship is not formally psychoanalytic, containing elements of support and attachment, but there is also sustained work helping the patient understand the nature and meaning of his illness and its origins rather than simply seeing it as a biologically determined 'disease'. Meanwhile, other research has revealed the widespread nature of psychotic symptoms, and role of childhood adversity and trauma as precursors to the development of psychotic illnesses (Bhavsar and Murray, this volume, pp. 45–63), strongly suggesting that environmental factors such as the family and wider social environment may crucially determine whether particular thinking styles become psychiatric illnesses. While formal psychoanalytic therapy for psychosis remain ethically and practically questionable, psychodynamically informed therapy on a long-term basis, incorporating elements of support, symptom management and, where appropriate, interpretation, are now part of any civilized service for people suffering from schizophrenia and manic depression.

Conclusion

Had this essay been written in the early 2000s, its conclusions about the future of PP might have been far more pessimistic. The ubiquity of neuropsychiatry, the dominance of CBT and psychology, the ascendancy of psychopharmacology, and increasing multi-professionalism within mental health, increasingly combine to confine psychiatrists to a forensic and prescribing role. A decade later, the picture looks very different. PP has a significant contribution to make to mainstream psychiatry in three main areas. First, it has much to offer in developing diagnosis-specific therapies, particularly in the domain of complex personality disorder. Second, PP enables psychiatrists to understand the transferential and countertransferential thoughts, feelings, and enactments aroused by the clinical work, thereby helping to avoid the ever-present iatrogenic dangers implicit in psychiatric practice. Third, through greater understanding of the nuances of the therapeutic relationship, PP-oriented psychiatrists can empathize and communicate effectively with their patients, even when the focus of treatment is not primarily psychodynamic. In conclusion, Leon Eisenberg's famous principle that psychiatry should be neither brainless nor mindless remains valid. In parallel with the impressive growth of neuroscience, PP offers an unrivalled and comprehensive clinical account of the mind's troubles, and how they can be understood and alleviated.

References

1 **Panksepp, J.** (1998). *Affective neuroscience: the foundations of human and animal emotions.* New York: Oxford University Press.

2 **Shore, A.** (2003). *Affect regulation and the repair of the self.* New York: Norton.

3 **Vaillant, G. E.** (1992). *Ego mechanisms of defense: a guide for clinicians and researchers.* Washington, DC: American Psychiatric Press.

4 **Barker, P.** (1991). *Regeneration.* London: Viking.

5 **Malan, D. and Della Selva, P.** (2006). *Lives transformed: how psychodynamic psychotherapy works.* Oxford: Butterworth.

6 **Balint, M.** (1957). *The doctor, his patient and the illness.* London: Pitman Medical. (2nd edn 1964, reprinted 1986, Edinburgh: Churchill Livingstone).

7 **Holmes, J.** (1993). *John Bowlby and attachment theory.* London: Routledge.

8 **Parkes, C. M.** (1996). *Bereavement: studies of grief in adult life.* London: Penguin.

9 **Main, T.** (1989). *The ailment and other essays.* London: Routledge.

10 **Meares, R. and Hobson, R.** (1977). The persecutory therapist. *British Journal of Medical Psychology* **50**, 349–59.

11 **Ryle, A** (1990). *Cognitive analytic therapy: active participation in change.* Chichester: John Wiley and Sons.

12 **Parry, G., Roth, A., and Kerr, I.** (2005). Brief and time-limited therapy. In: Gabbard, G., Beck, J., and Holmes, J. (eds.) *Oxford textbook of psychotherapy*, Oxford: Oxford University Press.

13 **Lemma, A., Target, M., and Fonagy, P.** (2011). *Dynamic interpersonal therapy: a clinician's guide.* Oxford: Oxford University Press.

14 **Bateman, A. and Fonagy, P.** (2006). *Mentalisation based treatment for borderline personality disorder.* Oxford: Oxford University Press.

15 Holmes, J. (2010). *Exploring in security: towards an attachment-informed psychoanalytic psychotherapy.* London: Routledge.

16 Stepansky, P. (2009). *Psychoanalysis at the margins.* New York: Other Press.

17 Paris, J. (2005). *The fall of an icon.* Toronto: University of Toronto Press.

18 Luhrmann, T. (2000). *Of two minds.* New York: Viking.

19 Kandell, E. (2006). *In search of memory: the emergence of a new science of mind.* New York. Norton.

20 Leichsenring, F. and Rabung, S. (2008). Effectiveness of long-term psychodynamic psychotherapy: a meta-analysis. *JAMA* **300**, 1551–65.

21 Abbass, A., Sheldon, A., Gyra, J., and Kaplan, A. (2008). Intensive short-term dynamic psychotherapy for DSM-IV personality disorders: a randomized controlled trial. *Journal of Nervous and Mental Disease* **196**, 211–16.

22 Solms, M. and Turnball, O. (1992). *The brain and the inner world.* New York: Other Press.

23 Steele, H. and Siefer, L. (2010). An attachment perspective on borderline personality disorder: advances in gene-environment considerations. *Current Psychiatry Reports* **12**, 61–7.

24 Diamond, D., Stovall-McClough, C., Clarkin, J., and Levy, K. (2003). Patient-therapist attachment in the treatment of borderline personality disorder. *Bulletin of the Menninger Clinic* **67**, 227–59.

25 Shedler, J. (2010). The efficacy of psychodynamic psychotherapy. *American Psychologist* **65**, 98–109.

26 Kandel, E. (2000). The future of psychiatry. *HHMI Bulletin* **13**, 6–8.

27 Busch, F., Milrod, B., and Sandberg, L. (2009). A study demonstrating the efficacy of psychoanalytic psychotherapy for panic disorder: implications for psychoanalytic research, theory and practice. *Journal of the American Psychoanalytic Association* **57**, 131–48.

28 Leichesenring, F., Rabung, S., and Leibing, E. (2004). The efficacy of short-term psychodynamic psychotherapy in specific psychiatric disorders: a meta-analysis. *Archives of General Psychiatry* **61**, 1208–16.

29 McGlashan, T. (1988). A selective review of North American long-term follow-up studies of schizophrenia. *Schizophrenia Bulletin* **14**, 515–42.

30 Alanen, Y., González de Chávez, M., Silver, A-L. et al. (2009). *Psychotherapeutic approaches to schizophrenic psychoses, past, present and future.* Hove: Routledge.

Index